The Insanity of Place/
The Place of Insanity

This book brings together many of the major papers published by Andrew Scull in the history of psychiatry over the past decade and a half. Its historiographic essays provide a critical perspective on such major figures as Michel Foucault, Roy Porter, and Edward Shorter, and subsequent chapters examine some of the major substantive debates in the field from the eighteenth century to the present. Chapters on psychiatric therapeutics and on the shifting social responses to madness over a period of almost three centuries add to a comprehensive assessment of Anglo-American confrontations with madness in this period and make the book invaluable for those concerned to understand the psychiatric enterprise.

The Insanity of Place/The Place of Insanity will be of interest to students and professionals of the history of medicine and of psychiatry, as well as sociologists concerned with deviance and social control, the sociology of mental illness, and the sociology of the professions.

Andrew Scull is Distinguished Professor of Sociology and Science Studies at the University of California, San Diego. He received his BA from Oxford University, and his PhD from Princeton. He taught at the University of Pennsylvania and at Princeton prior to coming to UCSD. His books include *Museums of Madness*; *Decarceration*; *Madhouses, Mad-Doctors, and Madmen*; *Durkheim and the Law* (with Steven Lukes); *Social Control and the State* (with Stanley Cohen); *Social Order/Mental Disorder*; *The Most Solitary of Afflictions: Madness and Society in Britain, 1700–1900*; *Masters of Bedlam*; *Undertaker of the Mind* and *Customers and Patrons of the Mad Trade* (with Jonathan Andrews); and *Madhouse: A Tragic Tale of Megalomania and Modern Medicine*.

Routledge Studies in Cultural History

The Insanity of Place/ The Place of Insanity

Essays on the history of psychiatry

Andrew Scull

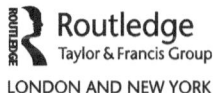

Routledge
Taylor & Francis Group

LONDON AND NEW YORK

First published 2006
by Routledge
2 Park Square, Milton Park, Abingdon, Oxfordshire OX14 4RN

Simultaneously published in the USA and Canada
by Routledge
711 Third Avenue, New York, NY 10017

First issued in paperback 2014
Routledge is an imprint of the Taylor and Francis Group, an informa business

© 2006 Andrew Scull

Typeset in Garamond by
Newgen Imaging Systems (P) Ltd, Chennai, India

British Library Cataloguing in Publication Data
A catalogue record for this book is available from the British Library

Library of Congress Cataloging in Publication Data
A catalog record for this book has been requested

ISBN 978-0-415-77006-4 (hbk)
ISBN 978-0-415-76212-0 (pbk)

Contents

Acknowledgments

I am grateful to Sage Publications for permission to reprint Chapter 2 and portions of Chapter 9 that were previously published in *History of Psychiatry*.

Chapter 3 previously appeared in Arthur Still and Irving Velody (eds), *Rewriting the History of Madness: Studies in Foucault's Histoire de la folie*, and is reprinted with the permission of Routledge.

Some portions of Chapter 4 previously appeared in the *London Review of Books*, and are reprinted with the permission of the publisher.

Chapters 5 and 7 first appeared in the *Times Literary Supplement* and are reprinted with permission.

Chapter 6 first appeared in *Social History of Medicine* and is reprinted with the permission of Oxford University Press.

Chapter 8 first appeared in the *Milbank Quarterly* and is reprinted with the permission of the publisher.

Portions of Chapter 10 appeared in T. Hamanaka and G.E. Berrios (eds), *The History of Psychiatry, East and West, on the Threshold of the Twenty-First Century*, Tokyo, Gakuyu Shoin, and are reprinted with the permission of the publisher.

Chapter 11 is reprinted from *Research in Law, Deviance, and Social Control* with the permission of JAI Press.

Chapter 12 first appeared in German Berrios and Hugh Freeman (eds), *One Hundred and Fifty Years of British Psychiatry II: The Aftermath* with the permission of Athlone Press.

1 Musings about madness

It comes as something of a shock to realize that I have been researching and writing about the history of Anglo-American psychiatry for well over a quarter century now. It scarcely seems possible that more than three decades have passed since I first begun burrowing around in the archives of those Victorian museums of madness that in the early 1970s were still the all-too-concrete legacy of the enthusiasms of an earlier generation, those warehouses of the unwanted whose distinctive buildings for so long haunted the countryside and provided mute testimony to the emergence of segregative responses to the management of the mad. I can still vividly recall my first encounter with those structures: the vast and straggling character of the old, then-decaying county asylums; and the elegant façades (and the not-so-elegant back stage features) of the bins catering to a more affluent clientele. It is hard to forget the sense of constriction and confinement that oppressed one's spirit on crossing the threshold of one of these establishments. At a slightly deeper level, one recalls that there was a frisson of fear playing at the edges of one's consciousness, an almost daily emotion I then tried to dismiss as irrational, and now recognize was a subterranean anxiety that reflected, not any sense of physical danger from one of the pathetic, drug-addled patients who still haunted the hallways, but the barely suppressed nightmare that one might find oneself trapped permanently in one of these barracks-asylums (whereas, in fact, of course, I was always able to retreat gratefully back into the "real" world once night fell). Above all, perhaps, I remember the smell, the fetid odor of decaying bodies and minds, of wards impregnated with decades of stale urine and fecal matter, of the slop served up for generations as food, the unsavory mixture clinging like some foul miasma to the physical fabric of the buildings. Small wonder that the English alienist, George Man Burrows, once proclaimed that he could unerringly identify a madman by the peculiar odor that emanated from him (Burrows 1828: 296–298).[1]

Nowadays, such encounters with the physicality of mass segregation and confinement, with the peculiar moral architecture which the Victorians constructed to exhibit and contain the dissolute and degenerate, are increasingly fugitive and fast-fading from the realm of possibility. This was brought home to me a few years back when attending a conference in the South-West of

England, when the delegates had occasion to tour the asylums that once served the county of Devon and the borough of Exeter. Their fates were various. One was still clinging to an ever more tenuous existence as a treatment facility; another was in the process of conversion to luxury housing (its developers coyly disguising its stigmatizing past); and the third, the old county asylum where the eminent English alienist, John Charles Bucknill, launched his career (Scull *et al.* 1996: ch. 7), and one of the most striking and original pieces of moral architecture I have encountered, was derelict and deserted, contaminated by asbestos and hence left to molder away, the prey of vandals intent on stripping the last vestiges of its integrity in the pursuit of items to resell at a profit. All three institutions were clearly destined in short order to find themselves consigned to the dustbin of history.

My first encounters with the sights, the smells, the sense of despair that enveloped these total institutions ought to have been enough to put any sane person off any lingering attachment to research in such settings. A few months of this should surely have sent me scurrying off in search of more salubrious subjects and objects with which to concern myself. After all, as any sociologist worth his or her salt could tell you (and as every psychiatrist ruefully knows), one of the dubious rewards that flows from trading in lunacy is a share in the stigma and marginality we visit on those unfortunate enough to lose their wits.

But, as the essays collected here testify, I have resisted the temptation to abandon madmen and their keepers to their fate. The irrational, and what I am sometimes tempted to think are our culture's equally irrational responses to craziness, have continued to hold me in thrall. I remain as intrigued as I was, as a callow graduate student, by the puzzles that are posed by what we variously call madness, lunacy, insanity, psychosis, and mental illness, and by the elaborate social institutions we have created to manage and dispose of the mad.

Fortunately, I am not alone in sustaining these obsessions. When I began to explore the world of madhouses, mad-doctors, and madmen, the territory was largely unoccupied, save by a handful of administrative historians, and by a few clinicians who trespassed, with varying degrees of skill and chutzpah, on the historian's turf. And in those days, I too was an interloper. As an alien representative of a discipline then embracing a societal reaction theory that seemed tempted to dismiss mental illness as purely a socially constructed category, and to romanticize the mentally ill as the victims of unspecified but apparently arbitrary "contingencies" and labels, I was given a suitably suspicious welcome by both clinicians and professional historians. Lacking the union card provided by a PhD in history, I was initially presumed to share my discipline's disdain for the intricacies of the historian's craft. And in speaking of lunacy reformers and psychiatrists in less than reverential tones, I naturally incurred the latter's wrath. For a time (sometimes for a very long time indeed), whatever I wrote was viewed through the distorting mirror of my disciplinary origins. Even to this day, virtually every professional historian reviewing my books feels compelled to remind the reader, usually as early as possible in the review, that I am a sociologist by training (and I suspect the reference is not intended to be complimentary); and the dean of American psychiatric historians has dismissed me as a Marxist *enfant terrible*. (Grob 1990). (Sadly, the "enfant" part of his characterization is now about as accurate as his depiction of me as a Marxist.) As for psychiatrists and clinician-historians, well, though some of my very best friends fall into those categories, others have seemed tempted to view me as Satan himself. For one Canadian psychiatrist, my work is riddled with "astonishing misrepresentation and distortion" and amounts to little more than "sophisticated mayhem" (Merskey 1994); while one of his British counterparts attempted to dismiss my history of insanity in nineteenth-century England as little more than "impassioned denunciation" that was "historically wrong" (Crammer 1994). Perhaps, my favorite example of this sort of fraternal assault is the occasion when the former editor of the *British Journal of Psychiatry* used the pages of the eminent scientific journal *Nature* to denounce my interpretation of his discipline's history as comparable to the version of reality provided in the pages of Joseph Stalin's *Pravda* at the height of the Great Terror (Freeman 1993).

One doesn't have to be a Freudian (and those familiar with my work will know I most certainly am not) to suggest that something beyond simple scholarly disagreement must surely lie behind such explosions of apoplectic fury. It is perhaps as well, however, at least so far as my scholarly reputation is concerned, that not everyone has been disposed to side with such savage critics. At the risk of seeming narcissistic, I naturally prefer the verdict set forth in the opening paragraph of a recent survey of the state of the field, which terms my *Museums of Madness* "arguably the most influential monograph on the history of psychiatry in Britain" (Bartlett and Wright 1999: 1). To be sure that compliment rapidly proves a double-edged sword, for it turns out, in the eyes of this younger generation of historians, I have now passed from the status of the arch-revisionist of the field to the remarkably different position of being the very embodiment of orthodoxy, the Aunt Sally figure against which a new generation of iconoclasts seeks to prove its mettle. Still, in this context at least, on the whole it is better to be Aunt Sally than Uncle Joe, and for someone with a sense of irony, the situation is not without its amusing side.

As its subtitle announced, *Museums of Madness* attempted a comprehensive examination of "the social organization of insanity in nineteenth century England." Looking back a quarter century after I completed the book, it occurs to me that my original training as a sociologist is reflected, not only in the kinds of issues and the intellectual resources I drew upon in the course of my research, but also in the cheek of attempting a grand synthesis of this sort, given the impoverished state of the then-extant historiography. A historian in the early stages of his or her career would almost certainly have chosen (or been counseled) to focus on a more manageable piece of the larger puzzle. In all probability, it was only my status as a disciplinary outsider that allowed and encouraged me, in my first foray into the field, to attempt to provide a global interpretation of such a vast territory: one that sought to encompass the rise of the asylum; the emergence and consolidation of what became the profession of psychiatry; the changing contours of insanity over the course of a century and more; and the relationship of all these to the nineteenth-century revolution in government, to the "reformed" Poor Law, and to the Great Transformation of English society.

I hasten to add that in speaking of the field as it existed in the early 1970s as "impoverished," I do not mean to imply that, before I wrote on the subject, it was bereft of scholarship of lasting value. That would be a claim of quite astonishing solipsism and conceit. Moreover, so far from seeking to denigrate the efforts of all those who went before me, I yield to no one, for example, in my admiration for the pioneering researches of William Parry-Jones into "the trade in lunacy" (Parry-Jones 1972); or the wide-ranging scholarship of Richard Hunter and Ida Macalpine, whether embodied in their remarkable series of introductions to the facsimile editions of nineteenth-century monographs (e.g. Hunter and Macalpine 1964a,b) in their provocative reinterpretation of the "madness" of George III (Macalpine and Hunter 1969), or their extraordinarily useful annotated compilation of texts *Three Hundred Years of Psychiatry* (Hunter and Macalpine 1963). Yet for all their virtues, these contributions examined only very limited portions of the terrain I sought to explore.

Whatever the merits of the particular answers it provided, I suspect that few would dispute the claim that the polemical edge of the arguments set forth in *Museums of Madness* have served at the very least as a provocation to other scholars. I think, too, that the range of issues addressed in that book has helped to encourage the sustained examination and interrogation of a much broader array of primary materials, as part of the attempt to understand just what was distinctive and different about nineteenth-century efforts to manage the mad. For regardless of my disciplinary origins, I have always shared the historian's commitment to original archival research, and from the very outset, I insisted on moving beyond the records of parliamentary inquiries and the minutiae of the statute book. Within a few years, Michael MacDonald and Roy Porter had joined the conversation making the seventeenth and eighteenth centuries the respective focus of most of their scholarship (MacDonald 1981; Porter 1987a). Gifted historians both, they drew upon a still broader range of source materials and brought to the fore still other issues that my own work had ignored or distinctly underplayed. The cultural meanings of madness, the role of religious ideas and of the fear of "enthusiasm," and the effort to recover the patients' perspectives were all especially notable aspects of their work, themes that one can now see being developed in work being done on the nineteenth and twentieth century, and issues of great importance that I have tried to respond to in some of my own more recent research and writing (Andrews and Scull 2001, 2003).

MacDonald, Porter, and I all, I think, exhibit a distinctly ambivalent attitude to the work of Michel Foucault (Foucault 1961), and yet it is also fair to add that in no small measure it was probably his wide-ranging speculations that attracted us to the field in the first place. Indeed, I suppose that the very ambition and sweep of Foucault's scholarship may have found some Anglo-Saxon echoes in our separate efforts to grapple across the centuries with the transformation of social ideas and practices *vis-à-vis* the insane. Even before his untimely death, though, Foucault had become something of a cult figure, in the eyes of the sectarians incapable of wrong. Quite obviously that is a notion from which MacDonald, Porter, and I sharply dissent, and my own critique of some of Foucault's failings appears as Chapter 2 below. More generally, I would add that it is easy, and all-to-too common, to over-estimate the influence of *Madness and Civilization* on subsequent scholarship in the field. Had that book never appeared, one suspects that the critical, revisionist tone of the writings that appeared in the 1970s and 1980s would have been little different, for the intellectual transformations the new historiography both reflected and represented had far broader sources in the general culture of the time, and were all-but-inevitable once the isolation and marginality of the history of psychiatry gave way to an invasion by the new social historians.

Certainly, anyone who looks back with an informed eye on *Museums of Madness*, *Mystical Bedlam*, and *Ming Forg'd Manacles* cannot help observing that this body of work was very much influenced by and responsive to trends in what was then quite literally "the new social history." Given the emerging emphasis on "history from below" and on recovering the perspectives of the poor and the powerless, it was quite natural that this should be so. And if my own early writing was more heavily indebted than MacDonald's or Porter's to the work of such marxisant scholars as Edward Thompson and Eric Hobsbawm, more than likely this once more reflected my sociological leanings. It is to my sociological training, too, that I would trace my persistent concern with trying to link the history of madness to broader changes in English society's political, economic, and social structures, and in the intellectual and cultural horizons of its people.

I think and hope that my perspectives on matters psychiatric have developed, deepened, and evolved in the years since that early book of mine first appeared in print, and I have naturally had occasion to reconsider some of my earlier intellectual positions. The alternative would be painful to contemplate. To the extent, though, that mine has remained a distinctive voice in the historiography of the field, I suspect that much of that uniqueness reflects my continuing underlying concern with these larger social, political, economic, and cultural phenomena. Even in turning, in recent years, to what some would regard as an oxymoronic category, the writing of sociological biography, I have sought to place individual lives firmly in their broader structural context. To be sure, in attending to the lives of individual alienists, one is observing people making their own history. But their actions are continuously constrained by and responsive to the wider social and cultural context within which they occur, so that capturing the idiosyncratic and the particular simultaneously requires the closest possible attention to the realm of the social. As I have noted elsewhere (Scull *et al*. 1996: ch. 1) in the process of confronting and coping with a given social reality, even in attempting to modify and transform the options available at a given historical moment, individuals may be making their own place in history. Yet their life courses are at once constituting and revealing the contours of the culture and social structure within which they exist and struggle, succeed and fail. The more, in other words, that we seek to understand the individual dimensions of someone's life, the more inescapably we find ourselves engaged in an essentially sociological enterprise.

The essays which are collected here constitute a selection from the work I have published in scholarly journals and anthologies over nearly two decades. During that period, by any measure the history of psychiatry has come of age as a discipline. Since 1990, it has possessed its own flagship journal *History of Psychiatry*, jointly edited for the first ten years of its existence, by distinguished clinical and social historians of psychiatry, and advised by a similarly eclectic and eminent international advisory board. (With Roy Porter's shocking and premature death, German Berrios now soldiers on by himself.) First rate scholarship has continued to appear in a whole range of other general medical historical and psychiatric journals – *Medical History*, *Bulletin of the History of Medicine, Social History of Medicine, Journal of the History of Medicine and Allied Sciences, Psychological Medicine, American Journal of Psychiatry*, to name only the most prominent examples – and important conferences and their published proceedings materialize with great regularity (e.g. Bartlett and Wright 1999; Melling and Forsythe 1999; Micale and Lerner 2001; Porter and Wright 2003). A spate of specialized monographs on the history of psychiatry continues to appear in two scholarly series, my own with the University of California Press and the Cornell University Press series edited by Sander Gilman and George Makari, and as individual titles from a broad range of scholarly and general interest presses. And on a triennial basis, the European Association for the History of Psychiatry has met, successively, in the Netherlands, Britain, Germany, Switzerland, Spain, and Scandinavia. With a steady stream of new doctoral dissertations, and an array of promising younger scholars entering the field, the institutional and intellectual foundations of the field seem assured.

In bringing together a number of essays in a collection such as this, I hope to achieve three interrelated goals: to contribute to some sort of sustained, methodological, and historiographic reflection upon major figures and developments in the field; to address a number of continuing controversies that have roiled the discipline; and to suggest some important future directions for research. Programmatic statements about the sort of work that needs to be done can easily amount to no more than a set of pious platitudes. In an effort to give some substance to my arguments, particularly with respect to my pleas for a more behaviorally oriented history of psychiatry, emphasizing more centrally what alienists have done for and to those who form the object of their attentions, I have included here some essays that seek to put my prescriptions into practice, looking directly at questions of psychiatric therapeutics and practice.

I begin, however, with a set of reflections about the place of madness and the mad in the social order. Too readily, sociologists, Szaszians, and others have embraced the romantic notion that insanity lies simply in the eye of the beholder, that mental illness is a myth, that were it not for the psychiatric labeling process, the very category of madness would somehow vanish from the map. On the contrary, unless we grasp just how deep and implacable are the havoc and disarray madmen and madwomen spread in their wake, how serious and calamitous are the misery they create and all-too-often suffer, we are unlikely to make sense of how profound and basic a threat, practical as well as symbolic, such persons pose to the social order. To suggest that our organized responses to mental disorder, whether at the level of the family, the community, or the larger society, are inevitably bound up with questions of social control is to take note only of a truism: that in the absence of any effective response to such looming turmoil and chaos, organized social existence itself would be called into question. The insanity of place (to borrow one of Erving Goffman's phrases) and the place of insanity ought surely to be at the center of our historical reconstructions.

The English title of Michel Foucault's first great book, *Madness and Civilization*, suggests some of the sweeping argument that is to come, and hints that he will engage more or less directly with these broad issues of the threat and the encapsulation of madness in the modern era. And so, in his idiosyncratic and extraordinarily ambitious way, he does. Ironically, though, the French title of his book implies a much less ambitious study: *Folie et déraison: L'histoire de la folie à l'âge classique* (Madness and unreason: A history of madness in the classical age, or the age of reason) sounds far more like a conventional historical monograph, which of course it was not. The irony extends further, for the French edition, while more modestly titled than its English counterpart, was far longer and more detailed, containing a mass of material that even now that Foucault has been deified in the academic Pantheon has never appeared in translation.

Some of Foucault's many followers have suggested that, in a largely Anglophone world, the original text has gone undiscovered and unread, even by those Anglo-American historians who specialize in the study of psychiatry, and, more damagingly still, even amongst those who have ventured into print to criticize their *maître*. Given Foucault's fame and the iconic status many attribute to his intervention into the history of unreason, these are anything but trivial claims, and they clearly deserve serious and sustained attention. More broadly, of course, there is the larger question of the status of his writings on madness as a piece of history: how well have his assertions stood up over the past forty years? How reliable are his historical claims? And on what sort of evidentiary base do his assertions rest? Chapter 3 represents an attempt on my part to grapple with these and related issues, and to reflect more broadly on the reception of Foucault's work on madness in an Anglo-American context.

Foucault's claims about an emerging "age of confinement" were challenged sharply, albeit, quite characteristically, only implicitly by Roy Porter's history of madness in England from the Restoration to the Regency. Much of the first generation of revisionist psychiatric historiography, my own included, had taken as its object the age of the asylum. Whether dealing with the United States (Rothman 1971), France (Goldstein 1987; Dowbiggin 1991), or England (Scull 1979), it was to the nineteenth century that this generation of scholars looked upon seeking to recast the parameters of psychiatric history. Gradually, that temporal restriction began to be lifted, and Porter's *Mind Forg'd Manacles*, and his more wide-ranging, if misleadingly titled patient-centered book, *A Social History of Madness* (Porter 1987b) marked the taking up of psychiatric themes by one of the late twentieth century's most prolific and widely read social and medical historians. Porter was always most at home in the eighteenth century, and it should come as no surprise that most of his best work on the history of madness focuses on England in the Augustan Age. Chapter 4 represents a first attempt on my part to assess the challenges he laid down to the existing historiography of English psychiatry. Subsequently, provoked in part by the conviction he radiated that there was more to be said about English madness in the age of Enlightenment than could be encompassed by the Manichean visions of nineteenth-century lunacy reformers and twentieth-century historians, I have devoted an increasing portion of my research to trespassing into "his" century (as Chapter 5 suggests), an intrusion to which Porter reacted with character-istic generosity (Porter 2001). It was deeply shocking, in the spring of 2002, to lose so prematurely an interlocutor with whom I had enjoyed so many spirited and friendly debates stretching over most of our respective scholarly careers.

I have spoken earlier in this introduction of the widening and deepening of my knowledge of the history of psychiatry in the course of my career. Only rarely does the opportunity arise to apply that broadened perspective to the subject matter that originally launched one's career, but when Yale University Press approached me in the early 1990s about the possibility of producing a revised edition of *Museums of Madness*, the book I had written based upon my 1974 doctoral dissertation, I seized the occasion to produce a much longer and more ambitious volume, one that ranged backward into the eighteenth century, and treated developments in the late Victorian period at far greater length than I had been capable of some fifteen years earlier. Just before the revised edition appeared in print under the title *The Most Solitary of Afflictions: Madness and Society in Britain, 1700–1900* (Scull 1993), I was invited back to Oxford (where I had begun my academic training in the mid-1960s) to address the Society for the Social History of Medicine as its President. Chapter 6, "Museums of Madness Revisited," is the published version of the address I then gave in the library of All Souls College. Because of the nature of the occasion, I have not, in this instance, modified the original text, though considerable new scholarship bearing on these issues has, of course, continued to appear over the succeeding decade and more, and my own positions of some of the issues discussed in this chapter have likewise continued to evolve.

Strangely, given the heightened attention bestowed on the history of psychiatry over the past three decades, attempts to synthesize the new scholarship and to produce a text that tries to make sense of the whole sweep of the Western encounter with madness in the modern world have been notable mostly by their absence. Two earlier studies produced in the heyday of the psychoanalytic dominance of American psychiatry, and written in the absence of a developed historiography among professional historians, are notable both for their historical naïveté and for their ideologically blinkered approach to the realities they purport to discuss. Teleological in the extreme, these books seek to tell a story of a profession blundering down biological blind alleys and then finally emancipating itself at the hands of a hero and a genius, the incomparable Sigmund Freud (see Zilboorg 1941; Alexander and Selesnick 1966). Hegel's dialectic has sprung to life, for the one attempt to challenge these overviews is Edward Shorter's recent volume (Shorter 1997), a book that puts forward a crude negation of their thesis as the new revealed truth. Shorter's shortcomings, I suggest in Chapter 7, are a function of his being blinded by biology, and his attempt to heap anathema on psychody- namic psychiatry and to praise modern biological psychiatry has produced a volume every bit as radically unsatisfactory as the Freudian histories he attacks. A profoundly disappointing work, his book is further marred by his total lack of sympathy with most of the scholarship produced over the last quarter century. Though these very faults have made his distorted version of the history of psychiatry appealing to the profession itself, they leave us badly in need of a more balanced and nuanced synthesis, one that grinds neither the psychoanalytic nor the biological axe, and takes seriously the preoccupations and contributions of contemporary scholarship.

In an American context, one of the most serious and sustained challenges to the whole generation of scholarly work that emerged from the 1970s onwards has been posed by the historian, Gerald Grob. Beginning in 1966 with a pioneering study of Worcester State Hospital in Massachusetts (Grob 1966), one of the first American asylums to adopt the moral treatment approach to mental illness advocated by Pinel and Tuke, Grob would spend almost his entire career (spanning nearly four decades) working on the history of American psychiatry. His major accomplishment was a trilogy of books examining the treatment of the mentally ill from the early national period through the late twentieth century (Grob 1973a, 1983, 1991). An indefati- gable researcher, over the years Grob acquired an unrivaled knowledge of the archival materials that bore upon his interests, and insisted that his was an approach that stressed "understanding the past on its own terms" (Grob 1977). Sometimes implicitly, but usually explicitly, he attacked most of his contemporary rivals for violating this injunction, rejecting the notion that asylums and psychiatry had anything to do with social control, and insisting that the primary driving force behind the evolution of American mental health policy was a concern with "uplifting the mass of suffering humanity" (Grob 1973: 109).

Grob's sophisticated reworking of the traditional meliorist interpretation of the history of psychiatry won him many plaudits from the profession, who naturally preferred his version of events to the considerably more critical interpretations offered by most other social historians. If few people outside the ranks of specialists read his work, put off by the grey mass of detail his insistence on the wholly incremental character of mental health policy led him to provide, and by his dull and plodding prose style, his weighty tomes are nonetheless widely (and rightly) seen as the most thorough and systematic alternative to the interpretations offered by the heterogeneous group of scholars he labels as "revisionists," amongst whose ranks he undoubtedly includes me. Psychiatric history, for Grob, is a history of good intentions often gone wrong, of the benevolent defeated by the once sort of historical inevitability he seems willing to countenance, the law of unintended consequences: "mental hospitals were not fundamentally dissimilar from most human institutions, the achievements of which usually fall far short of the hopes and aspirations of those who founded and led them" (Grob 1973a: 342).

Elsewhere (Scull 1989: ch. 2), I have criticized what I see as the fallacies and shortcomings of Grob's metahistorical assumptions, and tried to show how they undermine the account he offers of the nineteenth-century developments. I shall not rehearse those objections again here. But Grob has also turned his attention to the twentieth century, trespassing ever more nearly on the territory of the sociologist, and pioneering the exploration of a territory that still remains surprisingly lightly surveyed by modern scholars. As Grob has done so, he has borrowed increasingly heavily, though in ways he rarely acknowledges, from the work of social scientists he still overtly distrusts. His account of developments through 1940, for example, leans heavily on sociological models of the professionalization process, looking to the changing circumstances and interests of the psychiatric profession to account for much of what he observes. And when he turns to consider the reasons for the abandonment of the mental hospital and its replacement by what is euphemistically known as "community care," his invocation of the changing parameters of the welfare state and the role of cost shifting between levels of government – local, state, and federal – borrows, once more without acknowledgment, from my own work and that of other social scientists (Scull 1976, 1977, 1984b; Rose 1979; Lerman 1982; Gronfein 1985a,b). For the most part, however, those encountering Grob's account of developments since the Second World War will find themselves on familiar ground. The stated intentions of interested parties loom large, and professions of benevolence are taken largely at face value. The creation of social policy is presented as largely a rational process, and just as before, produces "irrational" and unfortunate consequences only because fallible human beings are unable to anticipate the impact of their well-intentioned interventions. And all is ultimately for the best in the best of all possible worlds. Chapter 8 examines these claims, and suggests why they ought to be found wanting.

It has always been anathema to Grob to suggest that the psychiatric enterprise had anything to do with social control. David Rothman had published his *Discovery of the Asylum* to considerable acclaim barely two years before the appearance of Grob's own general history of nineteenth-century developments. In it, he offered a bold interpretation of the rise of the asylum, the penitentiary, the orphan asylum, and the poorhouse in Jacksonian America as the product of a widely shared imperative to secure the social order in the new Republic:

> The response in the Jacksonian period to the deviant and the dependent was first and foremost a vigorous attempt to promote the stability of the society at a moment when traditional ideas and practices appeared outmoded, constricted, and ineffective... The well-ordered asylum would exemplify the proper principles of social organization and thus promote the safety of the republic and promote its glory.
>
> (Rothman 1971: xviii–xix)

Grob was scornful of any such attempt to attribute the emergence of the mental hospital to an attempt by dominant elites to restrain "deviant groups or largely lower-class elements, thereby ensuring some measure of social control (if not hegemony)" (Grob 1978: 4–5). Such claims, he insisted, illegitimately deduced original intentions from consequences, and ignored the benevolence that he was convinced had been the primary motor of change.

I share Grob's sense that Rothman's account of lunacy reform is deeply problematic, though for rather different reasons than those he adduces (Scull 1989: chs 2 and 5). And I would be the first to acknowledge that social control is a slippery concept, all-too-prone to abuse (Cohen and Scull 1983). Nor am I oblivious to the reality that referring to a profession and its associated institutions whose public persona is one of benevolence and therapy as instances of social control is a rhetorical move almost bound to provoke paroxysms of rage from the professionals, and those who identify with them. Still, as I shall argue at some length in Chapter 2, the profound threats posed by madness to the family, the local community, and the larger society at both the symbolic and the practical levels can be ignored by only the most willfully blind, and they all-but-require measures to constrain and contain the damage to the stability of social interaction, the routines of daily existence, the security of both person and property. The particular forms those measures of constraint and containment take, the conventions defining the kinds of behavior, attitudes, and emotions that exceed the bounds of the tolerable, are historically contingent and variable. Likewise, the boundaries between what counts as bad and as mad, what is dealt with in overtly punitive ways and what is handled more discreetly, and in ways that purport to operate (and at times do operate) in what most would agree are in the interest of the person restrained, are scarcely fixed and historically immutable. Psychiatry and psychiatric institutions are not *only* about the exercise of control over others. But they are not *incidentally* connected to the question of social control and to the defense of the social order either. Furthermore, the attractions of intervening under the doctrine of *parens patriae* in ways that are alleged to be always benevolently motivated and in the interest of the person affected, and the benefits of being able to claim that one's actions are driven by value free science, rather than moral, political, and prudential concerns, are scarcely disputable. The changing role of the psychiatric enterprise in the maintenance of the social order, at both the intimate and the macroscopic level, is thus in my view an entirely legitimate subject for historical inquiry. Its contours clearly vary over time, and there is nothing to be gained, and much to be lost, by failing to acknowledge that in these respects, it is both appropriate and legitimate to refer to psychiatry and its accoutrements as part of the apparatus of social control. How those contours have evolved is explored in a preliminary fashion in Chapter 9.

The three final chapters that make up this book are closely interrelated. I begin this section of the book with some historiographic reflections on the importance of examining the question of psychiatric therapeutics. Much of the work I have discussed in this introduction so far (and indeed this is true of the field more generally through the early 1990s), tended to shy away from any close encounter with the details of what psychiatrists did to and for their patients, or to treat such topics purely in passing. For two decades and more, the heightened interest in the history of psychiatry focused on such topics as the rise of the madhouse and the asylum, the emergence of what became the profession of psychiatry, and the shifting relationship between mad-doctors, madmen and madwomen, and the state. As was also true of medical historians more generally, the practicalities of psychiatric practice and questions of what counted as efficacious treatment and why at particular historical junctures were left largely unexamined.

Fortunately, this neglect has now begun to be remedied. As I suggest later, this is a salutary development not least because it may be the occasion for beginning to repair the schism that has marked the field almost from its inception, between clinician-historians and social historians. Some of the best and most interesting work on the history of therapeutics has been undertaken by psychiatrists who have taken seriously the need to master the historian's craft, and thus have been able to surmount the outmoded distinction between the internal and the external, the scientific and the social (e.g. Braslow 1997; Healy 1997).

The question of psychiatric therapeutics began to intrigue me in the early 1980s. Indeed, I have been at work on a larger study of that problem in the first half of the twentieth century for two decades now, with my editor at Yale University Press waiting with preternatural patience for me to complete a promised book on the subject. The general historiographic issues that confront those seeking to make sense of the history of psychiatric therapeutics are examined in Chapter 10. The two remaining chapters in the book then seek to explore some of the empirical substance that I have suggested warrants our sustained attention.

Though I question the conventional "wisdom" that mental disturbance is somehow gender-related, and though asylum records from the nineteenth century reveal that men and women went mad in roughly equal numbers, medical men (and the handful of medical women) frequently sought to account for female madness in ways that sharply differed from their etiological accounts of the madness of the male. These preconceptions manifested themselves not just at the level of the speculative etiology of insanity, but quite directly in the therapeutic arena, where interventions directed at female reproductive organs had few (though not no) counterparts where the male of the species was concerned. But the course and fate of sexual surgery, even restricting ourselves to the Anglo-American universe, turns out to vary from one society to another, as Chapter 11 shows.

The vulnerabilities of mad bodies to the desperate remedies of those who held them captive and claimed to cure them were scarcely confined to the nineteenth century. Indeed, the decades between 1910 and 1950 saw a veritable paroxysm of inventiveness on the part of some psychiatrists, and the introduction of a quite remarkable array of somatic treatments designed to root out the madness and restore the lunatic to sanity. Some of these have become the stuff of popular fiction and Hollywood movies – lobotomies, insulin comas, electric shock – while others have largely faded from our collective memory – deliberately inducing meningitis, chilling mad bodies into the low 80 degrees Fahrenheit, causing them to breathe an atmosphere of pure carbon dioxide. Chapter 12 examines one aspect of yet another of these forgotten therapeutic experiments, an attempt to surgically excise hidden reservoirs of infection that were allegedly releasing toxins into blood and lymph, and thereby poisoning the central nervous system and the brain. As I have shown elsewhere, the application of the notion that madness was the product of focal sepsis drew converts among some of the major figures in American and British psychiatry and general medicine (Scull 2005). Here I focus on the major British proponent of the theory, a veterinarian-turned-surgeon-turned-psychiatrist with the perhaps appropriate name of Thomas Chivers Graves. Taken as a whole, I suggest that this apparently bizarre episode should serve to remind us of some of the sorts of consequences that have not infrequently flowed from labeling our fellow human beings as being out of their minds.

Taken together, the essays that follow seek to provide a provocative and wide-ranging survey of many of the major intellectual issues and puzzles that have characterized the history of psychiatry over the past two decades. They are intended to serve variously as stimulus, provocation, and guide, alerting readers to on-going controversies in the field, and staking out a coherent and I hope plausible set of responses to them. For whatever changes and developments have occurred in my thinking on matters psychiatric, I would like to think that a characteristic intellectual stance underlies and gives unity to my work.

2   The insanity of place[1]

In a little-known paper published more than a quarter century ago under the ambiguous title "The Insanity of Place" (Goffman 1969) reprinted in modified form as an Appendix to Goffman (1971), the American sociologist, Erving Goffman examined at some length the character and extent of the havoc and disarray a mentally ill person provoked among his (or, we would these days add, her) nearest and dearest, the wider social circle he was embedded in, and the social order more generally. Explicitly criticizing the romantic excesses then current in his discipline, which saw in the mental patient little more than the put-upon victim of an almost arbitrary social labeling process, Goffman suggested that on the contrary, "the social signifi-cance of the confusion [the madman] creates may be as profound and basic as social existence can get." He insisted that

> Mental symptoms are not, by and large, *incidentally* a social infraction. By and large they are specifically and pointedly offensive ... It follows that if the patient persists in his symptomatic behavior, then he must cre-ate organizational havoc and havoc in the minds of members ... It is this havoc that psychiatrists have dismally failed to examine and that sociologists ignore when they treat mental illness merely as a labeling process.
>
> (Goffman 1971: 356–357)

Hence the need to develop strategies for limiting and encapsulating the threats, both symbolic and practical, that the mentally ill pose to their immediate interactional partners and to the social order more generally – strategies that have clearly varied across time and space, but ways of coping that of necessity must allow for the more or less continuous employment of techniques of containment and damage limitation. The lunatic may be seen variously as the embodiment of extravagance and incoherence; incomprehen-sibility and ungovernable rage; melancholy or menace. The various manifes-tations of Unreason – the rages of the raving, the dolor of the downcast, the grotesquely denuded mental life of the demented – each pose characteristic and to some extent distinct problems for society. But all these varieties of craziness serve to create almost unbearable disturbances in the texture of daily existence, disruptions that, the Szaszs and the Scheffs of this world notwithstanding (Szasz 1961; Scheff 1966), dictate, indeed *demand* some sort of organized and exclusionary response if organized social life is not to become chaotic or simply to collapse.

Necessarily, that is, in a desperate effort at self-preservation, families, the immediate interactional circle within which the disturbed individual is located, and the larger society itself must find ways to confine and contain the overwhelming chaos that the presence of such a person threatens to impose upon them all. Here is the social imperative that prompted some eighteenth-century consumers to opt for the perhaps not-so-tender mercies of the mad-doctor and the emerging "trade in lunacy" (Parry-Jones 1972); and the Victorians to construct their museums of madness (Scull 1979), those total institutions whose descendants Goffman (1961) had dissected so savagely and memorably in his earlier essays on *Asylums*.

As Goffman acknowledges, though all-too-briefly as was his wont, those physical and unmistakable measures of containment were in the process of changing rapidly even as he wrote. Where, for more than a century and a half, the Anglo-American societies with which he was most familiar had responded to this looming threat to the public order with overt attempts to segregate the insane, locking them up in social spaces that isolated and confined them quite apart from the rest of us, by the late 1960s, it was already evident that a sea change was taking place in these social arrangements. The traditional mental hospital was a crumbling institution, often quite literally a decaying one that was being supplanted by an ideology and a practice that emphasized containment in the community. The place of insanity was being transformed in ways that threatened, if one accepted the logic of Goffman's argument, once more to let loose havoc and disarray on society. Such a development, he suggested, must all-but-inevitably provoke novel and more subtle measures of isolation, encapsulation, and social exclusion. Otherwise the new place of insanity would provoke the insanity of place – a social order so disrupted and compromised as to constitute no social order at all.

As this preamble suggests, the social uses and deployment of space are necessarily of quite central significance to those who interest themselves in matters of the disorderly psyche, and who pay more than passing attention to the tinkering trade that makes its living from the psychiatrically disturbed – those mad-doctors or alienists of our recent past who now, perhaps not so perversely, prefer to embrace the only somewhat less stigmatized title of psychiatrists. Symbolically and, for much of the past quarter of a millennium, all-too-concretely, insanity has occupied some very special places in our society and culture. Their changing physical form, their mutable moral valence, have exercised the imaginations of the artist and the novelist quite as much as they now do the architectural and the social historian. They have formed the sites within which psychiatrists have plied their trade, around which politicians have practiced their evasions, and inside which patients have passed their often troubled existence. Small wonder that their changing forms and functions should at last form the focus of sustained scholarly attention.

For those of us in the English-speaking world, the symbol of a segregative response to insanity has long been that most famous/infamous psychiatric establishment, Bethlem Hospital or Bedlam. More than 750 years old, Bethlem's origins were as a monastic foundation, one of the many small medieval hospitals that were a familiar part of the feudal landscape. Its transformation into a specialized receptacle for the mad occurred over the succeeding centuries, and involved at least two changes in its location – a move to an old monastic building in Bishopsgate which Henry VIII had granted to the City of London after the dissolution of the monasteries that formed part of the English Reformation; and then a subsequent relocation to a newly constructed building in 1676, after the Bishopsgate site had grown dilapidated and boxed in by the encroaching metropolis. And into the eighteenth century, it stood as virtually the only space uniquely set aside to house the mad.

Robert Hooke's Bedlam – for it was the polymath experimental philosopher and Fellow of the Royal Society (see Hunter and Schaffer 1989; especially the chapter by Shapin 1989) who drew up the plans for the new establishment – was constructed (with little regard for the long-run integrity of the building itself, but with symbolic appropriateness) on the liminal space just beyond the old City of London wall, built upon the uncompacted accretion of discarded debris and effluvia that had gradually filled up the old moat. Here was a spectacular new palace (and there were few models for a building of this size save a palace), a space explicitly designed to show off the benevolence and solicitude of the capital's citizenry. (On the architecture of Hooke's establishment, see Stevenson (1996, 1997, 2000).) Constructed in the immediate aftermath of the Restoration of Charles Stuart to the throne, an event that signaled an end to the brief flirtation with regicide and republicanism, it marked the recreation of royal and civic unity which were thereby connected to the restoration of reason in civil society and the abandonment of the mad excesses of Puritan enthusiasm. Bethlem's size (680 feet long and 70 feet deep) and magnificence dominated Moorfields, one of the largest open spaces in London, and the asylum grew larger still from the late 1720s onwards, when wings were added at each end to enclose the incurable (or such of the incurable who were deemed too dangerous to leave at large, the element referred to by the governors as "incurably mad mischievous and ungovernable lunatics"). Those who strolled across Moorfields enjoyed a spectacular view of the hospital's palatial frontage.

Contemporaries took a special delight in pointing up the ironic contrast between the striking splendor of the hospital's exterior and the impoverishment and chaos that lurked within, and the curious provision, in Thomas Browne's (1730: 29) words of a building of "so stately a Fabric for Persons wholly unsensible of the Beauty and Use of it." Here, neatly reflecting the ambiguous place occupied by madness and the mad in early modern England, were a set of paradoxical juxtapositions between inner and outer, ditch and palace, deprivation and ornament. "The Outside," as Browne would have it, "is a perfect Mockery to the Inside," and prompted one to ask "Whether the Persons that ordered the Building of it, or those that inhabit it, were the maddest?" Yet for all that, Bethlem's governors could revel in their establishment's grand, not to say grandiose appropriation and display of benevolence, its inmates housed in a monumental structure that gave Bedlam "a new dignity among London's charitable institutions and international renown."

It was in the eighteenth century that Bethlem as "Bedlam" truly assumed its archetypical place as a byword for all things mad and chaotic. At the hands of a Swift, a Pope, a Hogarth, to say nothing of a whole host of more anonymous Grub Street scribblers, cartoonists, and pamphleteers, it became a vehicle for satirizing the follies of the nation, even as it began to generate its own internal history of scandal and vilification. Cast open to the prying eyes of the public through a policy that (at least till 1770) allowed outsiders virtually indiscriminate access and license as visitors to come and gaze at the insane, it became one of the sights of London, an ever more popular source of public entertainment. Its wards had become emblematic of Unreason, its very name synonymous with lunacy, and its crazed inmates reduced to a spectacle to which the masses responded with mirth, mockery, and callous teasing.

Yet even as insanity came to occupy so unenviable an ontological space, the tide began to turn. If more and more hoi polloi gathered to gawk and to laugh, to view inmates as animals in a peculiarly human sort of zoo, those who thought themselves their social superiors and moral betters began to parade their own sense of sorrow, mortification, and disgust, maximizing the distance between polite and popular culture, and in so doing, making manifest their own more refined sensibilities. Visiting Bethlem became one of a number of evocative symbols of barbarous insensibility and vulgar showiness, alongside public executions, public dissections, grandiloquent charity, and grandiose forms of burial. Significantly, when the renegade Bethlem governor and mad-doctor, the eponymous William Battie, took the lead in raising funds for a rival establishment to house yet more of the mad in the metropolis, his new charity asylum, St Luke's, embraced a stark architectural plainness that stood in evocative contrast to the opulence of the Bethlem building.

The contrast was all the more glaring since the new institution was deliberately and blatantly sited almost adjacent to its ancient rival, where its simplicity and regularity, its absence of decoration and ornamentation, provided a silent but forceful reproach to what were implicitly regarded as the excesses of an earlier age. (And sometimes not so implicitly: recall Ned Ward's (1709: 50–51, 54–55) dismissal of Bethlem as an "ostentatious piece of vanity," proof positive that "they were mad that built so costly a college for such a crack-brained society.") A move by St Luke's in 1784 to new premises in

Old Street that were designed by George Dance the Younger, served only to re-emphasize the Spartan design ethos embraced by its governors. Consistently, from the very outset, they had declined still another form of display, banning indiscriminate visiting as deleterious to the welfare of their institution's patients. If it took two decades for Bethlem to follow suit, the changing place of insanity was clear: the insane were not merely to be shut up in a specialized establishment, but the larger society was to be shut out.

Of course, the emergence of a rival charity asylum in London was but one aspect of what in hindsight has come to be regarded the beginnings of a major transformation in the place of insanity in English society. The eighteenth century saw the establishment of a number of other charity asylums in the provinces. At least as important, however, was the growth of the private, profit-making madhouse sector. In just the ways Goffman suggested some two or two-and-a-half centuries later, the presence of the insane provoked upheaval and uncertainty at every turn – commotion and disarray in the family; social embarrassment and exclusion; fear of violence to people and property; the threat of suicide; and the looming financial disasters that flow from the inability to work or the unwise expenditure of material resources.

In no sense, of course, were these problems novel. But the increased affluence of many segments of Hanoverian England, and the entrepreneurial character of a civil society in which people eagerly sought new opportunities to gain a living, prompted families with means to be willing to pay others to assume some portion of these troubles for them, and provided no shortage of volunteers for the task. Private care relieved the rich of the burden of their troublesome and unmanageable relations, and sequestered them far from public view. To an increasing extent parish authorities also got in on the act, paying small sums to those willing to provide places of confinement for difficult or impossible characters of a meaner sort – and in London, these establishments sometimes grew to a quite remarkable size, containing 2, 3, even 400 patients at a time. In Bethnal Green, in Hoxton, and in Hackney, men like Matthew Wright took leases on large old houses and converted them into places to which one could consign the most disturbed and disturbing. And west of the city, in the village of Chelsea, still another cluster of madhouses now emerged, just as others also began to appear in the provinces.

Such mansions of misery (Andrews and Scull 2001) rapidly acquired a visibility and cultural salience out of all proportion to their actual numbers. For although in theory madhouses might provide an invaluable mechanism for drawing a discreet veil over the madman's very existence, well-to-do families often recoiled from taking advantage of such sinister silences. At the other end of the social spectrum, public authorities were understandably loathe to expend tax moneys on incarcerating poor lunatics, save where the sheer extravagance of the mad's behavior, and the perceived threat they represented to the surrounding community, prompted a more interventionist stance. Demonstrably, most people preferred to seek other solutions to the problems their mad relations posed, and, if affluent, they possessed the wherewithal to do so. And yet the image of the madhouse, and the gothic fantasies about what transpired behind its high walls and barred windows, acquired an ever greater hold over the public imagination.

In the protest pamphlets of a Daniel Defoe (1728) or an Alexander Cruden (1739, 1754), the threats incarceration in such settings represented to the rights of the free-born Englishman (or woman) were prominently advertised. In the prose of the high-class novelist – Richardson (1754), Smollett (1762), MacKenzie (1771) – madhouse scenes and ruffianly characters like the eponymous Bernard Shackle served to titillate and entertain readers from the respectable classes. And for a larger mass-market, the sinister and corrupt possibilities of these miniature worlds were employed to still more melodramatic effect, in tales of "Pityless Monsters" who "delighted in inflicting Pain"; of females confined in "Chains, and Nakedness"; of sane persons locked up and abused, till they were driven mad by the torments of their keepers and the spectacle of their fellow inmates, with their "Howlings like that of dogs, Shoutings, Roarings, Prayers, Preaching, Curses, Singing, Crying,… Confusion" (Haywood 1726; Wollstonecraft 1788; Smith 1798). Even in the more mundane setting of the law-courts, suits brought for wrongful confinement, particularly by wives whose husbands evidently saw in the madhouse a convenient place to stow away or dispose of an inconvenient spouse, now surfaced with some regularity. (See, on this point, the researches by Elizabeth Foyster (1999) into the King's Bench and other legal records.) Much of the testimony before the cursory House of Commons inquiry into the mad business that took place in 1763 likewise revolved around issues of wrongful confinement (House of Commons 1763).

If the public image of these new places to which to consign insanity was painted in uniformly lurid hues, the madhouse fared little better at the hands of nineteenth-century lunacy reformers or (till recently) twentieth-century historians. And yet, as *Museums of Madness* first stressed a quarter century ago (Scull 1979: 43), such spaces "provided a context within which, isolated from the community at large, the proto-profession [of mad-doctoring] could develop empirically-based craft skills in the management of the mad," including the various forms of moral treatment that emerged at the York Retreat, the Manchester Asylum, and elsewhere. Moreover, as Roy Porter (1987a) among others has argued, the very lack of regulation and oversight that a later generation would blame for the scandals and horrors they alleged were endemic in the trade in lunacy produced an extraordinarily wide variation in the regimes to which the inmates were subjected. Modern researches have shown that some madhouses, at least, had proprietors who took a personal interest in their patients, and were not the benighted and brutal places all were long portrayed as being (Smith 1992).

What was typical of almost all these places, however, good, bad, and indifferent, was that few were purpose-built. It was obviously cheaper to adapt existing buildings to the business. Most were small, often ephemeral, family-run enterprises, housed in ordinary dwellings adapted to the purpose.

Even the large London establishments catering to a largely pauper trade took over existing decaying houses, albeit those constructed on a larger scale. Thomas Warburton's White House, for instance, occupied a rambling Elizabethan mansion and packed more than 300 miserable inmates into the existing spaces, though, as Lord Robert Seymour commented before the 1815 Select Committee on Madhouses,

> the house having been built for a private family... [it] is very unfit for the great number of persons it now contains; the ceilings are extremely low, the beds are so closely stowed as to be nearly in contact with each other, and the airing or exercise yards are most inconveniently small.

With carceral and security concerns usually paramount, bolts and bars, gyves, chains, and manacles were enlisted to ensure safe custody.

Even the charity asylums – Bethlem, St Luke's, the Manchester and York Asylums, and so forth, which had been constructed from the outset with their peculiar purpose in mind were not "purpose-built" in the sense that came to characterize their nineteenth-century successors. To be sure, there was some limited attempt to adapt the buildings to the presumed needs of their inmates. Hooke's design for Bethlem, for instance, had made some effort to secure light, air, and space for the patients, and to exploit the advantages of its bright and airy Moorfields location, these requisites being seen as conducive to the restitution of its inmates' health. And George Dance the Younger designed the windows on St Luke's southern façade to shelter "the insane from the gaze of the curious" (Stevenson 2000: 105).

But these small gestures were a far cry from the thorough-going rethinking of the social spaces that contained insanity that marked the first reformed institutions of the nineteenth century. For what developed at the York Retreat, and at the institutions that modeled themselves on that Quaker establishment, was a growing conviction of the centrality of all aspects of the design of the physical spaces within which the lunatic were confined, and the possibility of creating a curative environment for the mad. In gross and subtle ways, the buildings that contained the insane could contribute to or relieve their madness. Architecture itself was moralized.

Bars, for instance, sent the wrong message to the inmates – an impression of punitive confinement, so Tuke, as is well known, used iron dividers to separate the panes of glass that made up his windows – and painted them to look like wood. No high wall separated the Retreat from the road, sending a message to those who approached – the madman, his family, the casual passer-by – that here was not a place of confinement or a prison, but a home. Built on a hill to secure fresh air and invigorating views, the Retreat's airing grounds sloped away from the buildings, and so far as the eye could see, no barrier interposed itself between inmate and the countryside – in fact, a hidden ditch and wall (a ha ha) concealed the constraint that remained, but the emphasis on its concealment is new and important.

What was taking place, in the eyes of its proponents at least, was nothing less than "a total revolution in the opinions of medical men and legislators, respecting the insane, and in the principles upon which houses of detention are professed to be conducted" (Browne 1837: 138). Henceforth, "from darkness [the mad] passed into light – from savage ferocity into Christian benevolence" (Browne 1837: 139), a transformation made manifest in the concrete forms that rose up to contain them. The new institution, in the words of the patron saint of Victorian asylumdom, John Conolly, was the place where

> calmness will come; hope will revive; satisfaction will prevail; ... almost all disposition to meditate mischievous or fatal revenge, or self-destruction, will disappear; ... cleanliness and decency will be maintained or restored; and despair itself will sometimes be found to give place to cheerfulness or secure tranquility. [This is the place] where humanity, if anywhere on earth shall reign supreme.
>
> (Conolly 1849: 143)

On Conolly, see Scull (1989: ch. 7). Physically, the reformed asylum could scarcely be more remote from the old madhouse. Designed from the outset to facilitate "the comfort and cure of the inmates," and providing spacious and aesthetically pleasing accommodations, the building itself made vital contributions to the "moral training" of its inmates, constituting one of the most powerful means of replacing "their morbid feelings ... [with] healthy trains of thought" (Browne 1837: 183, 191).

Not least, the new social setting within which madness was to be contained permitted the use of physical barriers to create and reinforce not just social boundaries (as between social classes and between men and women, for instance), but moral ones as well. The structural differentiation of space thus provided the asylum's guiding spirit with the means "to watch, analyse, grapple with insanity among the insane, and seek for his weapons of aggression in the constitution and dispositions of each individual and not in general rules or universal specifics" (Browne 1837: 181). Differentiating among the amenities and rewards particular spaces offered allowed one "to offer temptations to the lunatic to cooperate in his own restoration" (Anonymous 1836–1837: 156) – or at least to behave himself – and facilitated the use of every aspect of the environment as "a more powerful lever in acting upon the intractable" (Browne 1837: 156).

Classification rooted securely in physical structures thus allowed the careful separation of the tranquil and the raving, the convalescent and the incurable, and once "the patients are arranged into classes, as much as may be, according to the degree in which they approach to rational or orderly conduct" (Tuke 1813: 141)[2] – and note well the elision between the two – the asylum authorities had a powerful weapon at their disposal with which to prevail upon the patients to exercise self-control and self-restraint. "[The insane] quickly perceive, or if not, they are informed on the first occasion, that their treatment depends in great measure on their conduct" (Tuke 1813: 141). If a patient misbehaved, he was simply demoted to a level "where this conduct is routinely dealt with and to a degree allowed" (Goffman 1961: 361), but where the social amenities were sharply curtailed. Only by demonstrating a suitable willingness to control his disagreeable propensities was he allowed to obtain his former privileges, always with the implied threat that their grant was purely conditional and subject to revocation. As Goffman (1961: 362) was to point out a century and a half later, "What we find here (and do not on the outside) is a very model of what psychologists might call a learning situation – all hinged on the process of an admitted giving in." The importance of this approach as a mechanism for controlling the uncontrollable is perhaps indicated by the persistent employment of architecture to permit classification, long after its use for other purposes the reformers had in mind had been abandoned. Here, within the asylum's tightly controlled environment, alienists boasted extravagantly that "the impress of authority is never withdrawn, but is stamped on every transaction" (Crichton Royal Lunatic Asylum 1846: 35).

All too soon, of course, the utopian dreams of the reform asylum's advocates collided with the recalcitrant reality that mental disorders would not yield so readily to the blandishments of the moral treatment regime. Though the invention of a more benevolent image for the madhouse was a vital piece of ideological work for those who sought to construct publicly funded asylums, the social space that was the new county asylum could not long sustain the illusions its projectors had so sedulously constructed and promoted. The sheer numbers that flocked into the asylum quickly ensured the transformation of the built forms that contained the lunatic into those massive mausoleums of madness whose relics still litter the countryside – some, like the remarkable piece of moral architecture that is the old Devon County Asylum near Exeter now stand empty, vandalized, and decaying; while others, refurbished, remodeled, and disguised, are resurrected as domestic retreats for affluent yuppies who remain blissfully ignorant of the very different uses to which the structures they inhabit were once put.

Before inquiring further into those miniature worlds wherein so many of the deranged now found themselves confined, it is well to remind ourselves of an important corrective to an older historiography that a new generation of scholars has recently provided. (For some points of entry into this emerging field of scholarship, see Melling and Forsythe (1999); Bartlett and Wright (1999); Wright (1999).) The very visibility of the asylum, and its centrality to both the reformers' schemes and the legislation of the Victorian age, too readily seduces us into an oversimplification of the place occupied by madness in this period. It is by now apparent, however, that even at the height of the preoccupation with segregative responses to mental disturbance, a more complex portrait is warranted. To be sure, one major alternative to the asylum was the scarcely less institutional workhouse, where despite the nominal opposition of the Commissioners in Lunacy, a sizeable fraction of the more tractable, less-threatening patients continued to be confined by cost-conscious Poor Law authorities. The 1871 census, for example, reveals that of the 69,019 officially certified lunatics, idiots, and imbeciles, only 39,734 were to be found in licensed asylums, and we know that many of the remaining 30,000 souls were consigned instead to workhouse wards. Many, but by no means all, and a major challenge for future historians will be to explore the hidden recesses in which others still found themselves, some within the domestic circle, and some in the shadowy subterranean world of "single lodgings" and the like. (For some preliminary exploration of this generally illicit netherworld, see the discussion of Sir Alexander Morison's private practice in Scull *et al.* (1996: ch. 5).)

Victorian letters, diaries, and autobiographies provide ample evidence that, despite all the propaganda in favor of reformed asylums, upper and middle-class families feared them, and had low expectations about the kind of care their relatives would receive in confinement. (See, for example, Winkworth (1883, esp. Vol. 1, 67); and Ray (1945, Vol. 2, 81). Akihito Suzuki's monograph (Suzuki 2006) will provide the best and most sustained analysis of these issues.) And certainly only a handful of private asylums, such as Ticehurst and Brislington House, could offer a regime even remotely approximating the upper-class mode of life, meaning that institutionalization necessarily constituted a degrading experience for those exposed to it. (For one patient's protests that even the regimes at Brislington House and Ticehurst failed to protect his gentlemanly status and prerogatives, see Perceval (1839, 1840).) Single lodgings and other forms of domestic care avoided the damaging labeling process (and possible publicity) associated with private asylums; and they approximated more closely to the aristocracy's preference for treating illness of all sorts at home. (For examples of the lengths to which these families might go before capitulating and sending a relation to the asylum, see the discussion in Scull (1994: 356–361), which draws upon the casebook records of Ticehurst and Manor House, Chiswick private asylums.) Perhaps the most striking demonstration of this point is Lord Shaftesbury's response to the madness of his own son. Chairman of the Lunacy Commission from its inception in 1845 to his death in 1885, and principal cheerleader for the asylum system, Shaftesbury disingenuously insisted to Parliament that if his wife or daughter were to become deranged, he would at once dispatch her to an asylum, and he exhibited a vociferous and lifelong public opposition to extra-institutional care. Yet when his own epileptic and insane son became unmanageable at home, he surreptitiously shipped him abroad to private lodgings in The Hague, and subsequently in Lausanne, Switzerland. (For details, see Shaftesbury's unpublished diaries, especially the entry for September 5, 1851, and the discussion in Scull *et al.* (1996: 313, n. 80).)

For the poor and unlettered, the surviving evidence about attitudes to the asylum is much more circumscribed and indirect. On the one hand, their straightened social circumstances, the narrow margin many of them experienced between subsistence and starvation, and the crowded character of their living arrangements intensified the difficulties they must have faced in coping with the disruptions and depredations of the mad. On the other hand, the asylum's associations with the hated Poor Law and its stigma, and its reputation in many quarters as "the Bluebeard's cupboard of the neighbourhood" (Anonymous 1857: 353) must have acted as a deterrent to the utilization of its services. Still, once tolerance had reached the breaking point, it seems likely that ties of blood may well have tended to accentuate rather than diminish the desire for seclusion, as families sought to hide what was unquestionably a source of profound shame and potential disgrace from public view and knowledge. Even here, however, there were pronounced regional differences in habitual practices, with the Celtic fringes, in particular, exhibiting quite different responses from those characterizing the English heartland. Ireland, for example, its semi-colonial status making the imposition of centralized schemes from Westminster much easier than elsewhere in the British Isles, witnessed a far greater reliance upon institutionalization (Finanne 1981); whereas Scotland continued to rely heavily on its "boarding out" system to supplement its institutions (Parry-Jones 1981; Sturdy and Parry-Jones 1999); while the inhabitants of rural Wales continued to resist the seductions of the asylum, with as many as 60 percent of the known lunatics in Carmarthenshire, Cardiganshire, and Pembrokeshire still residing at home with relatives as late as 1872, and as many as 72 percent in Anglesey, compared with the 5 percent or less in the most highly urbanized English counties like Lancashire, Middlesex, and Surrey (Hirst and Michael 1999; Michael 2003). Special investigations by the Lunacy Commissioners, a group professionally wedded to the asylum solution, revealed vehement resistance among Welsh families to any attempt to institutionalize their relations. (See Commissioners in Lunacy (1876: 74–76, 346–349).)

Perhaps, as we have suggested elsewhere (Scull 1993: 364–365), the distinct lack of enthusiasm in the periphery for consigning troublesome relatives to the asylum reflected their economic "backwardness," which brought with it a certain insulation from the corrosive effects of capitalism on the strength of family ties. Be that as it may, and notwithstanding the need to recognize the existence of a number of alternative mechanisms for coping with insanity, it was the brooding presence of the barracks-asylum which dominated both the physical and the symbolic landscape of madness. It remained the lynch-pin of social policy toward mental illness till past the mid-twentieth century. It grew to an average size of more than a 1,000 by 1900, and the total number of inmates incarcerated within its all-embracing walls increased to over 150,000 by 1954. And, though modern researchers have striven to dispel the image, protesting that even in the asylum's bleakest years, there was much trafficking to and fro, as a substantial fraction of each year's intake found itself returned to the community (Ray 1981; Crammer 1990; MacKenzie 1985), contemporaries were increasingly convinced that it served as "a mere house of perpetual detention" (Francis Scott, testimony before the House of Commons (1877: 388), "a system," in the words of James Crichton-Browne, "providing convenient storage of heaps of social debris" (West Riding Lunatic Asylum 1873).

Here was a fertile field for melodrama – the money-spinning pastiche of Charles Reade's (1864) *Hard Cash*; the protests of obstreperous patients like Louisa Lowe (1883) against "the Bastilles of England"; even the telling of tales out of school on the part of temporary professional participants in the mad-doctoring scene, like Montague Lomax (1922). Meanwhile, for public consumption at least, the guardians of these cemeteries for the still breathing periodically offered Panglossian portraits of their merits, informing any who would listen that all was for the best in the best of all possible worlds. In his presidential address to his assembled brethren in the Medico-Psychological Association, Joseph Lalor denounced the "exploded principle" that patients required individual attention, and announced that more extended experience had shown, on the contrary, that

> large are preferable to small asylums, no less on scientific principles, and from benevolent considerations, than from motives of economy... [So far] from producing... general turbulence and confusion... the association of large masses of insane people is found to be highly conducive to good order and quietude.
>
> (1860)

And some three decades later, Dr Urquhart, superintendent of the Perth Asylum, echoed his sentiments, praising,

> the quiet, chronic patients who give stability to the asylum microcosm,... the phalanx of failures, whose well-considered routine constitutes the force majeure of an ordinary asylum, into whose orderly ways the newcomer of ill-regulated brain drops by sheer force of superior numbers.
>
> (quoted in Burdette 1891: 255)

Naturally enough, such a parlous place in the moral landscape of the community left the insane and their governors at the mercy of the cheese-paring economies of the public authorities – economies that at times pushed beyond the boundaries of community acceptability, as when semi-starvation at the Buckinghamshire County Asylum in 1918 helped to push mortality rates up to one-third of its patient population (Crammer 1990: 76–77, 113, 126–127). The perceived failures of the asylum ensured a dismal place for psychiatry in the hierarchy of medical specialisms, and brought complaints from some of the profession that "The monotony of asylum life is of such a nature that there is every danger of those who constantly associate with the inmates themselves becoming mad" (Winslow 1910: 26–27).[3] It brought new attempts to justify the mental institution's place in the defense of the social order – not, any longer, as retreats for the cure and restoration of lost souls, but as repositories for the biologically unfit specimens who might otherwise breed uncontrollably and worsen the already anxiety-provoking increase in insanity (Greene 1889; Strahan 1890; Maudsley 1895; Mercier 1914). And it ensured the periodic eruption of scandals that further blackened the institution's reputation without fundamentally threatening its continued existence or undermining its social legitimacy.

That legitimacy seems to have evaporated remarkably rapidly, however, from the late 1950s onwards. And once fundamentally questioned, the empire of asylumdom proved only slightly more durable than the evil empire that was the Soviet Union, or the Shah's regime in Iran. To be sure, many of the first skeptics were sociologists, not ordinarily the most influential of actors in the political arena. Academic studies of the social organization of the mental hospital spoke at first of "institutional participation in psychiatric illness" (the sub-title of Stanton and Schwartz's (1954) collaborative study). Soon, however, there were dark mutterings to the effect that mental hospitals "are probably themselves obstacles in the development of an effective plan of treatment for the mentally ill" (Belknap 1956: xi), and suggestions that "in the long run the abandonment of the state hospitals might be one of the greatest humanitarian reforms and the greatest financial economy ever achieved" (Belknap 1956: 212)[4] – a process culminating in Goffman's (1961) denunciation of these places as irredeemably flawed "total institutions," engines of degradation, misery, and oppression resembling, in their central structural features, nothing so much as concentration camps or prisons. They were, he would insist a decade later,

> hopeless storage dumps trimmed in psychiatric paper. They have served to remove the patient from the scene of his symptomatic behavior, ... but this function has been performed by fences, not doctors. And the price that the patient has had to pay for this service has been considerable: dislocation from civil life, alienation from loved ones who arranged the commitment, mortification due to hospital regimentation and surveillance, permanent post-hospital stigmatization. This has not merely been a bad deal; it has been a grotesque one.
>
> (Goffman 1971: 336)

Such negative commentary was by no means confined to the ranks of the sociologists. To the contrary, from within the ranks of organized psychiatry itself came a growing chorus of criticism directed at the policy of shutting up the mad in Victorian piles – the very institutions that had given birth to their specialism. Pioneer social psychiatrists like T.P. Rees wondered openly whether

> The time has come when we should ask ourselves seriously whether the interests of the mentally ill are best served by providing more psychiatric beds, building bigger and better mental hospitals. Perhaps we should

concentrate our efforts on treating the patients within the community of which they form a part and teach that community to tolerate and accept their idiosyncrasies.

(1957: 527)

From the Institute of Psychiatry, the center of the English psychiatric universe, John Wing and George Brown (Wing 1962; Wing and Brown 1970) wrote at length about the perils of *Institutionalism and Schizophrenia*. And, in a classic psychiatric maneuver, Russell Barton (1965) even invented a new disease entity, "institutional neurosis," to sum up the dire iatrogenic effects of the mental hospital on the patients it purported to treat.

Politicians were now slow to jump on the bandwagon. In his inimitable style, the Minister of Health in the Macmillan government, Enoch Powell, pronounced mental hospitals to be "doomed institutions," spoke eagerly of his own role in setting "the torch to the funeral pyre," and urged the need for boldness, "erring [if at all] on the side of ruthlessness" (Powell 1961). And, as is well known, successive political regimes of a variety of ideological stripes have enthusiastically followed his lead, periodically producing Orwellian bleatings about "Better Services for the Mentally Handicapped" (Department of Health and Social Security 1971) while systematically adopting policies designed to produce precisely the opposite effect.

The place of insanity has thus been radically transformed in the past half century. Our contemporary techniques of containment and damage limitation when it comes to the severely and chronically mentally ill bear little relationship to the segregative policies we once pursued so sedulously. Rather, with the ambiguous assistance of the miracles of modern psychopharmacology (which serve to damp down florid symptomatology in some, but by no means all of the lunatics left at large), we have opted for a regime that in some respects mimics the place of insanity in the Augustan age. Many psychiatric casualties have been thrust back into the arms of their families. Here, largely bereft of official support or subsidy, unpaid carers (usually female) are left to cope as best they can, though, predictably, the upshot has been that "the burden on relatives and the community was rarely negligible, and in some cases it was intolerable" (Wing and Brown 1970: 192. See also the early study by Grad de Alcaron and Sainsbury (1963), and Creer and Wing (1974).). After all, as Goffman pointed out,

the compensatory work required by the well members [of the family] may well cost them the life chances their peers enjoy, blunt their personal careers, paint their lives with tragedy, and turn all their feelings to bitterness. But the fact that all of this hardship can be contained shows how clearly the way has been marked for the unfortunate family, a way that obliges them to close ranks and somehow make do as long as the illness lasts.

(1971: 353)

For families cannot or will not absorb all of the burdens the new policies impose, and so examinations of the place of insanity in our own era must look also to the sidewalk psychotic, the boarding house, and the gaol, to grasp the range of our current provision (or lack of provision) for the mentally ill. Over the past four or five decades, as Britain, like the United States, has sharply curtailed its reliance on the traditional mental hospital, the state has systematically neglected to build up the infrastructure of services and financial supports essential for any workable system of community care. During 1973–1974, for example, while 300 million pounds was spent on the mentally ill still receiving institutional treatment, a mere 6.5 million pounds was spent on residential and day care services for those "in the community." Local authority spending on residential facilities for the mentally ill was a derisory 0.04 percent of their total expenditure (Sedgwick 1982: 251). Three years later, 116 out of 170 local authorities did not provide a single residential place for the elderly mentally infirm. (*The Guardian* (London), January 13, 1976, cited in Sedgwick (1982: 105).)

The pattern has apparently become even more deeply entrenched as the years have passed. Throughout the Thatcherite and Major years, increasingly powerful pressures were brought to bear from the center to control and curtail local government expenditures – if necessary by simply abolishing particularly recalcitrant local authorities. As central subventions to local government increasingly took the form of block grants, it became even more unlikely that new community based services would be forthcoming – and so it has proved. In the words of Sir Roy Griffiths (1988), in his 1988 report on the state of the mental health services, community care is "a poor relation: everybody's distant relative, but nobody's baby." During Major's (mis)rule, statistics from his health minister's own constituency, Surrey Southwest, indicate rather precisely what the place of insanity was in the government's hierarchy of priorities: in 1992, in this affluent area, "476 pounds a year was spent on average on individuals with learning difficulties, and only 67p. on those with mental illness" (Jones 1994: 239, quoting Martin Eede, Chief Executive of the National Schizophrenia Fellowship). Or as the *Times* put it in the aftermath of the Silcock case,[5] in the last four decades of the twentieth century, "Plans were laid to empty the hospitals, but no plans were made to provide alternative care...the accelerated run-down of the hospitals sent into the community people with severe conditions whose needs were never met, and are still not being met" (quoted in Jones 1994: 240).

To mask the human consequences of the policies they pursued, the Thatcherite and Major regimes quite deliberately avoided funding any systematic study of what was happening. Indeed, they appear to have done their best to systematically impede such studies, not least by curtailing the availability of basic statistical information: a tactic justified by invoking the Rayner Report's (1981: Annex 2, paragraph 17) remarkable recommendation that "information should not be collected primarily for publication... [but] because the Government needs it for its own business." Evidently, the

Government decided that it did not need to know (or preferred not to know) what its policies in this area have meant in practice. It is perhaps better for the politicians (if not the rest of us) if they do not know in detail what has happened to those no longer confined in mental hospitals, when and how existing provision fails to meet the basic needs of impossible and vulnerable people, and so forth. After all, in the absence of systematic data, individual scandals can be dismissed as "anecdotal"; and local authority protests that they are being assigned an impossible burden (and given no additional resources to meet even part of the need) can be met with obfuscation, or with advice about how to avoid their apparent legal obligations under the Chronically Sick and Disabled Persons Act of 1970. (See the memorandum from one of Mrs Bottomley's bureaucrats, quoted and discussed in Jones 1994: 251–252.)

Are matters much different in Blair's Brave New Britain? Given the Blairite emphasis on controlling public expenditures and the low priority of the psychiatric services for a government desperately grappling with the problems of a grossly under-funded National Health Service, it seems doubtful. Over the past half century, the place of insanity in our social order has been radically rethought and revamped, and seemingly permanently so. If the upshot has been to spread insanity into places which were once somewhat protected from its damage and depredations, that appears to be a price our political masters are willing to pay – and thus, by default, so we must presumably be. For those of us concerned to study the interrelationships of space, psyche, and psychiatry, the spilling out of psychosis into the larger society, the multiplying sites within which madness is contained (or not contained) must surely move us firmly beyond our earlier fascination with Bedlams and Retreats. A much messier reality awaits the mad, and those who would make sense of their place and their fate.

3 A failure to communicate?

On the reception of Foucault's *Histoire de la folie* by Anglo-American historians

In view of some of the critical things I shall have to say about *Madness and Civilization* (Foucault 1965, 1972), I think that it is appropriate to begin by acknowledging that almost all those who have worked on the history of psychiatry during the past two decades and more owe multiple debts to the late Michel Foucault. On a purely mundane level, it was surely the reception accorded to Foucault's work and the stature he came to occupy in both the academy and cafe society, that played a major role in rescuing madness from the clutches of drearily dull administrative historians and/or psychiatrists in their dotage, giving the whole topic the status of a serious intellectual subject and thus attracting us to it in the first place. More broadly, whatever else he may have suffered from, Foucault did not lack for intellectual daring, and most of the best recent work in the field for the past 15 or 20 years can be seen as responding, at least in part, to the intellectual challenges he threw down.

That said, how well has *Madness and Civilization* stood the test of time? And how far is its clearly mixed-to-negative reputation among most Anglo-American scholars a reflection of their lack of acquaintance with the full text of Foucault's argument? How far, to put it another way, are complaints in English-speaking academia about deficiencies in Foucault's scholarship objections that can be turned back with interest on the complainers, whose starting point may not be the complete and authentic version of Foucault's own argument, but rather the severely truncated (and occasionally inaccurate) English translation?

Regrettably, one must concede that there is some truth to these allegations. Foucault's defenders can point, for instance, to Lawrence Stone's (1987: 274) attack on Foucault in the *New York Review of Books* for being "unconcerned with historical detail of time or place or with rigorous documentation." Remarkably, for criticism emanating from so eminent a quarter, this turned out to be an assault which was itself so carelessly constructed as to leave Stone open to a quite devastating riposte, one which Foucault himself hastened to deliver.[1] Alternatively, Foucault's supporters can cite the treatments of *Madness and Civilization* in Peter Sedgwick's *Psychopolitics* (1982) and in J.G. Merquior's volume on *Foucault* (1985) for the Modern Masters series, both of which rely unapologetically on the abbreviated English text and on rehashing the criticisms of others.

The implication seems to be that the publication of a complete version of Foucault's argument, references and all, would suffice to alter the verdict of most Anglo-American specialists that *Madness and Civilization* is a provocative and dazzlingly written prose poem, but one resting on the shakiest of scholarly foundations and riddled with errors of fact and interpretation. To the contrary, I predict the reverse would happen: access to the complete text would serve to strengthen conventional historians' doubts, and to remove the most effective defense mounted by members of the Foucauldian cult. And this would not be (as Foucault's more sophisticated supporters would have it) because one could anticipate persistent mis-readings of the master's *oeuvre*, the product of the ignorance of an audience unacquainted with the subtleties of continental scholarship and in consequence condemned to view his work "literally out of context, [as] an isolated archipelago of studies lost in a sea of staunch empiricism and pragmatism" (Guédon 1977: 245; see also Leary 1976). Rather, the problem is the very genuine deficiencies and vulnerabilities of Foucault's historical scholarship, defects which would only become all the more visible in a complete version of his text.[2]

Claims that

> [Foucault's] erudition, if one challenges its authenticity (e.g. on the selection of sources) is at least as authentic as anything one will find employed anywhere else to back up more orthodox theses in the history of ideas.
>
> (Peters 1971: 637)[3]

can perhaps persuade the credulous and give the monolingual critic some pause, so long as one can wave airily in the direction of a 1,000 and more absent and untranslated footnotes. They are likely to lose their protective powers when one realizes that the whole of Foucault's discussion of lunacy reform in the nineteenth-century England, for instance, rests on essentially two sources, Samuel Tuke's *Description of the Retreat* of 1813 (S. Tuke 1813), and Hack Tuke's 1882 *Chapters in the History of the Insane* (D.H. Tuke 1882); or again, that virtually his only source for his discussion of English and Irish poor law policy in the sixteenth, seventeenth, and eighteenth centuries is the dated and long-superseded work of Sir George Nicholls (1781–1865).[4]

Erik Midelfort's objection that Foucault has wrongly assumed "that confinement of the mad by the state was uniform all over Europe [in the classical age]" (Midelfort 1980: 257) and Lawrence Stone's similar complaint that Foucault had ignored the "enormous differences in the degree and organization of incarceration from country to country" (Stone 1987: 271) have been dismissed by Foucault and his followers. The master himself retorted that, in the unabridged French edition of his book, "on pages 67–74 and 483–96, I insist on the pronounced differences between a country like France and a country like England" (Foucault in Stone 1987: 285). Similarly, Colin Gordon (1990a: 15) cites a brief passage on pp. 405–406 of the French edition (Foucault 1972) to "prove" that Foucault was aware and took adequate account of the differences between France, Germany, Austria, and England. Again, the existence of a complete English translation will only expose the threadbare quality of these defenses. Of the two passages Foucault himself cites, one is devoted solely to a comparison of the Pinelian and Tukean versions of moral treatment, and is simply irrelevant to the issue at hand; while the other contains a few desultory comparisons of responses to poverty and dependency in Protestant Europe and France, essentially tangential to the larger argument Foucault is bent on constructing.[5] The passage to which Gordon refers simply regurgitates a list of names and dates on which various institutions were founded – for England, drawn from Hack Tuke (1882) and Tenon's (n.d.) contemporary report on English hospitals and prisons, and for Germany and Austria from a similarly restricted group of nineteenth-century sources. The notion that this brief listing, which is coupled with some misleading comments about the absence of a medical presence in eighteenth-century institutions like St Luke's,[6] constitutes a satisfactory discussion of the issue of cross-national variation in the resort to confinement simply won't stand scrutiny. A full translation of *Histoire de la folie* would make this only too apparent to an English-speaking audience. Moreover, and contrary to the impression most readers would derive from Gordon's commentary, Foucault's remarks entirely fail to mention the phenomenon of the growth of private madhouses in eighteenth-century England, though this is precisely one of the major developments which Midelfort had criticized Foucault for overlooking.

In any event, Foucault and his followers are caught in a bind here, because for years, not just his critics, but also his supporters had cited his discussion of the Great Confinement of the classical era as one of the more original and important contributions of his study. As one can scarcely avoid noticing, there are all-too-many passages in *Histoire de la folie* which insist on the sudden emergence and the universality of the impulse to confine: the spread of "an entire network" of places of confinement "across Europe..."; an associated shift in meaning, which had

> so hastily, so spontaneously summoned into being all over Europe the category of classical order we call confinement.... There must have formed, silently and doubtless over the course of many years, a social sensibility, common to European culture, that suddenly began to manifest itself in the second half of the seventeenth century; it was this sensibility that suddenly isolated the category destined to populate the places of confinement...Confinement, that massive phenomenon, the signs of which are found all across eighteenth-century Europe...Throughout Europe, confinement had the same meaning
>
> (Foucault 1965: 45–47, 49, 1972: 66–67, 75, 77)

and so on.

Critics like Erik Midelfort and sympathetic voices like Ian Hacking (1986: 29) have scarcely erred when they complained of Foucault's "predilection for French examples projected on to European history..." Nor are they mistaken to see in this cavalier propensity to over-generalize a source of grave interpretive errors. (For some further discussion of this point, see Scull 1989: ch. 1.)[7]

Foucault's discussions of the periods before and after the classical age are at least equally vulnerable to criticism, and, once again, the appearance of a complete translation is unlikely to help his defenders. Tuke and Pinel play a central role in his account of the era of moral treatment, which has as its crucial sub-text the changing nature and extent of medical involvement in the management of the mad. As Colin Gordon (1990a: 8) recognizes, a vital part of Foucault's analysis is his attempt to represent the concept of mental illness as being comparatively recent in historical origin, constituted and made possible by a set of changes in thought and practice dating from the end of the eighteenth century.

In Foucault's own words, the world of the asylum which Tuke and Pinel created constituted "l'apothéose du personnage médical." Of all the changes they instituted,

> elle est sans doute la plus importante, puisqu'elle va autoriser non seulement des contacts nouveaux entre le médecin et le malade, mais un nouveau rapport entre l'aliénation et la pensée médicale...L'oeuvre de Tuke et celle de Pinel, dont l'esprit et les valeurs sont si différents, viennent se rejoindre dans cette transformation du personnage médical.

Where, on Foucault's account at least, the physician till the late eighteenth century "n'avait pas de part à la vie de l'internement[, o]r il devient la figure essentielle de l'asile." Indeed, the asylum itself now becomes "un espace médicale" (Foucault 1965: 269–270, 1972: 523–524).

It is, of course, in a distinctly Foucauldian sense that the master concludes (Foucault 1965: 271, 1972: 525) that it was "Tuke et Pinel [qui] ont overt l'asile a la connaissance médicale." Where earlier medical accounts of the origins of madness had been of a piece with medical theorizing about disease in general,[8] their accomplishment was to create a novel and quite separate species of mental medicine: "apres Pinel et Tuke, la psychiatrie va devenir une médecine d'un style particulier... pour la premiere fois dans l'histoire de la science occidentale, [la médecine de l'esprit] va prendre une autonomie presque complète..." (Foucault, 1965: 274–275, 1972: 527). And within the new realm of a madness subordinated to a reconstituted medical authority, the specialty they created was one "dont les pouvoirs n'empruntaient a ce savoir que leur déguisement, ou, tout au plus, leur justification"; an enterprise whose true powers "sont d'ordre moral et social..." (Foucault 1965: 271–272, 1972: 525).

But, notwithstanding all the qualifications Foucault introduces here (including the claim that "[c]e n'est pas comme savant que l'*homo medicus* prend autorité dans l'asile, mais comme sage" (Foucault 1965: 270, 1972: 524), the central thrust of this line of argument is to assert an intimate, essential, and positive linkage between the new reforms and the consolidation of medical jurisdiction over the treatment of the mad. And one must immediately object that, as it stands, this whole discussion is fundamentally misleading, obscuring – indeed threatening to render completely invisible – what I take to be perhaps the crucial contemporary implication of moral treatment for the relations between medicine and the insane. For Tuke was a layman, and the whole burden of his version of moral treatment constituted "a rather damning attack on the medical profession's capacity to deal with mental illness" (Bynum 1981: 43). Moral treatment, at least in its English guise, was a *threat* to pre-existing medical involvement in the mad-business, and, as I have shown elsewhere (Scull 1989: 118–161; see also Bynum 1974), it took a concerted effort on the part of interested medical men to put down the challenge it posed to their emerging hegemony.

Similarly, although Pinel was an eminent physician, his experience convinced him that medicine was all but useless in madness, and he concluded that the success obtained in applying exclusively a moral regimen "gives great weight to the supposition that, in a majority of instances [of insanity], there is no organic lesion of the brain nor of the cranium" (Pinel 1962: 5). Dora Weiner's (1984, 1999) and Jan Goldstein's detailed reconstructions of the circumstances surrounding Pinel's "discovery" of moral treatment has demonstrated quite conclusively "its non-esoteric, lay origins – which Pinel [himself] so proudly and defiantly proclaimed" (Goldstein 1987: 72–119). By his own account, his contribution was to convert this "charlatanistic" technique developed by the lay *concierges* who had day to day charge of the insane "into a respectable tenet of official medicine," a scientizing project he accomplished through philosophical specification of the mechanisms of both cause and cure, and through the application of statistical methods to measure and confirm quantitatively "the efficacy of the treatment" (Goldstein 1987: 105, 101).

In Pinel's eyes,

> the lay *concierge*, as diligent, perceptive, and talented as he might be, was inalterably the intellectual inferior of the *médecin-philosophe*. The latter would take the rough-hewn commonsensical knowledge of the former and transform it into something refined, scientific, and esoteric; the elite professional confraternity, at one moment threatened with dissolution by Pinel, was thus fundamentally – and quickly – restored by him.
>
> (Goldstein 1987: 77)

But not always securely: as Ian Dowbiggin (1986) has shown, in France, too, moral treatment's implied or explicit denigration of the value of medical treatment on occasion threatened the legitimacy of the physician's presence in the asylum, a problem which long persisted and, even after it had apparently been solved, subsequently recurred, much to the discomfort of later generations of alienists. So the role of Pinel and Tuke in ushering in the Golden Age of psychiatry (Castel 1976, 1988) is at the very least far more complicated and indirect than the reader of *Histoire de la folie* would realize.[9]

Famously, in assessing moral treatment, Foucault stands Whig history on its head: this nineteenth-century "reform" constitutes, in his eyes, the imposition of an ever-more thorough going "moral uniformity and social denunciation" – the historical moment at which the medical gaze secured its domination over mental illness, launching "ce gigantesque emprisonnement moral, qu'on a l'habitude d'appeler, par antiphrase sans doute, la liberation des alienés par Pinel et par Tuke" (Foucault 1965: 259, 278, 1972: 514, 530). Such ringing denunciations embody a rather complex set of assertions, some of which I think are defensible and correct, others quite dubious or wrong. Be that as it may (and the issues are too many and complex to deal with in a paper as brief as this one),[10] Foucault's claims about the silencing of the mad under the dominion of alienism carry all the more force as polemic, since they contrast so pointedly with his portrait of the openness of mediaeval and early Renaissance society toward folly and unreason.

Foucault's floridly rendered portrait of a Continental equivalent of Merrie Olde England, an era in which folly flourished largely free of pernicious social restraint, is the last aspect of his discussion in *Histoire de la folie* to which I wish to give some attention. Erik Midelfort made these lyrical passages, with which Foucault launches his inquiry into the vagaries of the Western response to madness, the focus of some of his harshest and most dismissive criticism. And Colin Gordon (1990a: 17, 16) has now tried to debunk this whole line of argument by suggesting that it is the compound product of the mistranslation of a single phrase and a refutation of something "not actually asserted by Foucault."

The phrase in question is Foucault's claim that, in the Middle Ages, "Les fous alors avaient une existence facilement errante" (Foucault 1965: 8, 1972: 19). In his text, Midelfort quotes Richard Howard's English rendering, that the mad "led an easy wandering life," while quoting the French original, together with the related passages which follow it ("Les villes les chaissaient volontiers de leur enceinte; on les laissait courir dans des campagnes éloignées, quand on ne les confiait pas à un groupe de marchands et de pèlerins.") in a footnote. Gordon (1990a: 16) pounces: here is a "piquant illustration of the scholarly hazards of translation." The phrase, it seems, should rather be rendered: "the existence of the mad at that time could easily be a wandering one." Whether that wandering life would be an easy one, Gordon then claims, "is on Foucault's account of the matter, extremely dubious" (1990a: 17). Thus, Midelfort's whole line of criticism is vitiated by his neglect of the French text.

What could provide a better demonstration of how a complete and accurate translation of *Histoire de la folie* would serve to disarm the misplaced criticism of Anglo-American academics? Except that Gordon's whole line of argument places a weight on "facilement" that it simply cannot bear. Foucault's chapter on the mediaeval and early Renaissance period extends for more than 40 pages, and Midelfort's rendering of his views ranges across this whole text. As a complete translation of *Histoire de la folie* would make clear, and as Midelfort correctly concludes, the dominant thrust of Foucault's analysis is to emphasize the real presence of madness *within* society, in daily life as in art and literature, "au coeur même de la raison et de la vérité" (Foucault 1965: 14, 1972: 25). It is the openness of mediaeval society to folly and unreason, not its harshness and cruelty, that is at the center of Foucault's account,[11] notwithstanding the glancing references to whipping[12] and to *Narrenhäuser*. And it is in this context that one is asked to attend to "un object nouveau [qui] vient de faire son apparition dans le paysage imaginaire de la Renaissance; bientôt il y occupera une place privilegiée: c'est la Nef des fous" (Foucault 1965: 7, 1972: 18).

The myth of the Ship of Fools is quite crucial to the image of the mediaeval response to madness which Foucault wants us to embrace, and quite naturally, in consequence, *Stutifera Navis* is the title of his opening chapter. Before he turns to the plastic and the literary arts for evidence of a wide-ranging cultural fascination with Folly, it is in the *Narrenschiff* that Foucault sees and seeks to capture the essence of the mediaeval response to madness. The Ship of Fools is, he recognizes, "une composition littéraire, empruntée sans doute au vieux cycle des Argonautes, qui a repris récemment vie et jeunesse parmi les grands thèmes mythiques" (Foucault 1965: 7, 1972: 18–19), and in literary circles, it has plenty of company:

> La mode est à la composition de ces Nefs dont l'équipage de héros imaginaires, de modèles éthiques, ou de types sociaux, s'embarque pour un grand voyage symbolique qui leur apporte sinon la fortune, du moins, la figure de leur destin ou de la vérité.
>
> (Foucault 1965: 7–8, 1972: 19)

But there is a major difference: unlike, say, the fashionable Ship of Princes, the Ship of Virtuous Ladies, or the Ship of Health, the Ship of Fools is something more than a literary or an artistic conceit.

Indeed,

> de tous ces vaisseaux romanesques ou satiriques, le *Narrenschiff* est le seul qui ait eu une existence réelle, car ils ont existé, ces bateaux qui d'une ville à l'autre ménaient leur cargaison insensée.
>
> (Foucault 1965: 8, 1972: 19)

Having made this claim, Foucault then launches on a lengthy discussion of the practical and symbolic significance of these "real" ships, with their floating cargo of madmen off in search of their reason, parading up and down the Rhine, haunting the imagination of the entire early Renaissance, living symbols of "la situation *liminaire* du fou a l'horizon du souci de l'homme médiéval" (Foucault 1972: 22, emphasis in the original, 1965: 11).

Unfortunately for all those enamored of this romantic and delightfully delineated landscape, reality must be rendered in rather darker hues. As Erik Midelfort has pointed out, the ship of fools (like Foucault's other striking image of the mediaeval leprosaria, waiting across three centuries, "solliciter par d'étranges incantations une nouvelle incarnation du mal, une autre grimace de la peur, des magies renouvelées de purification et d'exclusion" (Foucault 1965: 3, 1972: 13) till they were populated by the mad) is simply a figment of the latter's over-active imagination: "Occasionally the mad were indeed sent away on boats. But nowhere can one find reference to real boats or ships loaded with mad pilgrims in search of their reason" (Midelfort 1980: 254; see also Maher and Maher 1982). Where the mad proved troublesome, they could expect to be beaten or locked up; otherwise, they might roam or rot. Either way, the facile contrast between psychiatric oppression and an earlier almost anarchic toleration is surely illusory. And in the face of the magnitude of Foucault's distortions, and the significance of these passages for his argument, it is more than a trifle disingenuous for Colin Gordon (1990a: 16) to concede, grudgingly, that "as far as I know . . . the denial that riverborne deportation was a systematic practice in the medieval treatment of the insane . . . may well be correct"; and then to attempt to minimize the importance of this concession by asserting that "the contrary is not actually asserted by Foucault."[13]

Where does all this leave us? It is an interesting (and deplorable) variation on Gresham's Law that the appearance of an abbreviated or otherwise defective translation of a major scholar's work seems to preclude or greatly delay the issue of a good one. Foucault is hardly the first to suffer such a fate,[14] and he is unlikely to be the last. Of course, then, one would welcome the appearance of a complete and accurate rendering of *Histoire de la folie* in English, and one gathers that Routledge are planning to issue a revised edition of this sort, if the copyright issues can be resolved (which to date, unfortunately, they have not been).[15] If such a translation eventually appears, it will doubtless provoke a reassessment of Foucault's work on the history of psychiatry. For the reasons I have sketched here (and not just among the adherents of the liberal public relations school of psychiatric history), I would wager a quite substantial sum that the judgment rendered in informed quarters will remain largely negative.[16]

4　Madfolk and their keepers

Roy Porter and the history of psychiatry

Roy Porter was a phenomenon. In a scholarly career spanning less than three decades – a life that was terminated all-too-soon by a heart attack – he produced a prodigious amount of scholarly and popular work, much of it original and important. Among general audiences, he is perhaps best known for his learned and dazzlingly entertaining history of London (Porter 1994), for his rich and rollicking social history of England in the eighteenth century (Porter 1982), and for his ambitious general history of medicine over two millennia (Porter 1997). For more than a quarter century, following his move from Cambridge to London, British audiences encountered him in a variety of other guises: as an astonishingly prolific reviewer of books on all manner of subjects and as an ubiquitous presence on television and radio, wittily discoursing on any number of historical themes. Scholars, however, knew that these manifestations were only the tip of a very large iceberg: for them, Porter during his lifetime loomed as an author and editor of positively Stakhanovite proportions, a veritable one-man publishing industry.

Editor for many years of major journals in both the history of psychiatry and the history of science and of scores of books and major works of scholarly reference, he was also the author of more than a dozen well-received, specialized monographs on topics ranging from the history of geology (Porter 1977) to the history of sex (Porter and Hall 1995); from the Enlightenment's deification of rationality (Porter 2000) to the history of madness and unreason (Porter 1987a,b, 2002); and from quackery and "the sick trade" in eighteenth-century England (Porter and Porter 1988, 1989; Porter 1990) to a biography of another famous scribbler, Porter (1988a). Only someone possessed of prodigious powers of assimilation and synthesis (to say nothing of preternatural intellectual talents and curiosity) would have been tempted to range so widely – not the least because these are territories populated by hosts of jealous academic specialists, each small sect ill-disposed to trespassers from outside their own narrow little guild.

A man of protean energies and appetites, Porter also did much to encourage and stimulate the researches of others. He served as a mentor to a stream of students, and as a magnanimous and anything but dogmatic scholar, he provided venues for all manner of new work to appear in print – in a stream of edited books of his own, and through his work in founding and editing journals. His loss is still felt keenly by his legions of admirers, nowhere more so than in the history of psychiatry, to which he made a whole series of important contributions over the last quarter century of his spectacular career.

Porter began, of course, as a more or less conventional historian of science – or as close to conventional as he ever permitted himself to be. *The Making of Geology* sought to push back into what had hitherto been considered the pre-history of the discipline, suggesting that "attitudes towards the Earth and its investigation underwent great transformation in Britain between the mid-seventeenth and the early nineteenth century" – or in other words, during the long eighteenth century that was Porter's favorite terrain (Porter 1977). But a move from Cambridge back to the city of his birth only two years after the appearance of this first book brought a sharp shift in intellectual focus, from what he once referred to as "the body natural" (or Mother Earth) to the body *tout court* – from nature to self. Not that such a shift should occasion much surprise, for Porter was an intellectual magpie, always interested in the shiny and new, never keen to behave like the proverbial intellectual hedgehog who knows only one thing well, but happy to trespass wherever his wandering intellect found a topic worthy of his interest and talents. Besides, his new appointment was at the Wellcome Institute for the History of Medicine, about to enter upon its golden age, lasting two decades, when all manner of innovative and original scholarship issued from its academic staff and students, and from the myriad visitors attracted to the riches of its library, and the intellectual stimulation of its seminar rooms.

It was in this context that Porter first discovered the history of psychiatry, joining with the Institute's head, William Bynum, and with Michael Shepherd, an unusual and erudite academic psychiatrist who shared their interest in historical approaches to madness. For Porter, himself a working-class scholarship boy intimately familiar with social realities infinitely removed from those of the Oxbridge high tables and incestuous ivory-tower debates, here was a subject matter that ever after retained an intense fascination for him. The field was in ferment when he began to familiarize himself with it, as revisionist social historians entered the lists, doing battle with clinicians dabbling in the same subject matter, and with the administrative historians who had traditionally swallowed the psychiatric profession's Panglossian line about "reforms" in the treatment of the mentally ill. Renegade psychiatrists like Szasz (1961), Laing and Esterson (1965), and Laing (1969) (as odd a coupling as one could imagine) in these same years played the role of a fifth column within the profession itself. Sociologists proclaimed the romanticized notion that mental illness was all just a matter of labeling (Scheff 1966). And although Foucault had not yet become the intellectual icon he would be in a few years, his *Madness and Civilization* (Foucault 1961, 1972) had already helped to attract a legion of younger scholars into this highly contested territory.

For more than two years, between 1981 and 1984, under the joint sponsorship of Bynum, Porter, and Shepherd, the Institute ran a bi-weekly seminar that brought together the best of the new scholars and scholarship, and created a scholarly ferment that did much to institutionalize the new discipline of the history of psychiatry, and to set many of its agendas for research. For those unable to experience the intellectual excitement at first hand, the appearance in print of some of the best of the work that had been presented at this series of workshops helped spread the sense of what was being accomplished, and to inspire others to enter the fray. The three volumes of *The Anatomy of Madness*, whose editorial introductions are marked by Porter's punning wit and wordplay, have enjoyed a remarkably long half-life. Indeed, they have recently been re-issued by Routledge, albeit at a price that makes them accessible to only the richest of academic libraries (Bynum *et al.* 1985a,b, 1988). And news of the seminars in turn attracted an array of talented young students to the Institute, where they worked under Porter and Bynum producing some seminal new work in the field. In later years, Porter's gregariousness, his love of debate and social contact, led him to a whole series of conferences on matters psychiatric, as well as more sustained encounters with some of the stars interested in the subject. The upshot was a series of edited and jointly authored volumes, a number of them, it has to be said, of more uneven quality, and none of them approaching in influence the *Anatomy of Madness* series, but all playing their part in institutionalizing the new discipline (Gilman *et al.* 1993; Micale and Porter 1994; Berrios and Porter 1995; Gijswijt-Hofstra and Porter 1998; Porter and Wright 2003).

Of perhaps more lasting value was Porter and Bynum's short-lived success in persuading Routledge to publish a series of new editions of classic texts, complete with introductions by major scholars. Not content with riding herd on those who agreed to contribute to this enterprise, Porter himself took on some of the most interesting commissions. His editions of George Cheyne's *The English Malady* (Porter 1991), of Thomas Trotter's *Essay on Drunkeness* (Porter 1988b) and, most memorably, John Haslam's *Illustrations of Madness* (Porter 1988c), with its unforgettable portrait of the encounter between Bedlam's medical staff and the recalcitrant patient, James Tilly Matthews, are likely to remain essential resources for years to come.

Porter's indefatigable energies soon expressed themselves in other directions as well. He was one of the prime movers in establishing a continent-wide association of scholars working on the history of madness, the European Association for the History of Psychiatry and his platform presence helped to ensure the success of its meetings, from the first conference in the Netherlands down (almost) to the present. Virtually simultaneously, joining forces with the Cambridge psychiatrist, German Berrios, in a characteristic gesture aimed at breaking down the barriers between social and clinically trained historians that have marked (and perhaps marred) the field, Porter helped to found what rapidly became the discipline's flagship journal, the eponymously named *History of Psychiatry*, a periodical the two men edited in tandem for a dozen years till Porter's premature and ill-omened retirement.

All of these activities taken together played a major role in organizing, institutionalizing, and stabilizing a new field of scholarship. As important, however, were Porter's two most sustained scholarly interventions in the field: each of which in its own way reflected characteristic preoccupations that can be traced all through the work he undertook in the last quarter century of his life; and each of which exemplifies the strengths and weaknesses of his scholarship. In *Mind Forg'd Manacles* Porter (1987a) pushed back the temporal focus of the history of madness to embrace his favorite century, England's Augustan Age. *A Social History of Madness* (Porter 1988b), exemplified a theme that ran through all his work in medical history more broadly conceived, an interest in history from below, in recovering the patient's perspective, in moving beyond a passive portrait of those subjected to the medical gaze and the weapons in the medical armamentarium – and, we may add, Porter's attempt to reach out to a general rather than a purely scholarly audience. What, then, can we make of these two books? What are their distinctive contributions, their strengths and their weaknesses?

For nearly two centuries before Porter published *Mind Forg'd Manacles*, the treatment of the mad in Georgian England had been almost uniformly portrayed in the darkest hues. Nineteenth-century lunacy reformers pictured the preceding age as mired in ignorance and cruelty, conjuring up indelible images of monstrous madhouse-keepers beating their patients into submission, chaining them up like wild beasts in foul holding-pens filled with shit, straw, and stench; of the callous, jeering crowd – urban sophisticates and country bumpkins alike – thronging to Bedlam in their thousands to view the splendid entertainment offered by the spectacle of the raging and raving mad. Generations of Whiggish historians, celebrating the Victorian asylum as a triumph of science over superstition, the very embodiment of an aroused moral consciousness, sang variations on the same theme, seizing on the passage from the madhouse to the mental hospital as decisive evidence of our progress toward ever greater enlightenment and heaping opprobrium on the benighted denizens of an earlier age.

This comforting collective mythology came under savage attack a generation ago, when Michel Foucault launched his sustained assault on the Enlightenment and its values by writing a revisionist history of madness and (Western) civilization: a history that turned the Whigs on their heads and denounced "that gigantic moral imprisonment which we are in the habit of calling, doubtless by antiphrasis, the liberation of the insane by Pinel and Tuke." In the ideological atmosphere of the late 1960s, such radical criticism attracted many adherents, even (strangely enough) among politicians and public policy-makers, who were determined, for very different reasons, to turf the mentally ill out of the barracks-like bins the Victorians had bequeathed us and to subject them to the tender mercies of "care" in the community. Even among historians, Foucault's polemic prompted a wholesale reassessment of reform, and although few embraced the full fury of his onslaught on the machinations of bourgeois Reason, little of the earlier complacency and optimism about the Victorian era survived.

And yet none of this work fundamentally altered our view of the eighteenth century. Foucault himself had seen the Classical Age as the first decisive step in Reason's repression of Unreason. From his perspective, the period from the founding of the first *Hôpital Général* in 1656 to the events of 1789 was in essence the age of the Great Confinement, a movement which swept the idle and insane from the streets, severed their connections with society, and cast them into oblivion – an oblivion in which they were nonetheless compelled, lest they further offend bourgeois sensibilities, to work as a moral duty.

Those whom Foucault influenced tended to concentrate their attention on the dramatic nineteenth-century changes in society's responses to mental disorder, and to the extent that they cast their eyes back on the pre-reform era, saw little reason to dispute its unsavory reputation. Even Michael MacDonald, whose splendid *Mystical Bedlam* (1981) used the casebooks of the astrological physician and divine Richard Napier to illuminate the mental world of the seventeenth century, and to suggest that mental alienation and distress might then have been dealt with in surprisingly sympathetic ways, joined in the chorus of condemnation of the "medical brutality" which followed. "The 18th century," he confidently announced, "was a disaster for the insane."

It is this long-standing consensus of reformers and Whigs, Foucauldians and Anglo-Saxon revisionists, which Roy Porter's dazzlingly written *Mind Forg'd Manacles* aimed to upset. Examining the "long 18th century" from the Restoration to the Regency, he attempted to provide the first systematic account of the evolution of attitudes toward insanity; of the emergence of a medical discourse about madness; of changing social provision for the mad; and even of the experience of being insane, insofar as this can be reconstructed from the surviving writings of mad people themselves. The portrait of the eighteenth century as the psychiatric dark ages was, he suggested, a gross oversimplification, and in its place he sought to provide a richer, more nuanced analysis, albeit one drawn almost exclusively from printed sources and from such secondary accounts of limited portions of this territory as we already possess. On the whole he succeeded admirably, and the vigor of his prose, his skills at synthesis and his ingenious use of the materials to hand made the book something of a *tour de force*. He may at times have overreached himself in his desire to overturn the conventional "wisdom," and not all his claims will withstand critical scrutiny, but these are comparatively small flaws which scarcely detract from the magnitude of his accomplishment.

Foucault is among the first of his targets – in some respects, too easy a mark. For the notion of a "Great Confinement" applies poorly to England, where there was no substantial state-led move to confine the mad (or the poor, come to that) during the seventeenth or eighteenth century. Indeed, the management of madness on this side of the Channel remained *ad hoc* and unsystematic, with most madmen kept at home or left to roam the countryside, while that small fraction who were confined could generally be found in the small "madhouses" which made up the newly emerging private "trade in lunacy." There was no English "exorcism" of madness; no serious attempt to police pauper madmen (on the contrary, a sizeable fraction of the clientele of the new madhouses came from the affluent classes, necessarily so if the new entrepreneurial system was to flourish); and so far from attempting to inculcate bourgeois work habits, "what truly characterized" life in the handful of eighteenth-century asylums "was idleness."

Other demonologies of Georgian responses to madness postulate a benighted and brutal era, riddled with sadism; a period of therapeutic stagnation or even retrogression, in which a sympathetic therapeutic eclecticism that had earlier held sway was replaced by catastrophically cruel medicoscientistic and mechanical treatments. These notions, Porter successfully argues, are too one-sided. They fail to capture the diversity and confusion that actually characterized the eighteenth-century scene, and they distort and omit aspects of the changing social response to madness which cannot be assimilated to a Manichean world-view.

Madness, he rightly insists, was for eighteenth-century Englishmen an extremely broad socio-cultural category. Separately or simultaneously, its manifestations could be seen as medical, moral, religious, or even satanic. It belonged to the body or the brain, or to the mind or the soul. It extended and ramified in all manner of directions, and its boundaries were vague and uncertain, disputed and negotiable. Between Bedlam madness and the fashionable vapors and melancholy, no clear-cut lines of demarcation could be drawn. It follows that one must recognize the heterogeneity of the responses such diversity drew, and rather than resorting to simplistic generalizations, one should try to map the resulting complexity.

One important point needs to be made at the very outset: crude notions that attribute the discovery of madness to the machinations of professional imperialists are unworthy of serious attention. Porter has no difficulty demonstrating that madness was a real presence in the popular mind "long before psychiatry spelt independent professional expertise." Our efforts to reconstruct these popular *mentalités* are hampered, of course, by the limitations of the evidence that has survived, by the fact, above all, that our access to folk beliefs is necessarily mediated through the productions of the literate elite. But the limitations are not decisive ones, and with due caution we can uncover a good deal. Fundamental to most eighteenth-century views of madness was the belief that the condition was transparent, visible to all who had occasion to view the lunatic: a notion to be sharply contested in the following century, once a professionalized psychiatry succeeded in establishing itself and sought to make the expert diagnostic gaze central to the identification of insanity. Equally widespread was the notion that insanity necessarily involved a disorder of the body – a psycho-somaticism as common among the laity as in medical circles.

Nor can even the link of mental disturbance and the body be seen as directly deriving from the interested efforts of mad-doctors. It is tempting, of course, to attribute the insistence on a physical grounding for mental afflictions to the imperialistic activities of the medical profession, but Porter demonstrates that patients were every bit as eager as practitioners to incorporate mental disturbance into the realm of the body. Nowhere is this more evident than among those afflicted with the vapors, the spleen, hypochondria, and hysteria: that whole complex of mental unbalance and upset which became so fashionable in the 1720s and 1730s, and which George Cheyne christened "the English malady." For sufferer as for healer, an organic condition was a real condition, not a mere *maladie imaginaire*. Moreover, as long as "superstitious" causes and "magical" cures still had their popular currency, the thought that "these morbid distempers were monsters of disordered minds" was a terrifying one, suggesting the possibility either of diabolical possession or of the subversion of the soul itself, and rendering doubtful any prospect of cure. Faced, on the one hand, with ridicule for malingering and, on the other, with fears for one's immortal soul, it is small wonder that, for sufferers too, placing the blame on the body came to seem a preferable explanation for their travails.

The emergence of "the English malady" marked an important moment in the history of madness, a time when at least certain forms of mental imbalance became "not just acceptable but smart." These kinds of disturbance, at least, were not the peculiar province of the poor. On the contrary, Cheyne spoke for all his fellow physicians when he held that

> fools, weak or stupid persons, heavy and dull souls are seldom much troubled with Vapours or lowness of Spirits... [rather the victims are] those of the liveliest and quickest natural parts whose Faculties are the brightest and most spiritual, and whose Genius is most keen and penetrating, and particularly when there is the most delicate Sensation and Taste.

"Thus," as Porter says, "by a Mandevillian sleight of hand, fashionable physicians flattered melancholy, making the corruption of the oligarchy's brains as acceptable as the corruption of their politics."

If this gentrification of some forms of nervous disorder encouraged a certain degree of interest in the subject among fashionable physicians, the more violent and extreme forms of alienation remained beyond their clinical ken (at least until the second half of the century). There were, nonetheless, important developments even here. Over the period from the Restoration to the Regency, one can trace in medical speculations on the subject "a massive naturalization of the understanding of insanity. Disturbance ceased to be thought of largely in terms of sin or possession by Superior or Infernal powers," and the way was smoothed towards more "secular and social mappings of madness." In parallel with this, medical conceptualizations of mental disorder increasingly moved away from humoral accounts, toward more complex and rhetorically powerful (if no less speculative) iatro-chemical and physical explanations.

Such developments can only be understood as part of a wider movement to render everything natural and rational: a Weberian de-mystification and disenchantment of the world was taking place whose other ramifications included the rise of mechanical science, the extension of man's domination of nature, and the concomitant progress of material civilization. For a cosmopolitan elite intent upon replacing the kingdom of darkness by Enlightenment, traditional popular beliefs (especially popular supernaturalism and "enthusiasm") were a "deadly" compound of "credulity, superstition and fanaticism." Robert Burton's visions of religious madness as a satanic pandemic, a commonplace in Tudor and Stuart England, seemed increasingly incomprehensible to those "rational" eighteenth-century Christians unconvinced of direct divine (let alone diabolic) intervention in the world. More than this, religious transports – lusting after salvation, dreading damnation, searching for God's saving grace – "struck real fear into the polite and propertied, alarmed lest a popular religion of the heart should foment civil disorders, as in the bad old times of the Civil War." Medical theorizing about madness exercised a powerful attraction here, for one could move beyond ridicule and reasoned refutation of popular credulity and superstition, turning them instead into pathology, mere "Methodistical madness."

In less elevated social circles, the belief in madness as psychomachy survived and even, to some degree, flourished. Wesley himself "staunchly denied that madness was merely reducible to physical illness." Even though his *Primitive Physick* advocated the use of drugs and medical treatment (including electricity) in the battle against lunacy, he simultaneously "championed belief in a demonomania, and the practice of spiritual healing." As Porter confesses, we simply don't know how demonological allegiances shifted during the eighteenth century, but outside the ranks of the New Dissent and particularly among the more educated, one can clearly see that the literal belief in Satan, witches, demons and demonic possession was ever more firmly viewed as silly, superstitious, even sick.

All of this helped to humanize and domesticate the mad. Other developments, too, began to create the social space into which medicine moved as it sought to claim a monopoly over the treatment of the insane. Fragmentary evidence suggests that the practice of boarding out lunatics can be traced back into the years before the Restoration. Clearly, however, the "trade in lunacy" became far more visible and important over the course of the eighteenth century, being but "one aspect of the emergence of a thriving service sector in the *laissez-faire* economy at large." In a variety of ways, the nineteenth-century orthodoxy that segregation from the sane was in the madman's best interests thus had its roots in the growing resort to confinement in the Georgian age. Still, we do well to remember that the number of lunatics locked up in specialized places remained quite modest at the turn of the century (somewhere between 2,000 and 3,000 cases over the whole country). Reflecting the small scale of the trade in lunacy, Porter estimates that, by century's-end, somewhere between 30 and 50 practitioners were specializing in the business of treating the mentally disturbed, many of them operating madhouses. These establishments formed the matrix within which a set of practical skills in managing the mad could emerge, though one must immediately qualify this by noting that even by the close of the century, mental medicine remained "eclectic, pluralist and divided."

Most madhouses were small, informal, and ephemeral family concerns in the business of peddling discreet silences. Our information about their operations is correspondingly patchy, though Porter marshals enough fragments to show that there were great variations between such places in their clientele, the skill or otherwise of their proprietors, their size and their opulence. Contrary to the uniformly bad reputation madhouses acquired from the exposés of the early nineteenth-century lunacy reformers, Porter suggests that some of these establishments may have provided relatively humane care for their inmates. Certainly, the existence of a free trade in lunacy, virtually untrammeled by outside intervention, supervision or control, encouraged experimentation, and very probably contributed to the emergence of new technologies of treatment in the closing decades of the eighteenth century. At the same time, however, those laying claim to these skills had little sense of collective identity. Indeed, in such an inchoate, ill-organized marketplace, it was natural and unsurprising for each practitioner to emphasize his distinctive attributes and talents, and even his possession of "secret" remedies that made his operation preferable to those of his competitors.

Porter devotes a good deal of space to an examination of the theory and practice of these proto-psychiatrists, zealously seeking to rescue them from the neglect or contempt they have encountered at the hands of other historians. It is wrong, he asserts, to dismiss their writings as "either tedious or second-hand." He intends, as well, to emphasize the continuities between eighteenth-century practices and the Utopian programs of nineteenth-century lunacy reformers; to show that the practices of the new moral treatment regime cannot be represented as a distinct rupture with the past; to insist that "both in rhetoric and in reality, 'moral' forms of therapy were well tried and tested long before the close of the 18th century." There is perhaps a measure of truth to some of these claims, but Porter's eagerness to rescue the reputation of the Georgian age prompts him to some strained interpretations of the evidence and a serious overstatement of his case. I don't mean to imply that his attitude toward his favored period is wholly uncritical, he accepts, for instance, that "for pauper mad people, the Georgian madhouse was hell" (while quite rightly insisting that "as yet we know too little about how they were treated previously, to be able to say with confidence whether it was a worse, or just a different, hell"). On larger interpretative issues, however, his arguments and judgments strike me as distinctly more dubious.

Take, for example, his affirmative answer to his own question: "Was there a moral therapy in the 18th century?" Other revisionist historians (myself included) have long contended that Tuke's well-publicized program at the York Retreat was not an isolated achievement. The whole thrust of this body of work has been directed at demythologizing moral treatment, disabusing us of the naïve notion that it was the isolated product of individual genius, and tracing some of the broader social roots of the new ethic of rehabilitation which it exemplified. Moreover, such claims have necessarily accorded a crucial place to evidence of virtually simultaneous and multiple discoveries of the principles underlying moral treatment, not just the widely publicized examples of Pinel and Chiarugi on the Continent, but domestic parallels as well, such as the work of John Ferriar at the Manchester Lunatic Asylum in the 1790s, of or Edward Long Fox, from whose Bristol madhouse Tuke recruited Katherine Allen, the Retreat's first matron.

In what ways does Porter claim to go beyond this? First, by widening the circle of those entitled to be known as "moral managers" to encompass a much larger group comprising of William Battie, Thomas Arnold, William Perfect, Joseph Mason Cox, Francis Willis, Benjamin Faulkner, William Pargeter, Thomas Bakewell, William Hallaran, and others. But immediately problems arise. Of these figures, only the unfortunately named William Battie was active before the 1780s, and Cox, Bakewell, and Hallaran are nineteenth-century practitioners. As Porter concedes elsewhere, we know remarkably little about Battie's practice other than the fact that it made him a very rich man. Hence the only ground for asserting that Battie is somehow the "real" pioneer of moral treatment turns out to be the text of his 1758 *Treatise on Madness*, a book which Porter insists "contains (albeit in a rather schematic and theoretical ideas) the key ideas of Tukean moral therapy."

This simply won't do. Not least, it raises in an acute form the obvious problems of making inferences from theory to praxis. Porter assumes that the two conveniently coincide here because his argument requires it. Elsewhere, he exhibits a more seemly skepticism. Thomas Fallowes, for instance, was a quack who possessed a self-awarded MD and flourished in the early eighteenth century. He has the doubtful honor of being the first mad-doctor convicted for illegally confining a patient. Fallowes promised, in Porter's words, "a veritable pudding time to his clients ... curative therapy, gentleness and comforts – good accommodation, air, exercise and diet." The reality was, of course, very different but "every proprietor knew he could not cash in by harping on the severity of his treatments, or on his talents as a whip master." Quite so. But granting the point, why should we assume that Battie was different? Why, on this occasion, should we follow Porter in treating Battie's pious protestations about his practices as any more believable than his less reputable rival?

Battie's conviction that "management did much more than medicine" likewise did not distinguish him, even from what most historians have seen as the benighted practices of the Monro family at Bedlam, the doctrine being borrowed from the Monros' few public pronouncements on how one ought to go about managing the mad. (Recently, indeed, Jonathan Andrews and I (Andrews and Scull 2001) have shown just how similar the practices of the two rivals for prominence in the metropolitan mad-business really were.) And while Battie's insistence on the individual character of madness and its unresponsiveness to universal cures, together with his adoption of Lockeian associationism, did mark some tentative steps toward a fresh therapeutics, all of this remained a considerable distance from "moral treatment" as a later generation was to understand the term.

The closing decades of the eighteenth century witnessed a good deal of therapeutic experimentation among madhouse proprietors, including those Porter labels "moral managers." Deriving very different conclusions from Lockeian associationism than those underpinning Tuke's moral treatment, these men stressed that the madman's loss of contact with our consensually defined reality reflected how deeply the chains of false impressions and associations were engraved on his system – a conclusion which both licensed and required that extreme measures be taken to jolt the system back into sanity. Shower baths, rotating chairs, tranquillizing chairs, and other exotic forms of physical restraint and coercion were all employed in a Herculean effort to force the thought processes out of their erroneous pathways. And behind this technology lies the heroic figure of the mad-doctor himself, able, as Pargeter put it, to be at one moment "placed and accommodating in his manners, and the next, angry and absolute," willing to try "kindness and mildness" but never hesitating, in Joseph Mason Cox's words, to employ "irresistible control and coercion."

Contrast this with Tuke's insistence that attempts to compel patients to think and act reasonably were themselves irrational. He pronounced, "intimidation or coercion, "may make or modify the symptoms of insanity, but can seldom produce permanently good results." Besides, the tamed madman, like the tamed tiger, "is the result of treatment at which humanity would shudder." As even Porter is ultimately driven to acknowledge,

> management took on a very special connotation at the Retreat. For little store was set by the theatrical talents or verbal acrobatics of the doctor in breaking the will of, or outwitting, the lunatics. Instead of Napoleonic generalship or the "terrific system," the Retreat emphasized community.

Walking, talking, taking tea with their superintendent, patients were to be taught to restrain themselves by a regime which cleverly exploited their "desire for esteem" within the confines of a carefully constructed therapeutic environment. All of which, *pace* Porter, constitutes a distinct departure from the practices of Pargeter *et al.* even if it had its analogues elsewhere.

Alongside *Mind Forg'd Manacles*, in a typical manifestation of his notorious rate-busting tendencies, Porter simultaneously produced a companion volume, misleadingly labeled by its publisher, presumably in hopes of hyping its sales, *A Social History of Madness*. As happens all too frequently, the book's contents are more accurately conveyed by its subtitle *Stories of the Insane*. As much as possible, it is also a volume that tries to recapture these as stories *by* the insane, and in this respect, it is of a piece with some of Porter's best work in the broader field of the history of medicine. As he moved from his earlier incarnation as a historian of science to work on the social history of medicine,

Porter was one of the first to insist on the importance of recovering the patient's perspective on illness and its treatment. Such an endeavor is perhaps especially difficult in the case of the insane, for their status as moral actors is essentially erased once they have entered the ranks of the lunatic, and their words and actions are too readily dismissed as the ravings and importunings of the irrational, epiphenomenal noise of no interest or substantial significance. All-too-successfully, over the past quarter-millennium, society has sought to shut them up, literally and metaphorically, in the process invalidating and essentially eliminating their own voices.

As always, it turns out that Porter is a splendid spinner of tales, drawing on the autobiographical writings of two dozen mad people to recover their consciousness rather than their unconscious, "to explore what mad people meant to say, what was on their minds." The cast of characters includes Nietzsche, Cowper, and John Clare; Sylvia Plath, Laing's Mary Barnes, and Freud's Dora; Robert Schumann and Vaslav Nijinsky; and poor George III, in his declining years a living facsimile of Lear.

There are also other less familiar figures. There is, for instance, the remarkable Alexander Cruden, the self-styled Alexander the Corrector, an expatriate Scotsman, Protestant fundamentalist, author of a Biblical concordance published in 1737 and still in print today, proof-reader *extraordinaire*, who was consigned to a series of madhouses for such offences as his obsessional courtship of an affluent widow, Mrs Payne, and subsequently of the wealthy daughter of a former Lord Mayor of London, a woman whom he had never met, and never did manage to meet ("Like Freud, Cruden never took no for an answer"); and on a subsequent occasion, hauled off by his sister, Mrs Isabella Wild ("Cruden was plagued by names"), for taking a shovel and using it to whack a malefactor he saw profaning the Sabbath. Cruden's response to his assorted confinements was to launch a pamphlet war against madhouses, "English Bastilles" which robbed the free-born Briton of his liberties. A monstrous, wholly blinkered egoist, he was for ever "vindicating" himself. (For a recent biography of Cruden, see Keay 2004; see also Andrews and Scull 2001, ch. 3.)

As Porter proceeds to demonstrate, the patient as crusader appears in multiple guises. John Perceval, son of the last British prime minister to be assassinated, differed from Cruden in acknowledging that he was mad, not simply a sane man locked up by his enemies. But he found his asylum treatment "inquisitorial, inhumane, degrading," and he insisted that although religious terror had brought on his insanity, "the real cause of the appalling severity and prolongation of his condition was the medico-psychiatric treatment he had received." On his recovery, and to his family's distress and dismay, Perceval became a lifelong critic of Victorian asylumdom, and one of the prime movers in the wonderfully named Alleged Lunatics' Friend Society. (See Hervey 1986. For Perceval's own account of his illness and treatment, see Perceval 1839, 1840.)

Some of the most devastating passages in Porter's book deal with Freud and his follies. Porter never displayed much sympathy for psychoanalytic speculation, and here he examines, for instance, the case of Daniel Schreber, former chief judge to the Dresden court of appeal. Schreber's *Memoirs* of his madness were used by Freud as one of the props for his theory that there was an intimate connection between paranoia and homosexuality. Freud sees Schreber's fears of castration in terms of his "putative desire to be sodomized by Flechsig" – his physician – "and (by derivation) by his brother and father." Porter takes some pleasure in pointing out that Schreber's fear was well-grounded in reality, "for the neuro-anatomist Flechsig made therapeutic use of castration at his clinic." Similarly, he notes that Schreber's father was one of Germany's best-known pediatricians, a man who placed "overwhelming emphasis upon the values of duty, discipline, control, and 'unconditional obedience' " and who practiced what he preached on his own children. Yet Freud, who was most certainly aware of Schreber *père's* principles, saw no connection between the father's unremitting tutorial surveillance and the son's madness, though it turns out that the latter's delusions of persecution in middle age exactly reproduced bizarre physical contraptions his father had used and recommended.

Equally sobering are Porter's discussions of "Dora" (Ida Bauer) and the "Wolf Man," Sergius P., the person Freud helped turn into "the eternal patient, a nonagenarian proof of analysis interminable." Reading Porter's reconstruction of the events surrounding their "madness" and his examination of what Freud made of their symptoms, one is tempted to adopt his view that the founder of psychoanalysis all too closely resembled the obsessional theorist in Swift's *A Tale of a Tub*. Freud even picked up "Swift's trick whereby pseudo-confessions of ignorance are turned into a demonstration of omniscience."

Porter plausibly suggests that the words and actions of the "mad" can be seen as "the struggles of the despairing and powerless to exercise some control over those – devils, spooks, mad-doctors, priests – who had them in their power." Well yes, this may in part be what is going on here. But, as he himself admits, the evidence he adduces is "highly selective and episodic." An anthropological relativism that refuses to accord "the myths advanced by earlier mad-doctors and psychiatrists any privileged truth status" risks romanticizing the mad, and notwithstanding Porter's protestations that "it would be facile" to portray all of the insane "as victims pure and simple of psychiatry," his clever reconstructions of the patients' progress make it all too easy to do precisely that.

But if there are grounds for objecting that this first stab at reconstructing the patient's point of view is too glib, too quick to represent the mad as put-upon, too ready to construct clever readings that may or may not correspond to the lived reality of insanity and its interpersonal impacts, one must nonetheless acknowledge the heuristic value of this change of tack. For much even of the revisionist work in the history of psychiatry in the 1970s and 1980s, critical or even over-critical of the psychiatric enterprise as it may have been, had had remarkably little to say about the objects of professional attention, the mad folk themselves. Patients too-often remained all-but-invisible, or mere ciphers assumed to play no independent role in the drama that was being reconstructed. David Ingleby's witty objection (Ingleby 1983: 142) that these histories closely resembled "the histories of colonial wars [and told] us more about the relations between the imperial powers than about the 'third world' of the mental patients themselves" was unfortunately all-too-accurate when he raised it. If it is no longer a valid criticism of the field, Porter's *A Social History of Madness*, for all its limitations, deserves a significant share of the credit.

Still, the task of taking the perspective of the patient seriously is by no means easy, and the dangers of romanticization is great. Almost by definition, the experiences and consciousness of most of the seriously mad are largely inaccessible and difficult to recover, and the difficulty is further compounded by the predominance of the poor and illiterate or quasi-literate among their ranks, at least into the twentieth century. Generally, the surviving evidence is fragmentary, not representative (whatever that might mean in this context), and often filtered through the case notes and sensibilities of their confidants and captors. For the middle and upper classes the situation is a little better, not least because the power and privileges accruing to the well-to-do generally accorded them greater levels of individual attention, thus making it somewhat more likely that relevant evidence (correspondence, diaries, first-hand reports) will have survived. This is especially true if one widens one's focus from the inmate him or herself to encompass the immediate family, for the impact of insanity on the domestic circle almost inevitably was so great as to prompt commentary and discussion among the patient's intimates, often in written form.

The emerging interest in recovering the perspectives of mental patients and their families forms part, of course, of a wider interest on the part of professional historians in constructing a "history from below." Rather than viewing those who ended up in asylums (and their nearest and dearest) as mere ciphers, passive victims whose fortunes and fates are wholly at the disposal of those funding and running the institutions, a sustained effort is now under way to give voice to the voiceless, and to provide a more nuanced, less one-sided account of the interaction of magistrates, Poor Law officials, alienists, families, and patients. Families, it is now fashionable to argue, were not just put-upon submissive pawns pushed about by a Leviathan state and its minions, but actively used and manipulated the asylum system for their own ends. (See Forsythe *et al.* (1996); Wright (1998); Walsh (1999); Michael (2003).) Recent scholarship has suggested, for instance, that it was not so much the judgments of asylum superintendents, but rather the ability and willingness of patients' families to absorb particular individuals back into the household, regardless of continuing mental disturbances and infirmities, that must be seen as the central determinants of decisions over discharge or retention within the confines of the asylum (Wright 1999). On some accounts, too, patients are to be accorded a measure of agency. If not quite the masters or mistresses of their fates, neither, the new orthodoxy would have it, were they wholly incapable of resistance and of influencing the terms of their confinement (Jackson 2000).

Yet it is easy to push these arguments too far. For there are gross imbalances of power and resources at work here for families, and even more clearly for patients, where the problems of social subordination and economy powerless-ness are compounded to an extraordinary degree by the impact of the label of insanity. For the lunatic, the madman, the psychotic, the schizophrenic, call them what you will, suffer a sort of social and moral death. Their wishes and will, their very status as moral actors, as agents capable of expressing valid preferences, and exercising autonomous choice are deeply suspect in light of their presumed pathology, as the often dark history of their treatment under confinement abundantly shows. Erving Goffman's essays on the "moral career of the mental patient" and the "underlife" of the total institution (Goffman 1961: chs 2 and 3) long ago pointed to acts of distancing and resistance employed by inmates. But the pathetic and self-defeating qualities of the "make-dos" he describes, which serve only to reinforce others' sense of them as pathologically different and inferior, are powerful reminders of the profound power imbalances that structure the over-matched inmates' lives, and of their moral and political insignificance in the larger equation.

One last major issue remains to be flagged: as elsewhere in his historical writings on a wide variety of topics, one of the curious and often-overlooked features (and limitations) of Porter's scholarship on psychiatry and its history was his reluctance to spend much time in the archives, and his necessary dependence, in consequence, on printed sources as the primary building blocks from which he constructed his interpretations. On occasion, as in his introduction to Haslam's *Illustrations of Madness* (Porter 1988c) and in the jointly produced history of Bedlam (Andrews *et al.* 1997), one does encounter work based on original manuscript sources. But in the Bedlam book, these passages are based upon the archival labors of his collaborators, notably Penny Tucker and Jonathan Andrews, with Porter's interventions being concerned with matters of presentation and argumentation, not the process of discovery itself. And in reconstructing the *folie à deux* of Haslam and his patient, James Tilly Matthews, Porter relied entirely on the work of a paid assistant to peruse the abundant materials that survive in the Bethlem archives on the case. (The Bethlem archivist at the time informed me that she had never seen Porter on the premises.)

Those of us who find the role of historical detective exciting and rewarding may find ourselves baffled by this stance, particularly in someone as energetic and intellectually curious as Porter. Perhaps it reflected no more than his impatience, his constant drive to "scribble, scribble," and a sense that archival work was too time-consuming, too slow, and painstaking for someone of his temperament. Certainly, though, this odd lack of first hand acquaintance with the raw materials with which we all must ultimately work could not but invite error and omission. There are, for instance, mistakes of chronology and detail in the published account of Haslam and Matthews that might not have been made had Porter seen for himself the manuscript materials from which his account was constructed. More importantly, although Porter had the unparalleled riches of the Wellcome Institute library to draw upon, and his remarkable memory, skills at synthesis, and élan as a prose stylist with which to transform these texts into a bold new overview, he necessarily remained constrained by the limits these printed sources imposed, limits others have now begun to transcend.

It has taken, in some instances, more than a decade for Porter's attempts to stimulate new work on madness in the eighteenth century to bear much fruit and for new, archivally based work to begin to appear in print. The signs are, however, that the provocation he provided with his pioneering synthesis is at last provoking a serious re-examination of his favorite Georgian age. One of his very best students, Akihito Suzuki (1992a), produced a brilliant thesis challenging most of the received wisdom about the intellectual history of mental disorder in Augustan Britain – a work that yet awaits publication in a more accessible form. More recently, Paul Laffey has explored, in perhaps less sophisticated and subtle ways, some of the same territory (Laffey 2002, 2003). In still other publications, Suzuki has examined the domestic care of lunatics in eighteenth-century London (1998), and ransacked Quarter Sessions records (1991, 1992b) to provide a more nuanced portrait of the place of the mad in seventeenth and eighteenth-century England. Scholars like Leonard Smith have haunted provincial archives, and constructed more detailed accounts than we had hitherto possessed of the realities of the mad-business. And Jonathan Andrews and I (Andrews and Scull 2001, 2003) have made use of John Monro's long association with Bethlem, and surviving private papers, to construct a prism through which to view the emergence of the mad-doctor on the eighteenth-century stage, and to examine the interactions of doctor, patient, family, and the larger community. All of this new scholarship, if it sometimes takes issue with his arguments, and most certainly extends our knowledge into territories he gestured at but never sought to explore in depth, remains inevitably and profoundly in Porter's debt. For that and for many other reasons, one cannot help but mourn his untimely death.

5   The mad-doctor and his craft

What is Dr. Monro? A mad-doctor; and pray
what great matter is that? What can mad-
doctors do? prescribe purging physic, letting of
blood, a vomit, cold bath, and a regular diet?
How many incurables are there? ...
physicians ... are often poor helps; and if they
mistake the distemper, which is not seldom the
case, they do a deal of mischief.
> (Alexander Cruden, *The Adventures of*
> *Alexander the Corrector*, London 1754)

Rare is the doctor whose very name becomes synonymous with the practice
of a particular branch of the healing arts.[1] Yet, for eighteenth-century
Englishmen, the mere mention of the name "Monro" was sufficient to con-
jure up images of the imperious "mad-doctor" confronting and taming the
fancies and furies of the madman. Consulted by the richest and most powerful families in Georgian England, John Monro (1715–1791) stood at the very
head of his dubious profession, the target of satirical jests and gibes, and
simultaneously the repository of some of the "respectable class's" deepest fears
and most shameful secrets. Even his foibles and physique were matters of
common repute. When, in the aftermath of the election of 1784, Thomas
Rowlandson sought to skewer the pretensions of Charles James Fox, Whig
grandee and "man of the people," he drew him strait-waistcoated and driven
mad by his delusions of grandeur and the evanescence of his dreams of political power – and opposite him, peering through his quizzing-glass like a
connoisseur viewing some strange and suspect sculpture, the corpulent carcass of
"Dr. M(onr)o," dispensing his diagnosis with a dismissive aside "As I have not
the least hope of his Recovery, Let him be removed amongst the Incurables."

Who was this connoisseur of insanity, this high priest of the trade in
lunacy? How did he manufacture his fame and his fortune? What exactly was
it that this captain of confinement did to and for those who consulted him on
matters of madness? For, however familiar the man in his own time and place,
in ours he is largely forgotten. Nevertheless, his life and career provide us

with our own quizzing-glass – a prism through which we can peer at the patrons and customers of the mad-trade, and at the mad-doctor to whom, by necessity, they paid court.

John Monro succeeded his father James as physician to London's Bethlem Hospital in June of 1751, and his tenure there extended over nearly four decades, to within a few months of his own demise, with his son and his grandson then extending the Monros' monopoly of the post all the way until 1853. While medical dynasties by which whole families pursued the same profession from one generation to the next were by no means uncommon in the eighteenth century, and the proprietorship of particular private mad-houses was sometimes passed down through several generations of the same family, there seems to have been no equivalent to the Monros' domination of the Bethlem physicianship for 125 years at any other contemporary public institution – and theirs was a monopoly which did much to mire the hospital in a conservative and unadventurous regime.

At John's accession to the post, the family patronymic was already firmly identified with the treatment of the mad, partly through his father's long-standing association with the hospital, and even more because of the wide-spread disposition to employ madness and folly as metaphorical vehicles for satirizing the moral, social, political, and religious ills of the times. James, for example, had been rather dubiously immortalized in Pope's Dunciad (1729), as the main foe of the forces of folly that Pope (and other contemporary satirists) depicted as assaulting the British nation. Here he stands, a kind of Hippocratic King Canute, vainly attempting to emulate the mythical version of the monarch and to hold back the stormy seas of unreason:

> Close to those walls where Folly holds her
> throne, And laughs to think Monro would
> take her down, Where, o'er the gates, by his
> famed father's hand, Great Gibber's brazen
> brainless brothers stand.

Bethlem, at whose entrance Gibber's famous statues of raving and melancholy madness stood, was a monastic foundation dating from as early as 1247, and had been involved with the care of the lunatic since at least the fifteenth century. It has long occupied a singularly powerful place in our collective (un)consciousness. Not least it has served as the mythical and mystical Bedlam of our imaginings, the scene of riot, turmoil, and tumult – a veritable (or perhaps not so veritable) theatre of folly, where Reason wrestled with the demons of Unreason in a continuing drama of brutal beatings, callous cruel-ties, and the massive maltreatment of the mad. In John Monro's day, the institution was one of the sights of London, visited regularly and in substan-tial numbers by metropolitan sophisticates and country bumpkins alike. A staple of the stage at least since the age of Shakespeare and Ben Jonson, it sur-faced as a cliché in Grub Street novellas, as a satirical weapon in the poetry and prose of men like Swift and Pope and in the paintings and prints of Hogarth.

The inmates of Bedlam, literally in the eyes of those who came to gawp at them, and metaphorically in a variety of literary renditions of insanity, gave seeming substance to long-standing cultural stereotypes of mad behavior. They stood (or squatted) as an indictment of the lunatic seen variously as the embodiment of extravagance, incoherence, incomprehensibility, melancholia, menace, and ungovernable rage. The wards of the ancient foundation – ironically the smallest, most specialized, and least affluent of the great London hospitals of the Georgian age – were emblematic of Unreason, their occupants unwilling actors in a theatre where the throngs of visitors might inspect the product (and price) of immorality, the wreck of the human intellect, the dolor of the downcast, and the rages of the raving. Only in 1770 was public visiting finally curtailed, a shutting off as well as shutting up of the patients that, ironically, in time would expose them to yet greater abuse.

As the hospital's physician, Monro presided over this rather dramatic, if paradoxical, rise and fall of madness as spectacle. There is scant evidence, however, that he himself exerted or attempted to exert much influence over the practice. In any event, it may well be that, rather than his complicity in putting the inmates on display, what most indicts Monro's record at Bethlem is something else: the singularly unadventurous approach toward the treatment of patients which he and other medical officers continued to practice there for decades. Therapeutics at Bethlem was characterized by relatively uniform purges, vomits, and bleeding, administered seasonally to patients, with the occasional addition of tonics (such as alcohol) and cold bathing (or other cooling applications), warm or hot baths, all of these "heroic" interventions being supplemented by (a mostly "lowering" form of) diet and regimen. This model, whereby repletion in the system was countered by depletion and vice versa, was founded on an essentially humoral approach to mental diseases. Overlaid since the late seventeenth century by a new mechanistic brand of Newtonian science, older principles and even types of treatment had in reality changed remarkably little.

Like his father, and generations of Bethlem doctors before him, John Monro had only been appointed to Bethlem in a visiting, quasi-honorary capacity. Attendance at medical charities like Bethlem, as was the case with comparable positions at other London hospitals, was regarded as a part-time activity. Although posts were highly valued and often hotly contested, they most definitely were not meant to interfere with a physician's private practice and other gentlemanly pursuits. Hospital appointments were not a direct source of one's professional livelihood, but a means to a number of ends. Their primary value lay in the opportunities they provided for the widening of one's contacts among the affluent and socially prominent who served as the charity's governors; in the visibility they brought among the well-to-do more generally (the potential patients whose favor could help to establish a lucrative private practice); in the bolstering of one's own powers of patronage and social status; and in the securing of some small but stable source of regular income, while one pursued the less guaranteed, but higher, financial rewards available through private practice. Monro's hospital duties were thus understood by all to require nothing more than an intermittent attendance, leaving him ample time to prosecute a lucrative private trade in lunacy. And prosecute it he did, the wealth and property he accumulated in this fashion securing the family's fortunes for generations to come.

Physicians did not need to own a madhouse directly in order to profit from this new line of business. After all, to operate such an enterprise oneself was to court scandal, and many medical men preferred to share in the wealth as visiting consultants. As "professionals," they could thus collect fees for the disinterested provision of their skills and advice, rather than overtly relying upon the profits of a tradesman, those that derived from charging for the lodging and confinement of the afflicted. John's father James had chosen this mode of practice, combining the visibility and modest demands of his Bethlem physicianship with a pattern of providing attendance and advice to remunerative aristocratic patients confined in domestic settings, further bolstered by retainers and fees from independent madhouse-keepers who used his services. Status concerns thus played an important part in shaping the structure of the emerging trade in lunacy, and partially explain the numbers of lay proprietors of madhouses.

However, the rewards of speculating more directly in this variety of human misery could be considerable, and the temptation to do so correspondingly great. Anthony Addington's madhouse at Reading, for example, provided the foundation of the family fortune, and yet did not preclude his subsequent ascent to the role of court physician – besides helping to underwrite his son's rise to be Prime Minister of Britain. Monro's interest in the ownership of a madhouse was initially more secretive. He lurked as a silent partner behind the public pretence that the establishment he controlled, Brooke House in Hackney, was run by a layman William Clarke. Significantly, however, once the 1774 Madhouses Act instituted a requirement that the proprietor obtain a license from the College of Physicians, it was John who became the licensee. For almost a century and three-quarters thereafter, Brooke House remained at the core of the family's involvement in the mad business, though generally the grubby task of day-to day management was left in other hands.

Besides his income from Brooke House, and from another madhouse in Clerkenwell, Monro could count on substantial retainers from his contacts with a range of establishments owned and operated by others, and fees for providing advice and treatment to a wide array of nervous and distracted patients in more domestic settings. The fortuitous survival of Monro's private case book for the year 1766, handed down through generations of his descendants, allows a privileged peek into the multitude of settings in which he practised his trade, and at some of the travails of his patients and their families. It records details of the hundred private patients he treated that year, and provides, among other things, regular testimony about the close relationship of the Monros with many of the metropolitan madhouses and their proprietors. It frequently records the various madhouses where Monro visited patients and the names of the establishments to which patients were sent, often (presumably) on his recommendation, such as Miles's madhouse in Hoxton, Duffield's and Inskip's establishments in Chelsea, Matthew Wright's at Bethnal Green, and still others in Bloomsbury and Paddington.

The fact that almost 25 percent of the cases Monro attended (or heard about) in 1766 were sent to private madhouses does seem to provide some measure of the more frequent resort to private confinement that characterized the second half of the eighteenth century, and the enlarged carceral provision available for families in the private sector. Violence was especially difficult to manage within the home, and many of the cases Monro mentions as being confined in Hoxton and other private madhouses were described as extremely mad, violent, or suicidal, reflecting the importance of the containment function of early modern institutions for the insane. Yet if madhouses provided one mechanism for drawing a discreet veil over the madman's very existence, families often recoiled from taking advantage of such sinister silences. Demonstrably, most preferred to seek other solutions to the problems their mad relations posed, and (if affluent) they possessed the wherewithal to do so. Hence, those who sought to minister to minds diseased often found themselves treating the mad in family or community settings, and Monro's case book shows that he was no exception to this generalization.

Though a significant proportion of Monro's patients were plainly regarded as serious cases of madness – he refers to these cases using such terms as "violent," "raving," "furious," "lunatic," "mad," and so forth – many more were observed to be merely "bewildered," "nervous," "hysterical," "dull" or in "low/high spirits," or were fearful and anxious about being harmed themselves, rather than inclined to hurt others. This suggests that although the expertise of the mad-doctor was naturally thought to be necessary in cases of full-blown raving madness, his daily experience was more extensively preoccupied with the less florid and more harmless manifestations of mental disorder. Violence is, in fact, a rather rarer feature of John Monro's case book than perhaps one might expect, the illnesses of most of the cases he saw manifesting themselves in milder behavioral, emotional, and psychological difficulties. Most of the violence we hear about in the case book consists of "violent flurries" and anxieties. Patients were much more often prone to worrying about external (or internal, as in mental or physiological) threats to themselves and their loved ones than they were inclined to commit violence or murder themselves.

Part of Monro's clinical acumen, and almost certainly not the least of the services he provided to the families who consulted him, was surely his capacity to draw on his experience in order to render clear judgments about what was irrational or delusional, and what was understandable – and his authoritative pronouncements on such matters undoubtedly in themselves provided a measure of relief for relations confused and uncertain of how to react to disturbances of behavior, emotion, and cognition. He had, after all, seen so very many cases of mental upset, and could recognize patterns of behavior that were strange, upsetting, and unfamiliar to those who consulted him. Very often, he found himself called upon as something of a last resort, after the mentally afflicted had been ill for a considerable length of time. And yet Monro's attendance was not infrequently summoned in incipient cases too, as a preventive or early curative measure by families keen to ward off a worse mental explosion, or to avoid more serious consequences.

Much of the time, Monro's musings on his patients' outward manifestations of disease appear hesitant and vague, perhaps reflective of the elasticity of eighteenth-century medical theories. He was careful to record what he considered to be remarkable in each case, but quite evidently the minds and bodies of his patients were often something of a mystery to him. Monro was obviously influenced by mechanistic approaches that had encouraged contemporary physicians to attempt to pinpoint disease more specifically in various bodily sites. Yet the vigorous survival of ancient humoral medical models still frequently allowed him to situate derangement in non-localized physiological media and processes, such as the blood, the spirits, and the humors. He paid regular attention to any somatic disorders that might account for the mental disturbance that confronted him, and was equally diligent about searching for a family history of the disease, convinced that hereditary factors often played a large part in the aetiology of madness. However, rather than attending to the obscurities of the body's internal workings, Monro's diagnostic techniques were almost exclusively directed towards exterior physical signs that were observable by the naked eye at some remove: such things as demeanor, weight, grimaces, and pallor of skin.

In this, of course, Monro was entirely typical of the physicians of his age. Throughout the eighteenth century in metropolitan London, those claiming the title of "physician" clung tightly to what they asserted was their status as gentlemen engaged in the practice of a noble art. In general, they strove (to be sure with only limited success) to eschew their connection with the lower "tradesman-like" practices of their professional brethren, the surgeons, and apothecaries. Like the gentlemen they were, or rather were keen to be seen as, city physicians traveled about in carriages, carried swords and gold-headed canes, and wore wigs and robes – the external stigmata of superior status. Disposed to avoid the socially contaminating effects of anything that smacked of manual labor, they diagnosed essentially by symptoms rather than signs, rarely performed physical examinations, and avoided, so far as possible, the laying of hands on patients. Such menial tasks – inspection and interference with their patients' orifices, the bleeding, purging, and scarifying of their clients' bodies, along with the dispensing of the prescriptions they wrote – the lordly physicians left to the lesser branches of the noble art, those who worked with hand rather than head, and who performed, in somewhat servile fashion, at their direction. Theirs, as Trollope would later felicitously phrase it, was to be "a calling by which a gentleman, not born to a gentleman's allowance of good things, might ingeniously obtain the same by the exercise of his abilities" – so that considerations that bore upon social status and standing were at least as important as those with more direct economic consequences. The construction of "the art of physick" as a form of professional-gentility thus profoundly affected the very practice of medicine. It influenced the ways in which physicians diagnosed and prescribed, and manifested itself in even the most intimate details of the interaction between doctor and patient.

When patients consulted physicians about all forms of illness in John Monro's time, the clinical encounter thus bore little relationship to its modern counterpart. Conversation was as a matter of routine quite central to the diagnostic process, for patients' own accounts of the history of their disorders were considered of far more moment than anything that might be learned from the doctor's direct examination of the body before him. Those bringing their complaints to the physician expected and were expected to talk at length not just of their pains and their suffering, but to offer up vital information concerning their habits and regimen, and about any unusual events or behaviors that might have helped to precipitate their disorder. Within the broadly shared universe of discourse about disease that existed in the Augustan age, they often went further, and even offered their self-diagnosis of what was wrong. Physicians had learned to expect these features of the encounter with their patients; more than that, they were deeply dependent upon them for the performance of their most central tasks. Part of what marked off the skilful physician was in fact his ability to draw out his patient, and by subtle and sophisticated inquiry and inspired reading between the lines of what he was told, to elicit and interpret the evidence considered crucial to rendering an informed judgment about the nature of the malady in front of him.

Understandably, the diagnosis of madness differed somewhat from the approach to these other forms of illness. The mad-doctor was hardly disposed to place much credence in what he heard from what for him were evidently suspect sources. Yet even when Monro discounted his patients' aetiological ascriptions and prognostic musings, the fact that he recorded them presents us with some idea of the wide range of moral, supernatural, and mental processes (beyond or alongside the bodily realm) that contemporary lay people saw at work in reproducing and determining their afflictions. The delusions some patients suffered under were plainly terrifying to them, and to their nearest and dearest. Physical and mental discomforts often combined, patients expressing all kinds of worries about bodily ills and bizarre bodily processes which caused them pain or distress. Not infrequently in the pages of the case book, one encounters fears of material loss combined with kindred fears of a more metaphysical nature such as fears of loss of status or becoming a social outcast; or more threatening still, fears of loss of one's identity or very soul, and of being plunged into eternal damnation. Such anxieties often accompanied self-punishing and self-destructive impulses, self-harm, suicidal thoughts and acts, and other symptoms of depression. Several patients whom

Monro encountered in 1766 seem to have concluded that their melancholy, low spirits, and the like were punishments for their sins. Still others proffered supernatural explanations of their state: being bewitched by a mother-in-law, or possessed by the Devil. Psychological and emotional traumas, such as "a sudden fright," or "a sudden fit of Passion," or even the stress of "being upon the Jury at the Old Bailey the last Sessions," were invoked alongside a variety of environmental, circumstantial, and somatic events that were more or less directly connected to the loss of mental equilibrium, and it is quite apparent that it was accepted in this period that some predisposing psychological event could be crucial in the generation of nervous disorders and outright madness. Nor were such interpretations solely the province of patients and their relations. On the contrary, while keen to discern the physical causes behind emotional and intellectual disturbances, Monro was nonetheless far from being a materialist. His case notes demonstrate that he was willing to accept that madness might have strong intellectual or ideational origins. He was plainly convinced that the imagination might be dulled or "hurried" and the spirits demoralized or raised by mere upsets, shocks, exhaustion, accidents, and other psychological events.

Monro's case book reveals, as one might expect, that a significant number of his clients came from the "respectable" moneyed classes, including merchants, lawyers, journalists, and established tradesmen. Monro was called to attend, for example, on prominent city politicians and tradesmen, and at still higher levels of the social hierarchy; his services were sought by members of the aristocracy. But to assume that the aristocracy and the merchant elite were Monro's primary clientele would be mistaken. The case book suggests, on the contrary, that the majority of Monro's clients were from the middling and lower ranks of society – the shopkeepers, smaller tradesmen, and craftsmen who comprised the city's modestly heeled bourgeoisie – or else from the ranks of the nouveaux riches. Some of his customers, indeed, were from distinctly humble backgrounds, including servants, and even slaves. Among the sizeable number referred to as "poor," some at least must have been in the service of relatively well-off families, who presumably paid for their treatment, while a number of others in distressed circumstances appear to have suffered rather dramatic reversals in their fortunes, either precipitated by or precipitating their mental troubles.

All in all, Monro's socially heterogeneous patient population seems to suggest that, however lucrative and successful his practice became, he was never able to attain the kind of social status enjoyed by fashionable physicians from superior family backgrounds – those who became court physicians and who were regularly called upon by the uppermost echelons of society. Monro's social aspirations were compromised, perhaps, by his somewhat unorthodox family roots – his Scottish origins and his family's Jacobite sympathies – and by the ambiguous aura of respectability with which the specialist mad-doctor and physician of Bethlem was almost automatically endowed. Too close an association with him brought obvious perils in its wake, while the commerce the mad-doctor made out of madness left an indelible stain on his social pretensions.

Mercenary Monro may have been (and most certainly was seen as being). But it has to be said that his were interventions that, more often than not, were eagerly embraced by either the patients' families or the patients themselves, and often by both parties at once. The burgeoning fortunes of the mad-trade he did so much to establish were, when all was said and done, securely rooted in the demands and desires of its patrons and customers. The mad-doctor might be the butt of satirical commentary, his social standing diminished by the stigma surrounding his speculative trade and its sorry subjects, and his motives and clinical competence routinely questioned and lampooned in pamphlets and the popular press, but when mania and melancholia manifested themselves, increasingly it was his services that were sought, his institutions that were patronized, and his expertise that was implicitly or explicitly acknowledged. Here, after all, resided the essential foundations of the cultural authority of medical practitioners like Monro, the social roots of their economic success and their intellectual authority over the identification and treatment of the mad.

6   Museums of madness revisited[1]

Madness constitutes a right, as it were, to treat people as vermin.
(Lord Shaftesbury, *Diaries*, September 5, 1851)

What an awful condition that of a lunatic! His words are generally disbelieved, and his most innocent peculiarities perverted; it is natural that it should be so; and we place ourselves on guard – that is, we give to every word, look, gesture a value and meaning which oftentimes it cannot bear, and which it would never bear in ordinary life. Thus we too readily get him in, and too sluggishly get him out, and yet what a destiny!
(Lord Shaftesbury, *Diaries*, November 18, 1844)

As I write these reflections, two decades have passed since I first began the research for *Museums of Madness*. At that time, I most certainly neither expected nor intended to devote so much of my scholarly life to the exploration of the history of insanity. Still, the combination of choice and circumstance which first led me to take an interest in what Michael MacDonald has felicitously termed "the most solitary of afflictions to the people who experience it; but... the most social of maladies to those who observe its effects" (MacDonald 1981: 1) has never been an occasion for regret. Over the past twenty years, my initial fascination with this subject matter has, if anything, deepened, as I have continued to find new questions to pursue, new intellectual puzzles to worry over, and new archives to explore.

Of considerable importance in sustaining my interest in the field has been the increasing numbers of talented historians attracted to it. Their work has greatly expanded the range and depth of our knowledge, and has provided a far richer and more challenging historiographic context within which to work. Much of what I shall have to say here will necessarily be a reflection of the impact of this body of scholarship on my own. I should add, however, that I suspect that my own continued immersion in the relevant primary materials has been at least as important in the evolution of my work as the growth of a significant secondary literature. If not wiser, this experience has inevitably meant that I have become more knowledgeable than I was a decade and a half ago. Then, too, one hopes that the passage of the years bring a little maturity and broadening of intellectual horizons as some slight compensation for the encroachments of middle age.

If all this sounds as though I am laying the groundwork for a retreat from the major positions I staked out a decade and a half ago, or have repented youthful indiscretions, I hasten to dispel such hopes. In the eyes of some members of the psychiatric establishment and of adherents to various versions of the liberal public relations school of psychiatric history, my early work in the field marked me as a sort of Marxist *enfant terrible* of the discipline. I must confess that much of the criticism that has emerged from these quarters strikes me as misplaced, addressed to a crude caricature of my arguments, rather than what I actually wrote; and in other instances, it involves claims that I believe are not supported by the historical record (Crammer 1990; Grob 1990; Berrios and Freeman 1991). Furthermore, although I have changed or modified my positions on a variety of issues in response to other more well-founded criticisms, and to my own further explorations in the archives, I remain as uninterested as ever in producing the sort of sanitized and "responsible" history that seems indispensable if one is to secure a warm welcome in certain quarters; and I continue to believe that a central portion of the historian's task ought to consist in rescuing those portions of the past our collective memory seeks to repress, if not to cast into oblivion. It has never been my purpose to reduce the history of our responses to madness to an unrelieved parade of horrors, a nightmarish vision of a world of ever more inescapable Foucauldian repression. But I am no more comfortable with recycling stirring tales of the progress of humanity and science. Necessarily, what I have to say continues to have a critical edge, for I am convinced there is much to be critical about.

This presidential address provides an occasion to reflect on my own work in the context of the recent historiography of the asylum and of those who had charge of it. Coincidentally, perhaps, some eighteen months earlier, I had been approached by Yale University Press to prepare a new edition of *Museums of Madness*, a task I have recently completed. Obviously, the approach I have taken here will be relatively schematic, touching upon a handful of important interpretive issues, rather than attempting the more systematic overview of the territory that I have space for in the book. Still, I hope they will suffice to provoke debate, and to indicate where I situate myself in some important contemporary controversies.

I must begin by acknowledging that without question, in revisiting the Victorians' "museums for the collection of insanity," I have observed and recorded much that I overlooked or insufficiently emphasized when I first attempted to comprehend the rise of asylumdom. Over the past decade and a half, others have taught me to look at and for aspects of our responses to insanity that I had previously neglected, and to reassess the significance of some of those that I had observed. In a variety of ways, then – both large and small – I have found myself taking into account the correctives offered by a whole generation of revisionist and counter-revisionist historiography.

It would be an arrogant author indeed who would expect otherwise. And yet at the end of it all, I find myself offering a portrait of lunacy reform and its aftermath that is still, nonetheless, recognizably descended from the account I first offered fifteen and twenty years ago – necessarily so, for I remain convinced that many, perhaps most, of the central arguments I originally made have stood the test of time. I hope that this stance is something more than a stubborn persistence in error, but it is surely for others to judge whether I have succumbed to perils of this sort.

As its sub-title indicates, the primary focus of *Museums of Madness* was the social organization of insanity in nineteenth-century England. But if the Victorian bins were the dead weight of the past which constituted our particular nightmare, they themselves could not be understood in isolation from an earlier history of attempts to grapple with unreason. Fifteen years ago, with the exception of William Parry-Jones's pioneering work on "the trade in lunacy" (Parry-Jones 1972) and Hunter and MacAlpine's monumental anthology of early writings on insanity and their revisionist reinterpretation of George III's "madness" as porphyria (Hunter and Macalpine 1963; Macalpine and Hunter 1969) the history of madness in early modern England was, to borrow Sir Richard Blackmore's phrase, "an intellectual Africa" (Blackmore 1724: 263). Much exploration still remains to be done, but our maps of the territory are by now far more detailed and accurate, and in the light of the researches of Michael MacDonald, Roy Porter, and Jonathan Andrews (to name just a handful of major contributors to the expansion of our knowledge), we have moved decisively beyond the period of writing fables about a dark and dimly understood continent.

My own discussion of the early modern period could not but benefit from taking this work into account. We now have a much clearer picture, for instance, of the complex and convoluted paths by which we passed, between the seventeenth and the nineteenth century, from an eclectic fusion of the supernatural and the scientific – the religious, the magical, the social, the moral, and the medical – to a purely naturalistic and secular account of the overthrow of the precarious rule of reason. Michael MacDonald, in particular, has argued that the spreading influence in upper-class circles of medical explanations of insanity was to a significant extent a reflection of underlying political and religious conflicts. The English Civil War and its aftermath, if it achieved nothing else, vividly demonstrated to the ruling elite the perils of Puritan zeal and religious enthusiasm. Consequently, the upper classes were ever more inclined to repudiate popular supernaturalism, and with it the language of religious psychology and the practice of spiritual healing. Taking their objections to the pious emotionalism of the radical Protestant sects a step further, Methodism and other forms of enthusiastic Christianity, so far from being the source of healing miracles, were increasingly portrayed as prime producers of candidates for the madhouse.

This is an important set of insights, though one should not push them too far. At most, I think such fears functioned as a catalyst, helping to speed and facilitate the process of secularization, rather than forming an essential precondition of it. After all, similar shifts were under way elsewhere in Europe, without the special stimulus of a world turned upside down. More broadly and, I would argue, more significantly, efforts by physicians to define madness as a uniquely and exclusively medical problem and province were aided by and dependent upon the larger social changes which (for some segments of the population, at least) were bringing about the disenchantment of the universe; promoting a more secular outlook on a world increasingly seen as orderly and rational; and undercutting the earlier emphasis on a spirit-drenched cosmos. And those efforts only began to take on a sustained and systematic character alongside and in intimate relationship to the movement to segregate the mad into the specialized institutions that have been the primary focus of my attention.

Central to the process of reform in the nineteenth century, and to the attempt to transform existing practices, was the construction of a particular vision of the past, one which portrayed the treatment of the mad in Georgian England uniformly in the darkest of hues. Lunacy reformers in the new century pictured the preceding age as mired in ignorance and cruelty, conjuring up indelible images of monstrous madhouse-keepers beating their patients into submission, chaining them up like wild beasts in foul-holding pens filled with shit, straw, and stench; of the callous, jeering crowd – urban sophisticates and country bumpkins alike – thronging to Bedlam in their thousands to view the splendid entertainment offered by the spectacle of the raging and raving mad. Generations of Whiggish historians, celebrating the Victorian asylum as the triumph of science over superstition, the very embodiment of an aroused moral consciousness, sang variations on the same theme, seizing on the passage from the madhouse to mental hospital as decisive evidence of our progress toward ever-greater enlightenment, and heaping opprobrium on the benighted denizens of an earlier age.

With the early and honorable exception of William Parry-Jones' (1972) efforts to present a more nuanced view of the trade in lunacy, modern scholarship had done little till recently to disturb the unsavory reputation of the pre-reform era, or to alter in any fundamental fashion our view of the eighteenth century. English Foucauldians followed their master in seeing the Augustan Age as the first decisive step in Reason's repression of Unreason. And even so subtle and sophisticated a historian as Michael MacDonald joined in the chorus of condemnation. "The eighteenth century," he confidently announced, "was a disaster for the insane" (MacDonald 1981: 230).

There is unquestionably something distinctly odd about the spectacle of Victorian reformers and twentieth-century Whig historians standing arm-in-arm with Foucauldians and Anglo-Saxon revisionists to condemn the eighteenth century as the psychiatric dark ages. Indeed, the juxtaposition is so startling that one is tempted to conclude that the mere existence of such a peculiar intellectual alliance abundantly testifies to the truth of the propositions it advances, and simultaneously provides us with compelling reassurances about the ultimate triumph of fact over ideology. And yet, as Roy Porter has reminded us (Porter 1987a), the eighteenth-century madhouses did not form a monolithic system, and patient experiences varied quite considerably among and between them. More generally, in place of the rather simplistic and formulaic views of madness in the classical age which were accepted as recently as a decade ago, a subtler and more complex picture is now emerging.

It was Bedlam which dominated most of the eighteenth-century portraits of lunacy (most famously and vividly of all in Hogarth's didactic representation of madness as the wages of sin) and revisionists have recently been hard at work to rescue the hospital's reputation (Allderidge 1985; Porter 1987a; Andrews 1991). It would be foolish, of course, to reduce the classical encounter with madness to this single setting, and yet even for contemporaries, its wards became emblematic of Unreason and its very name synonymous with lunacy. Though it was "the smallest, most specialized and least affluent of the great London hospitals" (Andrews 1991: 353), its prominence in the eighteenth-century literary and journalistic discussions of insanity was matched only by its "immense popularity" as a source of "public entertainment" – for, until 1770, its doors were open to virtually all comers (Andrews 1991: 11).[2] Recent scholarship has demolished careless earlier estimates that the number of visitors thronging the galleries to view the patients approached 100,000 a year (Allderidge 1985).[3] But the number which came was undoubtedly large, and a wide variety of sources testify that "Londoners and tourists from the country flocked to Bethlem in droves, as one of the wonders of the city" (Andrews 1991: 39). For the nineteenth-century reformers, as for the twentieth-century historians, here was the quintessence of the classical response to madness, and the occasion for the most lurid retrospective reconstructions of the defects of the *ancien régime*.

The reality even here, as Jonathan Andrews has recently insisted, was somewhat more complex than this generalization allows. At least some of the visitors were the patients' families and friends, who were presumably activated by sympathy and affection, and the official rationalizations of the policy on visitation emphasized more defensible motives than mere "curiosity"[4] for allowing strangers access; Bethlem's value as a moral lesson, for instance, illustrating the product (and price) of immorality; the possibility that outsiders would act as informal overseers of the institution; and the usefulness of visitation as an incentive or stimulus to charitable giving. Clearly, too, all of these were operative at one time or another. Not least, the fee charged to those anxious to view the inmates made a quite substantial contribution to the hospital budget, and allowed the governors to economize on staff salaries – a factor which presumably explains their reluctance to abolish or restrict visits even after mid-century, when increasing numbers of the elite began to view the custom with discomfort or disdain (Andrews 1991: 14–17, 23–38, 70–71).

St Luke's, which was founded in 1751, forbade casual visitors from the outset, and its first physician, William Battie, as part of a scarcely veiled critique of the regime at Bethlem, urged that "the impertinent curiosity of those, who think it pastime to converse with madmen and to play upon their passions, ought strictly to be forbidden" (Battie 1758: 68–69). Differences of taste and sensibility provide a potentially invaluable mechanism for marking status boundaries, and accordingly, over the course of the eighteenth century, the emerging middle classes strove to maximize the distance between polite and popular culture. From mid-century onwards, public visits to Bethlem increasingly became the occasion for drawing invidious contrasts between elite refinement, rationality, and sensitivity, and the depraved attitudes, mindless superstition, and moral coarseness characteristic of hoi polloi. Samuel Richardson provides an early and striking illustration. In the course of discussing a visit to Bethlem, he comments:

> I was very much at a loss to account for the behaviour of the generality of people, who were looking at these melancholy objects. Instead of the concern I think unavoidable at such a sight, a sort of mirth appeared on their countenances; and the distemper'd fancies of the miserable patients most unaccountably produced mirth and loud laughter in the unthinking auditors; and the many hideous roarings, and wild motions of others, seemed equally entertaining to them. Nay, so shamefully inhuman were some, ... as to Endeavour to provoke the patients into rage to make them sport.
>
> (Quoted in Max Byrd 1974: 89)

Initially, as Andrews indicates, one observes a shift among the better sort away from "searching out and describing the most entertaining and brutish of the inmates [toward a concentration] on the most moving." Soon, however, broader objections begin to be voiced to the exhibition of the insane before the rabble. Compare, for instance, the objection raised by MacKenzie's fictional hero to a proposed visit to Bethlem:

> I think it an inhuman practice to expose the greatest misery with which our nature is afflicted to every idle visitant who can afford a trifling perquisite to the keeper; especially as it is a distress which the humane must see with the painful reflection, that it is not in their power to relieve it.
>
> (MacKenzie 1771: ch. 20)

But even those most concerned to place public visiting in its contemporary context concede, in the end, that Bethlem's primary attraction was as a freak show (Porter 1987a: 122).[5] The masses reacted with "mirth, mockery, and callous teasing" to the sight of the mad (much as they behaved at public executions, and when criminals were confined in the stocks); and their treatment of "the patients they encountered was often vicious in the extreme" (Andrews 1991: 45). Those from the upper echelons of society behaved a trifle more circumspectly, and looked down their noses at the behavior of "the mob"; but they, too, boasted about "the 'delight' Bethlem afforded them. [Till past mid-century,] amusing anecdotes concerning the antics witnessed during a day's visit were clearly considered thoroughly in keeping with 'the gaiety and good humour' of many a polite table" (Andrews 1991: 43).

In emphasizing the defects of an overly simplistic portrait of the eighteenth-century practices, therefore, one must be careful not to swing too violently to the opposite extreme. There is much evidence, some of it provided by patients themselves (Carkesse 1679; Stafford 1692; Cruden 1739, 1754; Metcalf 1818), which suggests that the proverbial brutality of the Bethlem attendants is a reputation justly earned. Andrews' inspection of the hospital archives has uncovered a plethora of examples of "exploitative and neglectful servants...misappropriation of funds, misuse of provisions, and cruelty," and he concludes that "Ultimately, the overwhelmingly negative assessments of contemporary visitors to the hospital are difficult to dispute...there is little evidence to contradict the general impression that it was 'terrific' discipline rather than care which epitomized treatment of patients by staff at Bethlem" (Andrews 1991: ch. 5). Clothing was "coarse and uncomfortable," the diet meager and inadequate to maintain health, idleness and inactivity the norm, the reliance on chains and other forms of restraint widespread and routine, the patients vulnerable to both physical and sexual abuse, and subjected to what Carkesse termed "Mad *Physick*": "drenching" with medicine which was at once "uncomfortable, painful and debilitating, producing voiding from both stomach and bowels, scarification, sores and bruises" (Andrews 1991: 301).

Predictably, given that most eighteenth-century madhouses were small, informal, and not infrequently ephemeral family concerns, engaged in the business of peddling discreet silences (Andrews 1991: 137), the information which survives about the operations of the trade in lunacy in other settings is distinctly patchy and incomplete. Certainly, though, enough is known to cast doubt on any claim that they constituted a uniformly benighted and brutal regime. The very existence of a free market, essentially untrammeled by outside intervention, supervision, or control, created a social space within which therapeutic experimentation could proceed; and while neglect may indeed have been the norm, individual madhouses seem to have made genuine efforts to secure their inmates' well-being and comfort. Nathaniel Cotton of St Albans, for instance, managed his patients (who included the poet William Cowper) without either violence or restraint, while many of his competitors relied heavily on chains, manacles, and physical coercion to manage their patients. (For Cowper's own account of his breakdown – 1763–1765 – and treatment by Cotton, see Cowper 1816.)[6] And the lack of uniformity in this regard was matched by variability in other respects as "in size, opulence, the social rank of their charges, the qualifications and skills of their proprietors, and their notions of treatment" (Porter 1987a: 140).

However, Porter and Andrews, among others, have sought in important respects to take their defense of the Georgian age a step further (Porter

1981–1982, 1983, 1987a; Andrews 1991: 204–218, 382–389). They urge us to see essential continuities between the eighteenth-century practices and the utopian programs of the nineteenth-century reformers. And they advance the bold hypothesis that the practices of the new moral treatment regime which was then established cannot be represented as a distinct break with the past.

This is to misconstrue, I think, the character of the changes we can observe emerging in the second half of the eighteenth century. It underestimates the extent to which, throughout the period they examine, methods of treatment continued to exhibit substantial continuities with the past. And it rests upon a misunderstanding of the degree to which the versions of moral treatment which begin to emerge at the turn of the century, most famously at the York Retreat, rested on a fundamentally different approach to madness, one which does, indeed, mark a distinct rupture or change in English responses to insanity.

Andrews rightly criticizes my own careless remark that "every" eighteenth-century treatise on treating the mad advocated the liberal use of the whip (Scull 1979: 63). On the contrary, as he points out, from mid-century onwards, some influential voices began to express doubts about the need to beat the mad. Richard Mead was among the first to urge that "it is not necessary to employ stripes or other rough treatment to bring [the outrageous] into order" (Mead 1751: 98); and he promptly found an unlikely ally in John Monro, who declared that the traditional belief in the salutary effects of whipping had been "deservedly exploded...as unnecessary, cruel, and pernicious" (Monro 1758: 38). More forcibly still, near century's end, William Pargeter announced that he "at once condemn[ed] this practice, as altogether erroneous, and not to be justified upon any principles or pretences whatsoever" (Pargeter 1792: 129–130).

Reality, however, is more complex than this line of argument allows. Although one must acknowledge that the greater reticence about openly acknowledging corporal punishment signals the onset of a not insignificant shift in sentiment, in certain circles at least, still there is a legitimate question about the degree to which principle and practice corresponded. Moreover, there was hardly uniformity on this point. William Battie, whom Porter portrays as the author "(albeit in a rather schematic and theoretical guise) [of] the key ideas of Tukean moral therapy" (Porter 1987a: 276), was one of those who continued to emphasize the utility of "bodily pain" and "fear" in the treatment of the insane (Battie 1758: 84–85). And two decades later, as eminent a man as William Cullen, professor of the institutes of medicine at Edinburgh, and the most influential medical teacher in the late eighteenth-century Britain, still more bluntly insisted that it was "necessary to employ a very constant impression of fear...awe and dread" – emotions that should be aroused by all restraints that may occasionally be proper...even by stripes [whipping] and blows" – and cautioned that where physical force was necessary, stripes, "although having the appearance of severity, are much safer than strokes or blows about the head" (quoted in Hunter and Macalpine 1963: 478).

In any event, most of those who began to argue against the use of the whip in the second half of the century did so, not from any principled opposition to the use of force itself, but rather because they had concluded that beating was superfluous and unnecessary, and therefore to be condemned. Mead's own objection, for instance, was not to beating as such, but only to it's being redundant for in his view, "all maniacal people are fearful and cowardly" (Mead 1751: 98). The observant mad-doctor would discover that "chiding and threatening" (supplemented, to be sure, by the various unpleasant weapons in the physician's therapeutic armamentarium) were in general amply sufficient to tame their excesses and restore a measure of tranquility (Mead 1751: 98–99. Mead's doctrine on the cowardliness of the insane was widely influential. See, for instance, MacBride 1772: 592; Falconer 1788: 83; Cox 1813: 34).

Sometimes, coercion and control continued to be quite straightforward, as on the occasion when Thomas Bakewell proudly boasted of using a handwhip to silence and subdue a particularly outrageous madman (Bakewell 1805). Rather than whips and cudgels, however, it was chains and other forms of mechanical restraint which continued to figure most prominently in this regime of coercion, being seen as useful, even essential adjuncts to the attempt to compel right thinking. The routine character of the use of restraint is equally evident whether one looks to the evidence on asylum practice or to the comments of outsiders who had occasion to view what went on inside madhouse walls; and the ready availability and regular use of these transparent means of repressing disorder and tumult provided powerful incentives for the patients to behave themselves. Famously, instruments of restraint were powerfully supplemented by the authoritative presence of the mad-doctor, whose ability to wrestle with and single-handedly subdue the demons of madness now acquired almost mythic proportions (Scull 1993: 69–70). Equally, however, the technological inventiveness of the age was adapted to the task of "eradicat[ing] false impressions by others still more violent" (Falconer 1788: 82; Cox 1813: 45) – Rush's "tranquillizing chair," various devices to employ near-drowning for its salutary effects, and Joseph Mason Cox's famous swinging device all being employed as agents of moral repression, capable, so their advocates asserted, of reducing the most violent and perverse to a meek obedience.

The fundamental basis of the approach to insanity thus remained the traditional one of subjugating the mad, of the breaking of the will by means of external discipline and constraint, as part of an almost literal battle between reason and unreason. By contrast, moral treatment was most strikingly characterized by the insistence on minimizing external, physical coercion, which might force outward conformity, but which could never produce what was now seen as the essential *internalization* of moral standards. Within what rapidly became the new orthodoxy at the turn of the century, attempts to *compel* patients to think and act reasonably would themselves be stigmatized as irrational; the very effort to *tame* madness would increasingly be seen as seriously misguided; and formerly respectable therapeutic techniques would necessarily be discarded with remarkable haste, ultimately, indeed, being regarded with an odd mixture of incomprehension and moral outrage.

Andrews, Porter, and their followers have certainly shown that traditional practices were elaborated and refined as the by-product of the growing resort to the confinement of the mad during the Georgian age. But moral treatment – with its insistence that inmates could be induced to collaborate in their own recapture by the forces of reason, its self-conscious deployment in this task of the invisible yet infinitely potent fetters of the sufferer's own desire to please others, and its reliance upon the purpose-built asylum, and the healthful influences of the new moral architecture – marked something far more important, and in a variety of respects amounted to a radical break with and critique of that previous tradition. The instruments now at the disposal of the managers of the mad constituted, if their proponents were to be believed, in every respect "a more powerful lever in acting upon the intractable" (Browne 1837: 156) than the fear and physical coercion that had previously been seen as indispensable.

One of the more controversial claims in the first edition of *Museums of Madness* was my effort to link these changing conceptions of madness and its treatment to larger transformations in the social conditions of existence. In particular, I suggested that in understanding both the genesis and the broadening appeal of new perspectives on the insane, one should place considerable weight on the influence of the rationalization forced by competition and by the ever-wider penetration of the marketplace. Recent work by John Brewer, Neil McKendrick, and J.H. Plumb on the commercialization of English society in the eighteenth century (Brewer *et al.* 1982) has only strengthened my conviction of the importance of these connections.

As these authors have stressed, the commercialization of society, the transformation and improvement of material life for large segments of the population, the massive reorientation and expansion of the economy, and the associated arrival of a world in which human invention and creation were all-pervasive phenomena – these developments necessarily altered the mental universe, not just of a privileged elite, but of increasingly sizeable portions of the population at large. As early as 1751, Henry Fielding had noticed some of the more obvious effects, complaining that

> the introduction of trade...hath indeed given a new face to the whole nation, hath in great measure subverted the former state of affairs, and hath almost totally changed the manners, customs, and habits of the people, more especially of the lower sort.
>
> (Fielding 1751)

Feverish commercial activity was matched (and necessarily so) by an almost frenzied propensity to consume, and the logic and dynamism of the marketplace reached into every crevice and corner of English society, bringing with it the taste for innovation, for novelty, and for "improvement." New attitudes to the world were being inculcated, often unconsciously and certainly unintentionally, and their effects ramified in all directions.[7]

Agriculture, of course, still absorbed the energies of the bulk of the workforce. Yet so far from rural society being immune to the changes I have discussed, they "spread through it like a contagion" (Forster 1767: 41).[8] Even the appearance of the countryside was dramatically transformed over the course of the eighteenth century, as the commercialization of agriculture accelerated the enclosure of the land; and as improvements in transportation and communication – the roads and canals that were at once produced by, and the precursor and precondition for further expansion of the market – changed the face of the landscape and brought peripheral communities into contact with a wider world (Brewer *et al.* 1982: 327–328). Most significantly of all for our present concerns, there was the importation of new flora and fauna, and the deliberate creation of new varieties of familiar forms, through selective breeding of animals, birds, fish, vegetables, and fruits – a process that accelerated markedly past mid-century. Earlier, these efforts had provoked some of the traditional concerns about the propriety of interfering in this way with God's creation, accentuated in this instance by the need to resort to inbreeding to fix desirable traits (seen by some as a violation of the divinely ordained prohibitions against incest). But the economic gains and the potential for creating rewarding novelties proved too great to resist, improved varieties of sheep, cattle, horses, pigs, and dogs; a cornucopia of new varieties of vegetables, flowers, and fruit. Even urban dwellers got into the act, concentrating on breeding songbirds, pigeons, and ornamental fish. Nature was revealed as anything but fixed and immutable, and the revelation of the truth of this proposition was well-nigh universal:

> in every town and in many villages, adults, and even children, were attempting to improve nature, indeed to control it.... The idea of experiment, of changing nature, was no longer a philosophic concept, but a widespread practical art.
>
> (Brewer 1982: 323 *et passim*)[9]

The development and acceptance of this new outlook were further accelerated and confirmed by the rise of manufacturing – a form of human activity in which nature is simply relegated to a source of raw materials, to be worked on and transformed via active *human* intervention. Taking things still another step further, in this sphere economic competition and the factory system were the forcing house for a thorough-going transformation in the relation of man-to-man. For industrial capitalism demanded "a reform of 'character' on the part of every single workman, since their previous character did not fit the new industrial system" (Pollard 1965: 297). Entrepreneurs concerned to "make such machines of men as cannot err" (Josiah Wedgwood, quoted in McKendrick 1961: 46) soon discovered that physical threat and economic coercion would not suffice; people had to be taught to *internalize* the new attitudes and responses, to discipline themselves. More than that, force under capitalism became an anachronism (perhaps even an anathema) save as a last resort. For one of the central achievements of the new economic system, one of its major advantages as a system of domination, was that it brought forth "a peculiar and mystifying... form of compulsion to labor for another that is purely economic and 'objective'" (Dobb 1963: 7).

The insistence on the possibility of radical transformations of nature, including human nature; the importance of securing the internalization of norms in order to reduce a recalcitrant population to order; the conception of how this was to be done; and even the nature of the norms that were to be internalized – in all these respects, I suggest that we can observe how the emerging attitude towards the insane paralleled contemporaneous shifts in the world at large, and even in the treatment of the "normal" populace. The new attitude coincided with and formed part of what Peter Gay has dubbed "the recovery of nerve" (Gay 1969: 6) – a growing and quite novel sense that people were the masters of their own destiny and not the helpless victims of fate. Likewise, it had obvious links with the rise of "the materialist doctrine that people are the product of circumstance" (Fine 1977: 431). "Is it not evident," said James Burgh (and certainly it *was* to an ever larger circle of his contemporaries), "that by management the human species may be moulded into any conceivable shape?" (Burgh 1775: 176). The implication, boldly proclaimed by the Enlightenment *philosophes*, was that one might "organize the empirical world in such a way that man develops an experience of and assumes a habit of that which is truly human" (Claude Adrien Helvetius, quoted in Fine 1977: 431).

This faith in the capacity for human improvement through social and environmental manipulation – summed up in Helvetius' classic dictum, "l'education peut tout" – was translated in a variety of settings (factories, schools, prisons, asylums) into the development of a whole array of temporally coincident and structurally similar techniques of social discipline (Ignatieff 1976; Foucault 1977). Originating among the upper and middle classes, for example, there emerged the notion that the education and upbringing of children ought no longer to consist in "the suppression of evil, or the breaking of the will" (Plumb 1975: 69). With the growth of economic opportunity and social mobility, the old system of beating and intimidating the child to compel compliance came to be seen as a blunt and unserviceable technique, for it ill-prepared one's offspring for the pressures of the marketplace. The child needed to be taught to be "his own slave driver," and with this end in view, "developing the child's sense of emulation and shame" was to be preferred to "physical punishment or chastisement" (Plumb 1975: 67, 69). John Locke, the theoretician of these changes, provided an early elaboration of their rationale:

> Beating is the worst, and therefore the last Means to be used in the Correction of Children.... The *Rewards* and *Punishments*...whereby we should keep Children in order *are* of quite another kind...*Esteem* and

Disgrace are, of all others, the most powerful Incentives to the Mind, when it is once brought to relish them. If you can once get into Children a Love of Credit and an Apprehension of Shame and Disgrace, you have put into them the true principle.

(Locke 1968: 152–153)[10]

The essential continuity of approach is equally manifest in the methods and assumptions of the early nineteenth-century prison reformers. Crime had been seen as the product of innate and immemorial wickedness and sin. Now, however, the criminal was reassimilated to the ranks of a common humanity. As Fine puts it,

> The prisoner was to be treated as a person, *who possessed a reason in common with all other persons*, in contrast to animals and objects. However hardened the prisoner was, beneath the surface of his or her criminality an irreducible reason still remained.
>
> (Fine 1977: 429)

In consequence, as lunatics were for Tuke, felons were "defective mechanisms" that could be "remoulded" through their confinement in a penitentiary designed as "a machine for the social production of guilt" (Ignatieff 1978: 213. See also Evans 1974.) And for such purposes (again the parallel with moral treatment is clear), prison reformers clearly perceived that "gentle discipline is more efficacious than severity" (Howard 1778: 8).

The new practices, which had their origins in the wider transformation of English society, were shared, developed further, and given a somewhat different theoretical articulation in the context of coping with the mad. In a society where self-interest was elevated to a law of human nature and where all people were subjected in a superficially equal fashion to the pressures of the marketplace, the notion that everyone shared a common humanity possessed an obvious appeal. By extension, the insane were now drawn into this community of mankind. At least among the more "enlightened" and increasingly self-conscious adherents to an elite culture, "the mad had become ... not merely 'creatures', but 'fellow creatures'" (Andrews 1991: 62, quoting the *London Chronicle* of May 1761 and the *Gentleman's Magazine* 18, 1848: 199)[11] – a development of manifest significance in bringing about the lunacy reform movement.

Elsewhere (Scull 1991), I have noted the strong utopian strain that ran through early nineteenth-century discussions of the asylum. In quite extravagant terms, and in sharp contrast to what were unambiguously portrayed as the horrors of the eighteenth-century madhouse, the first generation of reformers promoted the asylum as a reliable mechanism for manufacturing sane citizens from mad raw materials. Here were "miniature worlds, whence all the disagreeable alloys of modern life are as much as possible excluded, and the more pleasing portions carefully cultivated" (Anonymous 1836–1837: 697). Here, in an ideological vision of extraordinary resonance and attractiveness, was a social universe that constituted an organic, harmonious whole – a hierarchical order arrayed under its benevolent philosopher-king, in which everyone knew and respected his or her place; where even the rage of madness was reigned in without whips, chains, or corporal chastisement, amidst the comforts of an artfully recreated domesticity. Those promoting the new realm of asylumdom basked in the assurance that their creation marked a clear rupture with the coercion, fear, and constraint of an earlier regime, the replacement of "a moral lazar house" with the "moral machinery" through which the mind would be strengthened and reason restored. The principles of a rational, humane, and – most important of all – a curative treatment of the insane were at last to hand.

Much of *Museums of Madness* was, of course, devoted to dissecting the future of this particular illusion. Almost as soon as the system established itself, cures proved evanescent, and the asylum's newly refurbished image became tarnished, soon to approximate that of a cemetery for the still breathing. Embedded within moral treatment from the outset were structural tensions between repression and rehabilitation, between the imposition of moral discipline and the development of self-government and self-control; and over time, these tensions were systematically resolved in one direction only, in favor of an oppressive system of moral management, enforced conformity, and disciplined subordination. For those in charge, there then came the difficult ideological task of explaining therapeutic failure and rationalizing the collapse of the very expectations they themselves had aroused. Imprisoned within the walls of their own institutions, albeit on better terms than the inmates whose lives they supervised, asylum doctors had ample time at their disposal to reflect on a bleak and depressing situation as to what could and should be done for "a vast assemblage of incurable cases [trapped in] an unhealthy moral atmosphere...where delusion, and debility, and extravagance are propagated from individual to individual, and the intellect is dwarfed and enfeebled by monotony, routine, and subjection" (Browne in Crichton Annual Report 1857: 8). Most responded by reducing their contacts with their charges to a bare minimum; some by abandoning the asylum system entirely, choosing instead to graze in what were becoming the greener pastures of extra-institutional practice.

If the historiography of madness in the Georgian age was but poorly developed a decade and a half ago, the same may be said of the scholarly study of late Victorian psychiatry. Here, too, there have been salutary developments in recent years, a broadening and deepening of our knowledge that any synthetic overview must take into account. In a variety of respects – the processes by which the mad were cast out and, more rarely, brought back into society; the organization and operations of a whole range of Victorian asylums; the consolidation and development of the psychiatric profession itself; the activities of the central inspectorate and their bearing on the evolution of asylumdom; and the theoretical accounts and therapeutic responses directed towards the deranged – we now possess a much clearer view of the landscape.

Recent work has helped to establish, among much else, that the initiative required to launch the process of casting out the undesirable from the community and into the asylum rested mostly in non-medical hands – whether this meant the lunatic's own family, or those in authority (employers, police, magistrates, and workhouse masters, as well as the occasional workhouse doctor). Moreover, "their decision to commit did not follow from some objective measure of the patient's condition, but rather from an assessment of the family's financial and emotional resources to deal with the individual's mental disability" (Tomes 1988: 14). John Walton's study of asylum admissions in mid-nineteenth century Lancashire, for instance, has demonstrated the existence of considerable socially structured variability in the capacity of kinship networks among the lower orders to cope with burdensome forms of deviance and dependence, and parallel variations in the apparent incidence of insanity (Walton 1985: 137–139). At the same time, much remains opaque when it comes to understanding just how and why it was that people ended up institutionalized as mad, and for pauper lunatics at least, "we cannot reconstruct the circumstances leading up to the involvement of the officials in any regular or systematic way. We do not know what social processes lay behind the initiation of the administrative procedures" (Walton 1985: 137–139).

The richer and more detailed patient records for some private asylums make clear some of the ways in which wealth and social standing allowed certain families to circumvent or postpone the disgrace of incarcerating one of their nearest and dearest in the asylum. Upper and upper middle class families possessed the financial wherewithal to cope with the unproductive; the ability to employ large numbers of servants to manage their troublesome relatives; the capacity, if need be, to send them off to a quiet and secluded part of the country, or even abroad; and strong motivation to avoid the scandal and stigma that were still the inevitable consequence of having a relative officially certified as mad.[12] My own researches into the patient records of two elite establishments, Manor House Chiswick and Ticehurst, provide some striking examples of what might be endured in preference to institutionalization.

Miss Letitia Elizabeth W., for instance, a 46-year-old single "gentlewoman" admitted to Ticehurst on July 17, 1857, was sent only after the family had coped for an extraordinarily extended period with her peculiarities. Periodically, "for two or three weeks at a time," she would withdraw into her room and cut off contact with the household, exhibiting "great irritability if interfered with. She would afterwards of her own accord return to the family circle and resume her place and active duties as if no break had occurred." After ten years, the attacks grew "more prolonged and more serious" and she began to evidence "nervous excitement [and] a disposition to be violent if even slightly opposed," at other times refusing to eat and seeming depressed. The family tolerated these eccentricities for several months, before at length "by Dr. Conolly's advice" sending to an "Establishment" run by a Mrs Idea in St John's Wood. Returning home after exhibiting some signs of improvement, she relapsed and retreated to her room "for weeks together, . . . [when]

any endeavor to force society upon her seemed invariably to produce the worst results." After a year and a half of enduring this behavior, her family once more sent her off to Mrs Idea's establishment, and when that failed to produce any improvement, she was transferred to board with "a clergyman's family in the country." Only when it became apparent, after two even more trying months, that she required "more control than could be exercised over her in a private household" was she at length, after a dozen and more years of effort to avoid the stigma of certification, finally packed off to an asylum.[13]

Miss Hannah Julia K., a 40-year-old "gentlewoman" admitted on January 28, 1861 with "an imbecile expression of countenance" was reported to be "very quiet and silent" on her arrival at Ticehurst. Appearances were deceiving. For the previous six-and-a-half years, her family had coped with her "at home, being visited occasionally by a medical man," somehow dealing with someone prone to sudden outbursts of "violence and excitement" and periods of "unconnected chattering" with "imaginary voices," to say nothing of "destructiveness, pyromania, and indecency" – a tendency to "break tear or burn anything she can lay her hands upon, also tear her clothes off, and rush naked about the room, or stand at the window." It remains unclear what specific incident provoked her relatives into finally capitulating and sending her to Ticehurst, though the great difficulty the Newingtons subsequently experienced in managing her, even in an asylum, makes clear how much some rich families were willing and able to put up with before resorting to institutionalization. Within days of her arrival, repeated episodes of violence, hurling furniture around her rooms, throwing hot coals from the fireplace, stripping naked, and attempting to run out in the hallways, coupled with biting, scratching, and hitting her attendants led Charles Newington to complain that "Miss K's case has been falsely reported to us – her friends said she was generally quiet and tractable altho' occasionally violent – the reverse is the truth." Within a few days more, the asylum authorities were provoked into placing her under physical restraint. This, too, proved unavailing, and exactly a month after her admission, they "requested Miss K's friends to remove her." Though suitable alternative accommodation proved difficult to arrange, on March 17, she was finally sent under close guard to "Dr Monro's," with the admonition that "a more dangerous and violent person can scarce be met with" (Ticehurst Case Book 6, January 28, 29, February 2, 5, 16, 28, March 8, 17, 1861).

Trouble can come in many forms, of course. Mrs Anne F., another "gentlewoman," imposed a rather different set of trials on her wealthy husband. From 1844 onwards, after a fall during a pregnancy, she had gradually withdrawn into the role of an invalid, finally taking to her bed on a full-time basis some time in 1854 or 1855. Having a morbid dread of falling out of the "very large" bed to which she had retired, she piled "tables, sofas, chairs, etc." around it. Nor was this her only eccentricity:

> She has laid in bed for the last three years and not allowed herself to be properly washed or attended to – body and bed linen not changed for months – hands and arms begrimed with dried faeces – shutters and

windows tightly closed – curtains drawn around her bed – a large fire in hot weather, none in cold – covered with dirty shawls and old flannel petticoats ... sleeps the greater part of the day and keeps awake at night, takes her food, which she eats more like an animal than a human being at all hours night and day – generally chews her animal food and spits it out

and so on. All the while, "she has been either visited by or been under the care of the most eminent medical men in England" (Ticehurst Case Book 5, July 2, 1858).[14] without ever being officially labeled as insane.[15]

Not surprisingly, men who were active in business or the professions tended to be institutionalized more rapidly than their womenfolk. Where their peculiarities reduced or eliminated their earning capacity, or where their conduct threatened to dissipate the family's resources, confinement took on an obvious additional urgency. In other cases, their greater capacity for physical violence[16] – whether brought on by drink or other factors – must have exacerbated the problems of handling them by extra-institutional means.[17] Even in cases like these, however, the rich used their resources to avoid asylum treatment for as long as possible, sometimes succeeding completely.[18]

Albert S., for example, a 33-year-old admitted to Manor House Chiswick on January 20, 1885, had begun a business career in Manchester, but forsook this when the firm he had joined changed hands. Returning home to his parents, he soon abandoned thoughts of returning to the world of employment, looked after his aged father until his death, "was busy with home management, then ... took to the garden alone and then gave this up and read a good deal. Next this was greatly given up and he seemed to get weaker and weaker in mind." By 1882, he was expressing delusions that his parents had attempted to poison him and that he was being "mesmerized." Shipped off to India to see one of his brothers, he returned in some respects still more disturbed than before, convinced, for example, that he could "change his form at will and ha[d] travelled all over the world in different shapes." But he was "dull and listless" and his behavior was "sober and not given to any excess." His family therefore continued to provide for him at home for two more years, before his older brother, presumably tiring of the burdens this imposed, finally elected to have him committed as insane. Even then Walter S. took the precaution of writing to the proprietors to ask them to conceal Manor House's real character from his mother, since she objected to sending her son to an asylum (Manor House Chiswick Male Case Book 1884–1891, January 20, 1885).[19]

Charles V. de V.B., an old Etonian who later became Duke of A., had a still more variegated career prior to fetching up at Ticehurst. Sent off to Australia and New Zealand in the early 1890s while suffering from vaguely defined ill-health, he was subsequently commissioned into the army (though he was already claiming that his father and step-mother were bent on killing him, and a "brain specialist" brought in to treat him had pronounced him mentally unsound). Unable to manage his affairs, he ran up massive debts over the next three years. Once more his family stepped in, paying off his obligations on condition that he remove himself to India (where, extraordinarily, they had arranged for him to serve as aide-de-camp to Lord Elgin). A year later, he was back, like a bad penny, threatening to create a scandal by suing his father for causing him to go bald. His eccentricities now multiplied rapidly; he became wholly inactive, ate 4 or 5 portions at every meal, and spent most of his time asleep. Still, his family's great wealth allowed them to cope with his presence in the household, till on his father's death, his succession to the family title and estate forced their hand, leading to his confinement under certificates at Ticehurst in January of 1899 (Ticehurst Case Book 39, 1897–1903).

Such materials, I think, provide striking confirmation for my claim that the boundaries of madness in the nineteenth century were labile, and susceptible to a whole range of social influences. Once family tolerance and resources had reached breaking point, however, ties of blood may well have tended to accentuate rather than diminish the desire for seclusion, as families sought to hide what was unquestionably a source of profound shame and potential disgrace from public view and knowledge. Nor did the rest of the community evince any enthusiasm for the prospect of lunatics at large. As Bucknill put it, with pardonable bitterness, "The feeling and conduct of the British public towards the insane reminds one of nothing so much as that of the enlightened citizens of the free States of America. Noble and just sentiments are in every one's mouth, but personal antipathy is in every man's heart" (Bucknill 1860: 6).

Such attitudes doubtless contributed to the complacency with which so many segments of English society viewed the declining rate of cures in their asylums. The associated remorseless increase in the size of most nineteenth-century asylums; the rapid disappearance of an earlier therapeutic optimism; the deterioration of enormous receptacles for the insane into "museums for the collection of insanity," overcrowded and overrun by hopeless and decrepit cases; these were the paradoxical product of the curative regime lunacy reformers had thought they were establishing, and they constitute some of the central themes of my earlier work. To what extent should such a portrait now be modified?

In Gerald Grob's view, almost completely. It is, he claims, "a one dimensional view of mental hospitals that...often differed in fundamental respects." And he goes on to argue that "Before 1880 the proportion of chronic patients (Scull's description notwithstanding) was relatively low. Most patients were admitted and discharged within four to six months, and only a small minority remained for as much as a year or longer" (Grob 1990: 229).

That mental hospitals differed from one another in some respects is, of course, undeniable. How could it be otherwise? As I took some pains to emphasize, almost two decades ago, particularly significant in an English context were the differences between the county asylums (with their inevitable overtones of the Poor Law) and private establishments for the well-to-do (which varied considerably, of course, even among themselves, along such dimensions as size, opulence, and type of clientele). But to focus only on these differences, and to overlook the far more fundamental common features of these places is to put on display, in my view, an extraordinary myopia. I shall not attempt to marshal the relevant evidence here. That would exceed the patience of any audience for an address of this sort.[20] But I do not believe that it is simply my disciplinary background that leads me to opt for Goffman over Grob, and to see mental hospitals as sharing certain central characteristics as "total institutions" (Goffman 1961).

The claim that chronic patients were a "relatively low" proportion of asylum populations before 1880 is simply false, so gross a misreading of the relevant evidence that it scarcely requires refutation. I will cite just the experience of two not atypical asylums. On March 24, 1857, John Millar, the energetic and therapeutically oriented superintendent of the Buckinghamshire County Asylum, wrote in his private diary that he expected no more than 9 males and 11 females in the institution to recover their sanity. The condition of the remainder – 66 males and 100 females – was quite hopeless. His dismissal later that year failed to change this reality; his successor, Humphry, recruited from a Midlands workhouse, estimated a year later that "there is reasonable hope of recovery in only 13 of the 213 persons in the asylum." By 1876, he thought only 6 of 416 would recover (Bucks County Asylum 1853–1856, 1856–1879 Superintendent's Diary; Bucks County Asylum *5th Annual Report* 1858: 9; *23rd Annual Report* 1876: 7). At Lancaster Asylum, as John Walton reports the relevant statistics, "After 1850 the figure [for cures] never again reached 10 percent, and the death rate was almost always higher than the cures." And he notes that in cures and mortality rates, "Lancaster was not exceptional" (Walton 1985: 142). Even adding to the patients discharged cured, "relieved," or unimproved, the 10–18 percent who died within a year of admission, the *median* length of stay for any new cohort of inmates throughout the second half of the nineteenth century seems to have averaged more than a year, at public and private institutions alike (Ray 1981: 233; MacKenzie 1985: 152). And unless we live in an Alice in Wonderland world, that makes nonsense of claims that "only a small minority [of patients] remained for a year or longer."

More defensible and interesting are the arguments of Laurence Ray, Charlotte MacKenzie, and John Crammer that at the margin there was more turnover in asylum populations than has previously been realized (Ray 1981; MacKenzie 1985; Crammer 1990). Ray's study, for instance, which examines several cohorts of patients admitted to the Surrey County Asylum at Brookwood and to the Lancaster County Asylum, suggests that just over a third of them were released in under a year, and a handful more over the ensuing twelve months, and Crammer and MacKenzie report similar outcomes at the Buckinghamshire and Ticehurst Asylums respectively. To these, one must add the 10–18 percent who died, and the 6–17 percent who were transferred to other asylums (forming part of what Ray calls "a 'circulating' chronic population") (Ray 1981: 233).

This is an important addition to our understanding. Looking at admissions rather than the asylum population as a whole does demonstrate that there was a somewhat "more fluid interchange between the asylum and the outside world than is suggested by the emphasis on the accumulation of chronic cases" (MacKenzie 1985: 169). In certain instances, at least, temporary respite from the burdens imposed by the lunatic seems to have sufficed, and families resumed the attempt to cope with their presence even in the absence of cure. Each year, however, the patterns Ray, MacKenzie, and Crammer have identified meant that a very substantial proportion of the admissions remained behind to swell the number of long-stay, chronic patients, and as the size of county asylums grew remorselessly, annual admissions formed a smaller and smaller fraction of the whole. The effects of such processes, even at an elite private establishment where there was not the constant growth in overall patient numbers, are demonstrated by the outcomes MacKenzie provides for Ticehurst. Of those in residence on any given day, between 60 and 80 percent could expect to die in the asylum, and only between 2 and 11 percent could expect to be discharged as recovered. Put slightly differently, for those confined at Ticehurst between 1845 and 1895, the median length of stay fluctuated between 22 and 30 *years*. And it was this specter of chronicity, this horde of the hopeless, which (*pace* late twentieth-century revisionist historians) was to haunt the popular imagination, to constitute the public identity of the asylum in the second half of the nineteenth century, and to dominate Victorian psychiatric theorizing and practice.

One last respect in which I have substantially modified the analysis I presented in *Museums of Madness* is, in fact, the degree of attention I have given to psychiatric discourse and practice in the closing decades of the nineteenth century. In retrospect, I find my earlier discussion of these issues rather schematic and insubstantial, in need of considerable modification, extension, and elaboration. I have drawn here on the work of such people as Michael Clark, Elaine Showalter, Ian Dowbiggin, Stephen Jacyna, and Janet Oppenheim, but also on my own by now more extensive acquaintance with the relevant published and unpublished primary materials.

As Victorian asylums silted up with the chronically crazy, those W.A.F. Browne referred to as "the waifs and strays, the weak and wayward of our race" (Crichton Royal Asylum 1857: 5), so Victorian psychiatry moved steadily toward a grim determinism, a view of madness as the irreversible produce of mental degeneration and decay. Insanity, as the profession now came to conceive it, constituted nothing less than a form of phylogenetic regression – which accounted, of course for its social location and for the lunatic's loss of civilized standards of behavior. Patently, the mad were a defective and inferior lot, and psychiatric discourse now exhibited a barely disguised contempt for those "tainted persons" (Strahan 1890: 37; see also Maudsley 1870: 53; Tuke 1878: 152) whom it sequestered on society's behalf.

Such theoretical pronouncements were not without their practical effects. The profession's rigid and pessimistic somaticism, while it appeared to leave but little scope for expert intervention, had the compensating advantage of explaining away psychiatry's dismal therapeutic performance. More than that, however, it transformed its "failures" into a blessing in disguise, a demonstration that Nature herself embraced Hegel's "cunning of reason." The matter was clearly of some delicacy, since, of course, "it is the duty of every physician to exhaust all the sources at his command to cure or relieve disease..." (Greene 1889: 503). But perhaps one should not, after all, try so very hard, or lament very long one's therapeutic limitations. For, in truth, "No human power can eradicate from insanity its terrible hereditary nature, and every so-called 'cure' in one generation will be liable to increase the tale of lunacy in the next... [when all was said and done] it is evident that the higher the percentage of recoveries in the present, the greater will be the proportion of insanity in the future" (Greene 1889: 503).

Here, then, was an unimpeachable argument for an expanding system of mass segregation. The mad, it appeared, possessed an unbridled propensity to breed, their defects in will power and self-control encouraging them to "attend upon the calls of their instincts and passions as does the unreasoning beast" (Strahan 1890: 337), and thus to produce "every year thousands of children... with pedigrees that would condemn puppies to the horsepond" (1890: 334). For "these wretched creatures far down in the scale of degeneration,... only coercion" would suffice, a policy that should arouse no ethical qualms, since the lunatic had no more right to be left at large to procreate "than has the leper to mingle with the populace" (Strahan 1890: 337–338. Compare Maudsley 1879: 115 on the urgent necessity for the "sequestration" or "violent extrusion" of "morbid varieties or degenerates of the human kind.").

For the overwhelming majority of a profession that had begun with such elevated, even utopian hopes for the future, the nineteenth century thus ended on a note of quiet desperation and despair, as they confronted what they themselves now recognized as the Sisyphean task of wrestling with what one called "the most repulsive features of man's weakness, an atmosphere of moral miasma, an almost hopeless struggle, day by day, to retrieve or reset the broken fragments of reason" (Hawkes 1871: 32). The central mission of institutional psychiatry had been reduced to quarantining the incurable, rather than restoring the temporarily distracted to sanity. And by and large, asylum superintendents seem to have accepted the somewhat ambiguous professional status this brought them, working uncomplainingly within the limits of the authority granted by their employers.

Living as we now do in the twilight of the empire of asylumdom, we are aware that this isolation and somnolence were not to last forever.[21] As early as the 1860s, in fact, we can observe some members of the psychiatric elite seeking to escape the institution's stultifying grasp, and to carve out alternative career paths outside the walls of the asylum. To lavish consultation fees from cases they recommended for asylum treatment, they increasingly added income from a whole new class of "nervous" patients, the denizens of those shadowy regions Mortimer Granville labeled "Mazeland, Dazeland, and

Driftland," perilous territories others preferred to call "the borderlands of insanity." (Here, surely, is one source of historians' growing fascination with the rise of an extra-institutional psychiatry. See, for example, Showalter 1985; Stone 1985b; Oppenheim 1991; Shorter 1992.) Such "incipient lunatics," the carriers of "latent brain disease," included a whole array of neurotics, hysterics, anorexics, and sufferers from the newly fashionable "neurasthenia," or weakness of the nerves (Wynter 1877). Disproportionately female, and desperate to avoid the stigma and hopelessness associated with certification and confinement in an asylum, they provided a promising basis for an office-based practice, a financially lucrative if therapeutically frustrating clientele which was to be thoroughly exploited only in our own century. But here is a series of developments, however fascinating and worthy of sustained attention, that perhaps takes us too far outside the confines of the gloomy and isolated world to which I was asked to attend today, that "most blessed manifestation of true civilization" (Paget 1866: 34–35), the Victorian museums of the mad.

7 Blinded by biology

Whatever else he may lack as a historian, Edward Shorter is certainly not short of nerve. From *Strikes in France* (Shorter and Tilly 1974) to *A History of Women's Bodies* (Shorter 1982), from *The Making of the Modern Family* (Shorter 1975) to *The Cultural Origins of Psychosomatic Symptoms* (Shorter 1994), he has boldly (some would say recklessly) roamed across a dizzying array of times, places, and topics, pronouncing on a range of complex and often politically fraught issues with an air of dogmatic certainty other scholars have found alternately provocative or merely provoking. Having recently written two books that definitively dispose (in his eyes at least) of the mysteries of psychosomatic disorders (Shorter 1992, 1994), he now turns his attention to a broader examination of the history of psychiatry over the past two centuries.

It is, in his hands, a straightforward and uncomplicated story of triumphant progress, a tale of "smashing success" (Shorter 1997: vi) that has hitherto been obscured by the ideological posturing of Freud (or, as he doubtless ought to have been called Fraud) and his followers; and of a subsequent generation of anti-psychiatric "zealot historians" (this author prominent among them) who doggedly deny the reality of mental illness and the remarkable accomplishments of the profession they systematically seek to denigrate. Like a modern-day St George, Professor Shorter thus enters the lists, bravely setting forth to slay not one, but two sets of dragons, insisting as he rides off to do battle that the account he is about to provide "is not unabashedly apologetic but rather semi-apologetic" (Shorter 1997: viii). It turns out that he has much to apologize for.

Over the past quarter century, there has been an explosion of interest in the history of society's attempts to grapple with mental illness. Once the almost exclusive province of an odd mixture of plodding administrative historians and historiographical amateurs (psychiatrists themselves), the subject has finally become the focus of more serious and sustained attention, and the occasion for increasingly lively intellectual debates. Fairy tales about the great men of psychiatry and mythological portraits of our passage from the barbarousness of the past to the enlightenment of the present no longer substitute for a careful interrogation of the historical record. Remarkably, the intellectual transformation of the field has been international in scope – as apparent in France, Italy, and Germany as in Britain and North America; and while the greater depth and sophistication of our understanding obviously has owed much to the influx of social historians into the field, at least some of the psychiatrists-turned-historians have acquired a new respect for the demands of meaningful historical research and have made their own valuable contributions to the scholarly conversation. Viewed in this context, Edward Shorter's global history must count as an especially profound disappointment, embodying as it does a reversion to the simplicities of an earlier era, and serving as striking proof of the fact that degenerative impulses are not solely the province of the psychiatrically impaired.

It is, as Shorter notes at the very outset of his discussion, some thirty or forty years since anyone attempted an overview of the history of psychiatry. More recent scholarship has generally eschewed such grand ambitions. Portraits of key developments in a particular national context have more recently been supplemented by still more specialized studies of such issues as the interaction of law and psychiatry, the process of therapeutic change, the nature of the patients' experience, the process by which people got into (and out of) the asylum, the character of an individual psychiatric institution, or the career of an individual psychiatrist. In principle, therefore, there is certainly room for a new synthesis, a book that seeks to draw together the findings of this massive specialized literature and to provide a broadly comparative overview of the Western encounter with madness. It is deeply unfortunate, however, that the first person tempted to perform this task should be someone so dogmatically dismissive of the findings of most recent scholarship, and so concerned to fit the story he tells into a new Procrustean bed.

The general histories of an earlier generation were written by practicing psychoanalysts during the comparatively brief hegemony of so-called dynamic (Freudian) psychiatry in the United States. More than two decades apart, Gregory Zilboorg (1941) and Franz Alexander and Sheldon Selesnick (1966) took the lead in producing ideological tracts that presented the historical record as an odd combination of a series of serendipitous anticipations of Freud and more frequent blunderings down biological blind-alleys, till the dawn of the glorious Freudian revolution. Shorter has an equally simple tale to tell. His analysis, turning Zilboorg and Alexander's version of history upside down (or as he would doubtless put it, right side up), treats Freud and his epigones as the deaf and the deluded, and lavishes praise on everything that anticipates the acme of enlightenment, modern biological psychiatry.

Here, then, is still another Manichean version of history, a vision which sees only black and white in a fashion that is structurally identical to its long-discredited predecessors, save only for the reversed polarity. For Shorter, complexity and ambiguity scarcely exist, and the world operates throughout according to a crude and tendentious binary logic. Mental illness, for example, can be explained in one of two ways as the product of "the biology of the cerebral cortex," or "of the psychosocial side of patients' lives"; and both, he insists, "cannot be true at the same time" (Shorter 1997: 26). (The former, he informs us, is the province of "the tough-headed" and the latter of "the soft-headed.") (Shorter 1997: 287.) Psychiatry is either a completely self-interested enterprise, "its apparent good intentions . . . a sham, a pretense for gaining professional power"; or it is a noble, though for much of its history a tragic specialty, a community of dedicated scientists "whose good therapeutic intentions were [until recently] overpowered by events" Shorter 1997: 34). Historians who recognize the "central intellectual reality at the end of the twentieth century . . . [the triumph of] the biological approach to psychiatry" write good history; those who adopt a different starting point are "zealot-researchers" and know-nothings who torture the historical record to arrive at their pre-conceived conclusions, a malevolent bunch of "sectarians who have made the subject a sandbox for their ideologies" (Shorter 1997: vii–ix). And so on.

The judgmental tone and air of omniscience that even the most stone-deaf reader can detect in these passages are present throughout Shorter's discussion, and anachronistic assessments of particular events and individuals are legion. Shorter berates his fellow-historians for using terms like lunacy and madness, mad-doctor and alienist, accusing them of relying on "the very ludicrousness of these phrases [as a means of] discrediting the proposition that mental disorder exists as a natural phenomenon" (Shorter 1997: ix). Astonishingly, he never acknowledges that these are the categories and the language of the culture and period under examination, the ones used by the participants themselves. And he is oblivious to the point of obtuseness about the dangers of transposing modern concepts, terminology, and cognitive maps back on to a past where they fit uneasily if at all. Eighteenth-century madhouses are not in any sense the same sort of institution as late nineteenth-century German nerve clinics, though Shorter casually conflates the two. "Psychiatry" did not emerge on the historical stage fully formed, as one would conclude from his account of eighteenth and nineteenth-century developments. It was, on the contrary, the product of a long and complex series of changes, and the very term itself did not come into general usage in either the English-speaking or the Francophone world till the dawn of the twentieth century. Nor should nineteenth-century speculations about the hereditarian and degenerative origins of mental disorder be lent a spurious air of precision and science as he tries to do by associating them with the language of late twentieth-century genetics and neuroscience. To confound the two very different phenomena is to court precisely the kinds of confusion and misunderstanding historians ought to dispel.

In other respects as well, much of Shorter's narrative proceeds in a curiously old-fashioned way, lurching along from the contributions of one "great man" to another. Except that in Shorter's eyes, "greatness" is a function of one's approximation to or distance from the revealed truths of modern biological psychiatry. The early nineteenth-century French alienist, J.E.D. Esquirol, for example, is dismissed as a "romantic" for suggesting that the passions played a role in the etiology of mental disorder, and damningly dubbed the French

Jung (to Philippe Pinel's Freud) (Shorter 1997: 13). Jean-Martin Charcot's late nineteenth-century hysterical circus at the Salpêtrière meets with Professor Shorter's disapproval, and he is dismissed as a "mediocrity," someone who "understood almost nothing of major psychiatric illness" (Shorter 1997: 84). Then there is Adolf Meyer, the Swiss-born psychiatrist who dominated American psychiatry for the first forty years of the twentieth century. Meyer is blamed for putting "an end to the first biological psychiatry in the United States" and for embracing the siren song of the psychosocial. He gets his come-uppance in short order, being dismissed in a couple of lines as "a second-rate thinker and a verbose writer" (Shorter 1997: 93, 111).

By contrast, others are received with much pomp and ceremony into the company of psychiatric sainthood. Those canonized include the aptly named William Battie, physician to St Luke's Hospital in London in the eighteenth century; Wilhelm Griesinger, who spent most of his career as a specialist in internal medicine, but who is praised for linking psychiatry to the German university system and for advancing the claim that insanity was brain disease (but whose sainthood Shorter might have revoked had he been aware that Griesinger insisted that this brain disease was itself caused by psychological factors); and such central European luminaries as Theodore Meynert, Paul Flechsig, and Eduard Hitzig (all figures absorbed by the laboratory and the microscope, all heedless of the needs of their patients, and all completely uninterested in either the inmates' problems or their fate).

The wholesale neglect of those they purported to treat, and the fact that their entire program of research, as Shorter himself concedes, "produced almost nothing of concrete utility to clinical psychiatry" (Shorter 1997: 103) might be difficult enough to accommodate to a triumphalist narrative, but other aspects of late nineteenth and early twentieth-century psychiatry pose more serious problems still. The collapse of the asylum's reputation till it was seen as little more than a collection point for the chronic coincided with the rise of a heavily biological, deeply pessimistic account of mental disorder. Psychiatrists embraced a harsh discourse of defective heredity and degeneration that used the mantle of science to condemn psychiatric patients as tainted beings, impaired creatures who had regressed to the status of savages or sub-human brutes. And asylum doctors complained of misguided attempts to "prevent, so far as is possible, the operation of those laws which weed out and exterminate the diseased and otherwise unfit in every grade of natural life" (Strahan 1890: 331). The connections to eugenics, to proposals to sterilize the unfit, and to the genocidal impulses of the Nazis lie uncomfortably close to the surface, and Shorter engages in much sophistry and fancy footwork in an attempt to deny the obvious.

He is similarly disingenuous in discussing developments in institutional psychiatry in the 1920s and 1930s. Here was an era which saw an orgy of experimentation with a remarkable range and variety of physical treatments on vulnerable patients; experiments with barbiturate-induced narcosis; inoculations with rat-bite fever organisms; the deliberate induction of meningitis by injecting horse serum into the spinal canal; the surgical removal of teeth, tonsils, stomachs, intestines, colons, spleens, and uteri; the repeated induction of faradic shocks of up to 20,000 volts, deliberately aimed at creating fear and inflicting pain on resisting subjects; the use of carbon dioxide and nitrogen to produce anoxia and comas; injections of cyanide; insulin comas; metrazol (cardiazol) injections; lobotomy; and electroshock – to say nothing of paraldehyde and bromides by the bucketful. Here were biological treatments with a vengeance!

It is a story Shorter is naturally uncomfortable with, but cannot entirely avoid. While acknowledging as he ultimately must that "in retrospect, frontal lobotomy was indefensible for ethical reasons" (Shorter 1997: 229), he seeks for the most part to put the best possible face on things, uncritically accepting contemporary claims for the efficacy of some of these techniques and excusing much else by arguing that "this desperateness must be understood in the context of the time. The asylums were filling and psychiatry stood helpless in the face of disorders of the brain and mind" (Shorter 1997: 190). In parallel fashion, in a later chapter, he seeks to excuse the behavior of one of his heroes, Heinz Lehmann, who can perhaps take the credit for introducing the first modern anti-psychotic drug, Thorazine, to North America – but who had previously experimented with such harmful and useless treatments as injecting sulphur suspended in oil and typhoid anti-toxin into his patients, and with injecting turpentine into the abdominal muscles with the deliberate intention of producing huge abscesses. "The point," he would have us believe, "is not that researchers such as Lehmann behaved inhumanely with their patients. They were searching in the best of faith for something better to offer them" (Shorter 1997: 248). Indeed.

Some of Shorter's fiercest criticism, as one might expect, is reserved for Freud and the Freudians – those he holds responsible for an unfortunate interlude when psychiatry lost its way and blundered off into the swamps of pseudoscience. While I hold no brief for the Freudians, one has to wonder about a historian so prejudiced that he likens the spread of psychoanalysis to a "craze," or to "contagion" by a "dinosaur ideology of the nineteenth century" (Shorter 1997: 146, 159). Most commentators have suggested that the First World War, with its epidemic of shell-shock, played a vital role in calling into question the dominant somatic and hereditarian accounts of mental disorder. For Shorter, the war merits barely a paragraph, and the existence of combat-related neurosis is passed over in virtually complete silence. (It is accorded a single sentence in some 400 pages of text and notes.) Presumably, the whole business fits too awkwardly into a biological narrative, but given the vital importance of both World Wars to the development of psychiatry in the twentieth century, the omission of any sustained discussion of their impact is astonishing.

Errors of commission are at least as apparent as those of omission. There are the simple factual errors. *Pace* Shorter, Bethlem or "Bedlam" was not acquired by the City of London in 1547, or on any other date, and it most certainly did not remain "a city-run asylum until 1948." It was and remained a charity asylum throughout its history. John Haslam was not the physician at Bethlem in the early nineteenth century; Thomas Monro was. Conditions in eighteenth-century madhouses in England varied dramatically, so it is meaningless to claim that they were "little superior to those in the public ones." Nor can one accept the blanket assertion that "these private institutions offered custody, not therapy," some did, others didn't. Reasonably reliable national statistics of insanity in England became available in 1846, not 1826. All these howlers appear on a single page (Shorter 1997: 5).

Shorter's self-assurance and sense of having science on his side are most visible in his final chapters on modern biological psychiatry. But here, as elsewhere, he goes seriously astray. For example, when discussing the side-effects of the anti-psychotic drugs that were first introduced in the 1950s, Shorter conflates and confuses extrapyramidal symptoms (EPS) and tardive dyskinesia. Both are iatrogenic disorders brought about by the medication, and both originate in the basal ganglia. The difference is that EPS is a reversible, Parkinson-like syndrome (producing a stiff gait and a peculiar, mask-like face), but tardive dyskinesia is an often irreversible and grossly stigmatizing product of chronic exposure to anti-psychotic drugs. Shorter asserts that clozapine, one of these drugs, "was discovered in the mid-1970s" (Shorter 1997: 267). In fact, it was first synthesized in 1958, and its first clinical trials were conducted at the University Clinic in Bern in 1961–1962. So, far from entering psychiatry in the mid-seventies, its usage was sharply curtailed then, shortly after eight Finnish patients were reported to have died from drug-induced agranulocytosis. (Significantly, Shorter neglects to report or is ignorant of the agranulocytosis episode.)

Though the advent of the phenothiazines (like Thorazine or Largactil) is a central part of any history of psychiatry in the second half of the twentieth century, and particularly of one as biologically based as Shorter's, he consistently gets things wrong. He claims that "the drug's discovery owed nothing to serendipity." This is simply not true, for chlorpromazine was first developed as an anesthetic potentiator, and then tried as an anti-emetic, as a treatment for itching, and as a general sedative. Only at the last did attention focus on its value as an anti-psychotic, and this was indeed the result of "serendipity" – uncontrolled experiments on psychiatric patients by an obscure French naval surgeon (see Swazey 1974; Healy 1997).

Shorter further claims that "Chlorpromazine initiated a revolution in psychiatry comparable to the introduction of penicillin in general medicine. While it did not cure the diseases causing psychosis, it did abolish their cardinal symptoms so that patients with underlying schizophrenia could lead relatively normal lives" (Shorter 1997: 255). The comparison is inappropriate on its face – penicillin cures; phenothiazines provide at best a measure of symptomatic relief, in many instances at a heavy price in further iatrogenic illness. As for how extensive that relief is, Shorter's assessment can charitably be described as a serious overstatement. Kaplan and Saddock (1995), the editors of the major American psychiatric textbook, recently summarized the received professional wisdom, "The range of recovery rates in the literature is 10 to 60 per cent, and a reasonable estimate is that 20 to 30 per cent are able to lead relatively normal lives. Approximately 20 to 30 per cent of patients continue to experience moderate symptoms, and 40 to 60 per cent remain significantly impaired for life." So much for assertions that the outcomes of treatment with these drugs can properly be compared with the effects of antibiotics.

Shorter's claims for the role of genetics in the etiology of mental disorder are similarly tendentious and unbalanced, riddled with oversimplifications and overstatement. Though one would never guess it from his treatment of the subject, the whole field of psychiatric genetics is extraordinarily complex, shot through with methodological difficulties and uncertainties that make it extremely difficult to interpret particular "findings." Often, enthusiasts for genetic accounts have asserted that this or that chromosome is somehow "implicated" in bipolar disorder or schizophrenia – only to run aground because nobody could reproduce their results. And whatever position one ultimately accepts on the existence of a possible genetic contribution to the etiology of some forms of mental disturbance, almost no responsible scientist would imply, as Shorter strongly suggests is the case, that one can speak of a particular gene's actually "causing" schizophrenia.

A *History of Psychiatry* is by any measure a deeply unsatisfactory book. It is grossly misleading as a guide to the territory it purports to survey, and equally unreliable as an introduction to the modern historiography of psychiatry. The very shrillness and one-sidedness of Shorter's account may guarantee it a welcome of sorts among the more uncritical exponents of modern biological psychiatry. But those whose taste in historical writing is for something other than crude ideological tracts would do well to look elsewhere for intellectual sustenance.

8 "Nobody's fault?"

Mental health policy in modern America

> Whilst in ordinary life every shopkeeper is very well able to distinguish between what someone professes to be and what he really is, our historians have not yet won even this trivial insight. They take every epoch at its word and believe that everything it says and imagines about itself is true.
>
> (Karl Marx and Frederick Engels, *The German Ideology*)

During the past quarter century, a new generation of historical studies has provided us with rich insights into the rise of the nineteenth-century asylum, and the associated consolidation of mental medicine (see, for example Doerner 1969, 1981; Castel 1976, 1988; Digby 1985; Goldstein 1987; Scull 1989, 1991, 1993; Dowbiggin 1991). In an American context, two historians, Gerald Grob (1966, 1973a) and David Rothman (1971), have emerged as the two most prominent figures in the field, proceeding from radically different starting points to provide sharply contrasting assessments of the rise of segregative responses to madness. Where Grob provided a sophisticated reworking of traditional meliorist interpretations of the discovery of the asylum, and attempted in the process to rescue lunacy reformers' reputation for humanitarianism and benevolence, Rothman saw their schemes as fatally flawed from the outset, and embraced the Goffmanian vision of mental hospitals as inevitably disabling and dehumanizing "total institutions" (Goffman 1961), irredeemably awful and incapable of fundamental change.

Notwithstanding their fundamental intellectual differences, and the contempt and hostility the two men offered each other in print (particularly visible in Rothman 1976 and Grob 1973b, 1977), there are, oddly enough, some curious formal symmetries in their work, that is, both place major emphasis in their respective accounts on the stated intentions and more or less acknowledge motivations of the lunacy reformers themselves, while leaving under-examined the larger social and political order within which change occurs; and both offer remarkably solipsistic and ethnocentric accounts, apparently indifferent to European influences upon (and parallels with) American developments and almost equally neglectful of the relevant contemporary European historiography. (For elaboration of these points, see

Fox 1976; Muraskin 1976; Scull 1989: 95–117, 250–266). On another level, too, Grob's and Rothman's intellectual careers have remained closely inter-twined having examined its origins, both next proceeded to provide (inevitably contrasting) examinations of the fate of the asylum in the Progressive era (Rothman 1980; Grob 1983); and most recently, both have ventured into unfamiliar territory for historians, the sharply contested terrain of contemporary policy-making.

Significantly, Rothman did so as a historian turned public activist, convinced by his prior researches that the essential precondition for progress was the destruction of the dismal and decaying "museums of madness" that were our tainted inheritance from a prior generation of reformers. *The Willowbrook Wars* (Rothman and Rothman 1984) did not masquerade as a dispassionate and even-handed scholarly monograph. Rather, it provided an indictment of the horrors of institutional provision for the mentally retarded in contemporary New York, at once a piece of social *reportage* and a fierce polemic against seg-regative and institutionally based responses to mental disorder and deficiency. Gerald Grob, as one might expect, has not been tempted to stray down similar pathways. His new book (Grob 1991), as I shall show, provides the same sort of bowdlerized and "responsible" history that has won his previous work a warm welcome from the psychiatric powers-that-be – a book that, for whatever reason, curtails its temporal focus so as to avoid examining the worst failures of contemporary mental health policy; and in other ways averts its gaze from events that might force him to move beyond the trite conclu-sion that all human actions have unintended consequences which "tend to be complex and unpredictable" (Grob 1991: 303). As usual, Grob instead rushes to remind us (whenever critical assessment seems inescapable) that "[r]eality rarely corresponds with ideals sought" (Grob 1991: 239); that benevolent inten-tions are uniformly at work in the world; and that progress is unmistakable, whatever flaws and imperfections may yet remain.

In assessing Grob's contribution to our understanding of the post-Second World War era, I must stress at the outset that, for all the recent explosion of interest in the history of psychiatry, twentieth-century developments have remained largely unexplored territory, constituting in most respects "a wild and uncultivated region, an intellectual Africa" (as Sir Richard Blackmore (1724: 263) once termed the state of knowledge about madness itself). Even the least historically informed amongst us is aware, however, that the last half century has seen dramatic, even revolutionary changes in our society's basic responses to the problems posed by grave mental illness and disability. The Victorian bins to which we once consigned the mad, to be dealt with like so much human waste or detritus, have been substantially replaced by what were at first proclaimed to be new forms of community "care," but which now increasingly seem to be alternative yet quite possibly equally hideous policies of "privatized" malign neglect – at the hands of speculators in human misery in board and care homes; or on street corners and in gutters, the new resting place for our society's unwashed and unwanted. Those who bother to read the newspapers, or who involuntarily share urban public space with some of the "beneficiaries" of the latest triumph in the march of psychiatric progress, may be forgiven for wondering whether we have experienced still another twentieth-century revolution making only doubtful contributions to the sum of human happiness. Equally, of course, it may occur to them to ask what explains the emergence and – as important – the persistence of such radical departures in public policy, in the face of accumulating evidence of their disastrous impact on the lives of those they are allegedly designed to succor and save.

The third volume in Grob's trilogy (Grob 1973a, 1983, 1991) purports to provide us with a nuanced and historically informed answer to these questions. His book jacket promises us a careful analysis of "the post-World War II policy shift that moved many severely mentally ill patients from large state hospitals to nursing homes, families, and subsidized hotel rooms – and also, most disastrously, to the streets." And his opening paragraphs announce his fascination with "the ways in which public policy is defined, formulated, and implemented" and proclaim that "[t]his book ... is deliberately focused on the severely and especially the chronically mentally ill" (Grob 1991: xiv). On virtually all counts, I shall suggest that this is false and misleading advertising. In fact, the fate of the deinstitutionalized is accorded a scant dozen sanitized pages, toward the close of 300 pages largely devoted to the minutiae of intra- and inter-professional squabbles and bureaucratic infighting; no adequate account is provided of the policy shifts which prompted the abandonment of segregative approaches to the severely and chronically mentally disabled; and Grob's artificial and never justified decision to bring his account to a close in 1970 enables him to avoid the crucial question of why the massive reassignment of patients has persisted even as it would appear that the problems associated with deinstitutionalization grow ever more serious and impossible to ignore.

No one can doubt that the half century since the Second World War has witnessed some remarkable developments in American psychiatry. Mental illness, once almost exclusively a responsibility of the individual states, has increasingly attracted a substantial federal presence – directly, following the passage in 1946 of the National Mental Health Act, through the programs and activities of the National Institute of Mental Health; but also (and in many ways still more decisively), *indirectly*, through transformations in social welfare policies and the often unintended effects of the shifting character of the federal safety net. The psychiatric profession itself, after an intense romance with and a quarter century long period of domination by psychoanalytic theorizing and therapies, has grown weary of their charms, and has re-embraced the more medically respectable attractions of biological reductionism and psychopharmacology. Simultaneously, it has sought to broaden the market for its wares, reaching out beyond the clinically hopeless, socially deprived, often physically decrepit and always grossly stigmatized specimens who traditionally languished on the back-wards of the state hospitals to provide advice to the neurotic and to those who are well-to-do (or at least covered by insurance policies), but unfulfilled and unhappy; to the battered and to those doing the battering; to the divorced and the delinquent; and to the alcoholic and the drug addicted. (In the process, psychiatry has encountered increasingly fierce competition – intellectual and financial – from non-medically trained rivals, most notably clinical psychologists and social workers.) A federally financed flirtation with community mental health centers, temporarily underwritten by subsidies from Washington and linked to spurious claims about psychiatry's ability to utilize early intervention to forestall the development of psychoses, has come and gone, with neither the centers' construction nor their demise having any discernible relationship to the fate of the formerly institutionalized.

Meanwhile, state hospital populations, which had continued to rise, at least at the national level, from the mid-nineteenth century through the mid-1950s, have fallen precipitously in the decades since. The chronically crazy themselves, bereft of the social supports that might make their existence bearable, have suffered extremes of neglect. Organized psychiatry has increasingly handed over the task of coping with the permanently psychotic to the ill-regulated operators of nursing homes, board houses, and welfare hotels (where the ex-patients have not joined the ranks of the homeless sidewalk psychotics), limiting its own involvement with such unrewarding and dispiriting cases to the occasional prescription of anti-psychotic "depot drugs." And the political system has proved almost wholly unresponsive to the resulting crisis, notwithstanding the manifest and ever more visible failures of a policy of community "care."

For Grob, the explanation of this constellation of changes is ultimately to be sought in the transformative impact of the Second World War on what he portrays as a previously isolated and insular speciality, largely devoted to the institutional care of an increasingly geriatric and organically impaired in-patient population. The war, he suggests, marked "a watershed" in mental health policy, and in the evolution of the psychiatric profession itself. For the mental hospitals, it immediately brought further deterioration from the already attenuated support levels characteristic of the Depression years and consequent overcrowding, acute shortages of medical and other personnel, decaying buildings, abused and neglected patients. For the psychiatric profession, however, the war had very different effects. Previously marginal men whose "expertise" was lightly regarded by fellow professionals and laymen alike (where, indeed, it was acknowledged at all), American psychiatrists now hastened to put their talents in the nation's service, finding an apparently credulous audience in the war machine. Mass screening of military recruits, it was suggested, could identify those at risk of mental breakdown under the stress of combat, and largely obviate the enormous costs, psychic and material, of a new epidemic of "shell-shock." Subsequently, when such gains proved illusory, and neuropsychiatric casualties mounted anyway, psychiatrists instead proffered their services in the prevention of further outbreaks, and, where necessary, in the rapid treatment and return to action of soldiers afflicted with what was now called combat neurosis.

These developments coincided with, indeed helped to produce, a sizeable expansion in the number of physicians specializing in the treatment of mental disorders. More importantly, in Grob's view, they created a "basic intellectual shift" in psychiatry toward an emphasis on early intervention and treatment; the expansion of professional jurisdiction to capture an ambulatory albeit symptom-bearing population of neurotics, who could be dealt with in family and community settings rather than isolated and remote institutions; increased recognition of the seriousness of the public health problem which mental illnesses represented, along with greater optimism about the possibilities for effective intervention; and a growing fascination with psychodynamic theories and therapies. At the same time, the parlous state of the traditional mental hospitals left them vulnerable to scandal, a potential soon to be realized thanks to the efforts of muck-raking journalists and crusading reformers.

Clearly, there is something to all these claims. Just as surely, however, there are difficulties and problems even with this portion of Grob's analysis. In the first place, many of the transformations he attributes to the Second World War were already under way decades before. Attempts by elite specialists in "nervous disorders" to carve out office- and clinic-based practices, and to distance themselves from the deficiencies and failures of institutional psychiatry, were increasingly manifest on both sides of the Atlantic during the last third of the nineteenth century. In the United States, these efforts were often, though not always, closely associated with the development of the rival profession of neurology. (Sicherman 1977; Blustein 1979, 1981, 1991; Abbott 1982, 1988. For English developments, see Turner 1988; Oppenheim 1991; Scull 1993: chs 5, 6, and 8.) Such endeavors acquired additional momentum in the early twentieth century in association with the advent of new systems of "psychotherapeutics," most notably psychoanalysis (Sicherman 1967; Hale 1971; Hinshelwood 1991; Pines 1991). Far more important, however, was the impact of the *First* (not the Second) World War, for it was this militarily inspired epidemic of mass psychiatric illness which at once called into question the hereditarian and somatic approaches which had hitherto dominated institutional psychiatry, and brought the problems of psychiatric and emotional illness into new and startling prominence (Abbott 1982: 266–274, 459–470; Showalter 1985: ch. 7; Stone 1985a,b).

During the inter-war years, therefore, the intellectual center of gravity of American psychiatry was already shifting away from the institution. The concern with prevention, which had been a prominent theme among elite "nerve-doctors" from the late 1860s onwards (Rosenberg 1962; Sicherman 1967), acquired a new prominence in the 1920s. Spurred on by the Commonwealth Fund and by the National Committee for Mental Hygiene (founded by an ex-patient, Clifford Beers, in 1909, and directed by Thomas Salmon) (Dain 1981), psychiatry moved, for instance, to capture jurisdiction over the problem of juvenile delinquency (Salmon 1920) and to establish control over a new network of child guidance clinics (Stevenson and Smith 1934; Jones 1988; Horn 1989). Salmon was particularly vocal, but represented a growing constituency within the profession when he insisted on the need for psychiatry to reach out beyond the walls of the mental hospital and to involve itself in the treatment of alcoholics, the prevention of crime, prostitution, and dependency in the treatment of criminals, and in providing advice on eugenics and mental hygiene (Rosanoff 1917; Salmon 1917, 1924). And with respect to more conventional targets of psychiatric intervention, with the foundation of psychopathic hospitals, efforts were made to locate and treat, often as outpatients, the "not insane," the "not yet insane," and "early and incipient cases of mental diseases," all pictured as patients capable of being "restored to useful lives by early treatment" (Southard 1916; Lunbeck 1994). The blurring of the boundaries between the normal and the pathological, and the rise of the notion that mental health and illness formed a continuum (developments Grob is eager to attribute to the impact of the war with Hitler and Hirohito) were already taken-for-granted psychiatric beliefs decades earlier. As Cyril Burt testified,

> It was perhaps the First World War that most effectively brought home the artificiality of the distinction between the normal mind on the one hand and its abnormal conditions on the other. In the military hospitals the study of so-called shell shock revealed that symptoms quite as serious as the well-defined psychoses might arise through simple [sic] stress and strain and yet prove quickly curable by psychotherapeutic means. And thus, it gradually became apparent that much of what had been considered abnormal might be discovered in the brain of the average man.
>
> (1977: 5)

Psychodynamic ideas and psychotherapeutic approaches were already spreading rapidly in the 1920s and 1930s, particularly among the professional elite (Abbott 1982: 324–330, 377–387); and, led by Alan Gregg, from the early 1930s the Rockefeller Foundation was providing funding to institutionalize psychoanalytic training in the United States (Gregg unpublished; Brown 1987).

Nor was the involvement of psychiatry in the Second World War a resounding success. Mass screening of recruits angered the military apparatus, since the rejection on psychiatric grounds of some 1.75 million men interfered with the effort to maximize military manpower. Worst still, it did nothing whatsoever to stem the epidemic of war-related psychiatric disabilities, once the supposedly pre-screened soldiers eventually experienced combat. Efforts at prevention were similarly unavailing, and while Grob refers to the psychiatric treatment of war neuroses as a success, the evidence for this proposition is weak at best. Data collected at the time suggested, in fact, that the less psychiatric treatment a soldier received, the better his chances of avoiding permanent mental incapacity. Those dealt with at the front, who were given no more than warm food and a sedative to secure a night's sleep, typically recovered and resumed fighting; those sent back behind the lines for more extended psychotherapy for a few days were generally unable to return to combat, though often they were not totally disabled; but those sent to a rear echelon base hospital for more extensive treatment seldom reappeared, fewer than 10 percent returning to active duty. These outcomes were scarcely rousing testimony to the efficacy of psychiatric treatment, though, as Grob points out, military psychiatrists put the best face possible on these data, and tried to convince themselves and others that they were proof of the efficacy of early intervention.

Conditions in state mental hospitals during the war and in the immediate postwar era were undoubtedly appalling, and Grob devotes chapter 4 of his book to the exposes and withering criticism which these inspired. Novelists and film-makers vied with journalists and sociologists to document asylums' manifold failures as therapeutic institutions. Here again, however, one must ask what all these assaults amounted to, in what respects they were novel, and how far they contributed to the dissolution of the segregative approach to mental illness. Grob (1991: 71) himself sees a "crisis of unprecedented pro-portions" linked in part to the havoc wreaked on the system by the Great Depression and by the war itself; but deriving also from a transformation in the hospitals' functions and patient population which he claims began in the early twentieth century. "Throughout the nineteenth century," he argues, "patient populations were made up largely of acute cases institutionalized for less than a year... the bulk of patients were discharged in twelve months or less" (Grob 1991: 5). All this changed for the worse, he asserts, beginning around 1890, when the closing of almshouses precipitated the mass transfer of elderly and senile inmates, transforming mental hospitals into "institu-tions that provided long-term custodial care for an overwhelmingly chronic population..." (Grob 1991: 6).

This is an odd piece of revisionism. Careful recent studies of admission to and discharge from nineteenth-century asylums (both large public bins and elite private asylums) have certainly modified to a limited extent an earlier portrait which depicted them as little more than warehouses for the unwanted. We now know that a significant minority of each year's admissions tended to be released within the first twelve months after their arrival, rang-ing between 25 percent and perhaps 45 percent (though this fraction tended to decline over time). Adding in deaths and transfers, perhaps 50 or 55 percent of admissions were "resolved" within a year (for England, see Ray 1981; MacKenzie 1985; Walton 1985; for the United States, Dwyer 1987). But this is very far from being "the bulk" of a given year's admissions. Moreover, sim-ple arithmetic ensured that, over time, a larger and larger fraction of asylums' total population consisted of chronic patients, as each year's contribution of therapeutic failures lingered on to swell the hospital census. At Utica State Hospital in New York, for instance, recoveries calculated on total numbers of resident never rose above 16 percent after 1856, and by 1890 had fallen below 11 percent (Dwyer 1987: 150). Notwithstanding some turnover at the margin, therefore, by the last third of the nineteenth century, *pace* Grob the overwhelming bulk of mental hospital populations consisted of the chronically crazy, and the asylum had already been publicly identified – fairly or not – as an almost exclusively custodial institution. David Rothman's work (1971: esp. ch. 11, 1980: chs 9 and 10), for instance, has documented some of the dimensions of the "dramatic decline from a reform to a custodial operation" – most notably "overcrowding . . . the breakdown of classification systems, the demise of work therapy, and an increase in the use of mechanical restraints and harsh punishments to maintain order" even as early as the 1850s. Still more awkwardly for Grob's revisionist case, his own earlier study of nineteenth-century developments (Grob 1973a: 238, 306–308) reached essentially the same conclusions:

> After 1860, . . . the continuous rise in the number of chronic patients had all but obliterated the therapeutic goals of many hospitals . . . virtually every hospital in the nation was confronted with a problem whose magnitude was clearly increasing rather than diminishing . . . . Overcrowded conditions and the accumulation of chronic patients were increasingly the norm, as the transformation of mental hospitals into strictly welfare institutions as far as their funding and reputation were concerned solidified "their custodial character."

By the 1870s, moreover, mental hospitals were subjected to savage criticism being increasingly seen as actively harmful to those they purported to cure. Henry Maudsley (1871: 432), for instance, the leading English alienist of the age confessed that "I cannot help feeling, from my experience, that one effect of asylums is to make permanent lunatics." Spitzka (1878), Hammond (1879), and Weir Mitchell (1894: 19), among the leading American neurologists of the Gilded Age, were equally emphatic, complaining of the pernicious effects of incarceration, and of "the sadness . . . of the wards . . . [in which] the insane, who have lost even the memory of hope, sit in rows, too dull to know despair, watched by attendants, silent, grewsome [*sic*] machines which eat and sleep, sleep and eat." Lay critics were even less inhibited, denouncing the hospitals' failings, calling into question the superintendents' claims to expertise, and claiming that mistreatment and abuse were routine. (The short-lived National Association for the Protection of the Insane and the Prevention of Insanity was particularly vocal in this regard, but others (e.g. Packard 1873; Eaton 1881) were still more virulent in their criticisms.)

Neither the existence nor the content of the post-Second World War exposés was novel, therefore, as even Grob (1991: 72) ultimately concedes. In explaining why they mattered more on the present occasion, he is reduced to muttering vaguely about the changed setting in which the recycled critiques emerged. *This* time around, he asserts (Grob 1991: 72–73), with more than a trace of desperation, they counted, because "intellectual, cultural, and social currents converged to create a receptivity toward innovation."

Given that scandals about mental hospitals had routinely surfaced throughout their history, the more skeptical amongst us might be inclined to question how important new variations on this well-worn theme actually were in finally pushing the system towards massive change. Skepticism deepens when one scrutinizes the examples Grob provides. Take, for example, the most famous exposes of the late 1940s – Albert Deutsch's (1973) series on American mental hospitals for the New York newspaper, *PM* (subsequently reworked as the best-selling *The Shame of the States*); Albert Maisel's (1946) famous *Life* essay on "Bedlam 1946;" the revelations published by conscientious objectors "sentenced" to provide alternative service on mental hospital wards during the war (Wright 1947); and Mary Jane Ward's (1946) best-selling novel, *The Snake Pit* (serialized in *Reader's Digest* and made into one of the five most popular films of 1949) – all these texts shared a common stance towards the institutions of which they were apparently so fiercely critical. All portrayed the hospitals (and those who ran them) as making "a genuine effort to care for and heal the mentally ill" (PM, May 27, 1947, quoted in Grob 1991: 77), and, as Grob (1991: 74) concedes, each and every one of them was emphatically "intended neither to discredit mental hospitals nor to undermine their legitimacy." Quite the contrary, their explicit agenda was to pressure politicians to spend more money on the system, so as "to put an end to concentration camps that masquerade as hospitals and to make cure rather than incarceration the goal" (Albert Q. Maisel, quoted in Grob 1991: 75).

Grob is convinced of the importance of rhetoric and faith in producing social change and he repeatedly invokes their "power" as a major explanatory factor (e.g. Grob 1991: 92, 171, 176–177, 189, 224). But here, as elsewhere, this conviction lands him in the soup. For how can political speeches, reform propaganda, policy statements, and public relations prevarications be the motor of change, when they repeatedly propose and reinforce traditional notions about the necessity for funneling patients into mental hospitals? He grudgingly admits (Grob 1991: 92) that amongst the "curious coalition" of reformers he focuses on – "activist psychodynamic and psychoanalytic psychiatrists, journalists, political leaders, and lay and professional organizations" – "the long-standing commitment to an institution-based system remained outwardly unchanged." (Inwardly too, so far as we can tell that despite ransacking private papers and correspondence, Grob cannot demonstrate even a behind the scenes commitment to tear down the fabric of asylumdom.)

Three later chapters on developments from the mid-1950s to the mid-1960s are similarly unsatisfactory. Grob gives great prominence to the activities of the Joint Commission on Mental Illness and Health (1961), which appeared on the scene in 1955, and issued its final report, *Action for Mental Health*, in 1961. It is not clear why. Never adequately funded, operating with the vaguest of mandates and objectives, and riddled with internal ambivalence and confusion, the Commission sponsored an undistinguished series of monographs on a haphazard array of topics. Its own synthesizing final report was similarly unhelpful. Largely written by a specialist in public relations, it proclaimed (Joint Commission 1961: 295) with typically overblown and vacuous rhetoric that "the time is at hand and their courage is such that modern legislators may make history by adopting a new policy of action for mental health."

Leaving aside such shopworn phrases, however, the report was essentially an empty exercise, failing, as Grob (1991: 209) himself concedes, "to offer a precise blueprint that could serve as the basis for legislative action." Its call for further expansion of NIMH was doubtless appreciated by that agency (which had substantially underwritten the commission's costs), but high level officials at the Institute were privately scathing about the mouse that six years of labor had brought forth. Shown a pre-publication draft, Philip Sapir (chief of NIMH's Research and Fellowships Branch) dismissed it scornfully as "pedestrian, platitudinous, rehashes of previous statements, half-truths, or untruths...so incredibly bad that there seems almost no point in making specific criticisms" (quoted in Grob 1991: 217).

The one new federal policy initiative which post-dated the report derived, not from the Commission's recommendations, but from proposals independently put forward by the NIMH. The NIMH program involved the establishment of a network of community mental health centers, subsidized by the federal government, overseen and advised by the Institute. These were to be devoted to prevention and early treatment, a piece of empire building NIMH sold to its political masters by promising that their program would make it possible "for the mental hospital as it is now known to disappear from the scene within the next twenty-five years" (NIMH internal task force report, quoted in Grob 1991: 222).

Given the long-entrenched connections of traditional mental hospitals with the political system at the state level, it should come as no surprise that the emerging federal mental health bureaucracy from the outset attempted to carve out a different role for itself. It funded, for instance, a massive expansion of the involvement of the social and behavioral sciences in the mental health complex (by 1964, 55 percent of NIMH principal investigators were psychologists and a further 7 percent sociologists, anthropologists, and epidemiologists – who collectively spent 60 percent of the research funds awarded – while psychiatrists were 12 percent of the researchers, spending only 15 percent of the funds). It underwrote a similar expansion of programs to train professionals (most of whom promptly entered private practice). And it sought to create a new network of treatment facilities which depended upon federal dollars (and which therefore justified an expansion of the territory administered by federal bureaucrats). None of this, however, necessarily spelt the end of an entrenched reliance on segregative responses to serious forms of mental disorder.

In fact, we have known for many years now (see Chu and Trotter 1974; Kirk and Thierren 1975; Windle and Scully 1976; Rose 1979 and Gronfein 1985b) that the centers established under the Mental Retardation and Community Mental Health Centers Act of 1963, and successive legislation modifying this program, were quite simply irrelevant to the deinstitutionalization of the population of the traditional state hospitals. From the outset, those running these centers displayed a pronounced preference for treating "'good patients' [rather] than chronic schizophrenics, alcoholics, or senile psychotics" (Rieder 1974: 11) – in other words, a determination not to treat those being discharged from state hospitals. Unsurprisingly, this deliberate policy of discrimination against ex-state hospital patients and refusal to address their needs was, unlike most psychiatric interventions, highly effective in practice.

In the circumstances, it is surely misguided for anyone centrally concerned with the fate of "the seriously and especially the chronically mentally ill" (Grob 1991: xiii) to focus minute attention either on the internal politics of the formation and functioning of the Joint Commission on Mental Illness and Health, or on the bureaucratic and political maneuvering surrounding the passage of the Community Mental Health Centers Act. Ironically, Grob (1991: 420) himself concedes the essential point here:

> To be sure, resident populations of mental hospitals declined rapidly after 1965.... This dramatic change, however, was not related to the estab- lishment of [community mental health] centers. On the contrary, the transformation of the character and functions of mental hospitals was shaped by other developments.

Precisely. And yet these mysterious "other developments," which ought surely to be the primary focus of his analysis, receive only the most glancing of attention. Other data, moreover, confirm the centers' irrelevance, even to the profession itself. As Grob (1991: 256) notes, within just over a decade of the system's creation, "the relationship between the specialty of psychiatry and centers became problematical.... Centers were largely staffed by clinical psychologists, social workers, or non-professional staff – groups that had neither interest in nor experience with the severely mentally ill."

But this myopia, this failure to place developments in the mental health arena in a larger social and political context, is the defining characteristic of Grob's approach to the territory he has indicated he wishes to explore. Elsewhere, for example, he displays a similarly misplaced obsession with every twist and turn of professional and bureaucratic squabbles and conflicts which, his own account suggests, have quite marginal relevance to the cen- tral issues at hand. His second chapter, for instance, is largely taken up with surveying, in excruciating detail, the professional infighting in the years immediately after the Second World War between old line institutional psy- chiatrists, enraptured with lobotomies and shock therapies, and the psycho- dynamically oriented Young Turks who banded together to form the Group for the Advancement of Psychiatry (GAP). To be sure, this led to the public airing of some very dirty professional linen, but when "intraorganizational differences threatened to undermine public respect and confidence and thus destroy the very legitimacy essential to the well-being of any professional group" the reform movement fizzled, the schisms were papered over, and GAP essentially gave up on "the idea of transforming psychiatry, [and] became the vehicle for liberal and activist psychiatrists to express their views on a whole range of social and medical problems." Mysteriously, Grob (1991: 38–39, 41) claims that this outcome meant that GAP "may have lost the battle, but . . . surely won the war." He refers here to the growing postwar activism of psychiatry, the temporary increase in the influence of psychoanalysis among the professional elite, and to the disengagement of the specialty from the public sector. But the contention that the increasingly feeble apparatus of GAP was a precondition for (or even significantly related to) these developments is never demonstrated and seems highly doubtful.

Here, and in subsequent chapters on the politics of federal intervention and on conflicts between psychiatry and other mental health professions, Grob seems to believe that an exhaustive reading of internal documents and, more especially, of the private correspondence of psychiatrists, will somehow provide the key to understanding broad shifts in public policy. But this is to assume that deinstitutionalization flowed from conscious legislative efforts to accomplish this end, and involved rational planning to allocate the necessary resources for community-based care – assertions which find little support in either the literature or, more importantly, in the historical record itself (which suggests rather that expediency ruled) (see Lerman 1982). And it implicitly accords a larger and more determinative role for the opinions of professional experts than is remotely plausible.

Grob clearly wants to attribute the shift away from the traditional reliance on institutions to the activities and opinions of these elites. For him,

> the foundations for change [were, i]n effect, a curious coalition formed in the decade following the end of World War II. Composed of activist psychodynamic and psychoanalytic psychiatrists, journalists, political leaders, and lay and professional organizations, its members endorsed prescriptions for change.
>
> (Grob 1991: 92)

But this line of argument quickly collapses under any sort of scrutiny, for Grob's "curious coalition" were completely unable to agree on what sort of change to propose, much less muster the political muscle to secure enactment of a program of reform. Grob acknowledges as much: "This coalition was by no means unified around a common program." Unfortunately for his argument, however, its difficulties are graver still, for his "coalition" did agree on the continued necessity of the traditional mental hospital. (As Grob delicately phrases it, "the long-standing commitment to an institution-based system remained outwardly [*sic*] unchanged.") Having demolished his own case,

Grob is now reduced to clutching at straws. Desperately, he insists that "Nevertheless, by defining a problem and shaping an agenda, [the coalition's] members helped to set in motion a process that in the future would help to change the ways in which American society apprehended and responded to the problems posed by mental illness."

This is all rather sad. Grob (1991: 125, 179, 181, 216) may be willing to rest content with such banalities as the claim that these ruminations led to a "receptivity to community alternatives," and that, in turn, fueled by "the excitement, sense of urgency, and optimism characteristic of the postwar years...," such receptivity created dramatic changes in public policy when "the time was ripe." But to halt the analysis at this point is to beg the essential questions in a cloud of wishful and unconvincing rhetoric.

Though the reader of *From Asylum to Community* is never made aware of it, time must have been ripening almost simultaneously in many different national settings. In Britain, for instance, the mental hospital census peaked a year before this happened in the United States, and the central government was explicitly committed to running down in-patient treatment facilities by the early 1960s. To be sure, deinstitutionalization had a different pace and rhythm across the Atlantic, and some of the most distinctive features of the American mental health scene (most notably the growth of what I have elsewhere called (Scull 1981c) "a new trade in lunacy") have developed much more slowly and haltingly there. Still, the parallels are sufficient to cast serious doubt on a line of explanation that places most weight on parochial and personal factors.

The differences in the timing and intensity of the shift away from mental hospitals also provide us with clues about what has been driving the process. In both countries, admissions to mental hospitals were rising sharply in the postwar years. At the same time, the ramshackle barracks asylums inherited from the Victorian age were visibly decaying, potentially requiring massive infusions of capital for repair and expansion. Worse still, the tighter postwar labor market and the impact of unionization were sharply raising operating costs. Not surprisingly, therefore, policy makers in both countries were attracted by the possibility of shifting the locus of care away from increasingly costly traditional mental hospitals.

In the United States, however, the process of emptying out the mental hospitals proceeded far more rapidly than in Britain, and at an earlier stage the discharge of the senile and the elderly formed a much larger fraction of those decanted into the new community alternatives. Though there were marked variations from state to state in the timing of deinstitutionalization, national data make clear that there were two periods where the pace of discharges accelerated markedly in the United States, while no comparable shifts can be seen in the British data. The first of these occurred from 1965 onwards, and consisted disproportionately of inmates over the age of 65. The second, more broadly based and geographically widespread, dates from 1973, outside the self-imposed time limits of Grob's study, but after the major drawbacks of deinstitutionalization had begun to become widely apparent.

As briefly as possible, Grob (1991: 261) concedes that what he acknowledges was a "precipitous" fall in state hospital populations after 1965 occurred "largely because changes in funding patterns led to a sharp decline in elderly and chronic patients." It was, it transpires (Grob 1991: 267), "a series of far-reaching changes in the Social Security system [which] had a dramatic, though inadvertent, impact on mental health policy...," most especially the passage of Medicare and Medicaid. Elsewhere, his Rutgers colleague, Paul Lerman (1982: 209), has documented the intimate connections between the further acceleration in discharges from 1973 onwards and the advent of the Supplemental Security Income program in 1972, a change in eligibility rules which meant that "states [were] able to rely on non-matching federal grants to subsidize patient releases."

Lerman (1982: 79, 209) correctly points out that "the federal government could not – and did not – mandate that categorical grant-in-aid programs be used to depopulate state institutions. States had to discover and use this option." Inter-state variations in the pace of deinstitutionalization in substantial measure reflect how rapidly individual administrations grasped and exploited this opportunity: "States whose leaders exhibited entrepreneurial skills, and who were supported by executives and legislators willing to risk increased spending to gain long-term fiscal benefits via deferred construction and maintenance of facilities, displayed marked population reductions by 1969. Laggard states waited until Supplemental Security Income was passed in 1972 [allowing 100 percent federal financing]." It was developments of this sort, permitting the transfer of costs from the state to the federal level, and providing fiscal incentives for "community" treatment, which I and others (Scull 1977, 1984b; Rose 1979; Lerman 1982; Gronfein 1985) have previously identified as the key to understanding why governments at last proved receptive to criticisms of traditional institutions and eager to adopt alternative policies. (In Britain, of course, the unitary political structure meant that there were no such built-in incentives to transfer costs among levels of government, which helps to account for the different shape of deinstitutionalization policies there.)

The impact of these alternatives on the lives of the psychotic is by now only too apparent. Detailing the failures of community care as briefly and gingerly as possible, Grob (1991: 210) insists they are the unfortunate outcome of "a policy designed to improve the lives of the mentally ill," one which he reluctantly concedes "had unforeseen and sometimes [*sic*] unwelcome consequences." (Most observers would reverse this judgment: it is the *welcome* consequences that have *sometimes* been realized, and the *un*welcome ones which have been the norm.) Once again, as in the two previous volumes in his trilogy, Grob is reduced to insisting on the benevolence of policymakers' intentions, and the ironies of unintended consequences and historical accident: "The ideals that people pursue in seeking social change and the realities that subsequently emerge rarely correspond... The consequences of human activities... tend to be complex and unpredictable; ambiguity – not clarity or consistency – is often characteristic" (Grob 1991: 209, 303). To be sure, "The consequences of the innovations that transformed the mental health system, like those of all human activities, were at best mixed," and in some instances, "[t]he subtle shifts...were to have tragic consequences for many chronically and severely mentally ill persons most in need of assistance" (Grob 1991: 271, 304). But this merely reflects the one sort of historical inevitability Grob (1991: 304) seems ready to countenance: "Human triumphs invariably incorporate elements of tragedy as well."

I know of few other observers of the contemporary mental health scene who would associate the changes of the last thirty-five years with the idea of "triumph." Most would more readily concur with the complaints of a recent President of the American Psychiatric Association (Langsley 1980; see also Borus 1981; Mollica 1983), who denounced "the wholesale neglect of the mentally ill, especially the chronic patient and the deinstitutionalized." In the circumstances, I suggest that rather than uttering Panglossian platitudes about "reform" and "profound transformation[s] in mental health policy" (Grob 1991: 5), we might better occupy ourselves with the urgent task of understanding the full dimensions of "the demise of state responsibility for the seriously mentally ill and the current crisis of abandonment" (Gruenberg and Archer 1979). *From Asylum to Community*, notwithstanding its author's claims to the contrary, fails lamentably to advance us very far in that direction.

9 Psychiatry and social control in the nineteenth and twentieth centuries

To speak of psychiatry as a form of "social control" was quite common in the 1970s and 1980s, but has become increasingly unfashionable in the last decade or so. In recent years, historians of psychiatry, in particular, have shied away from such language, and have adopted a more benign perspective on the psychiatric profession and its institutions. Intentionally or not, they thus echo in their scholarship what have long been the reactions of the psychiatric profession itself to critics who have questioned its benevolence or doubted its devotion to the interests of those who serve as the objects of its attentions. Anxious to be seen as being in the business of helping and healing, psychiatrists can be (and have been) provoked to paroxysms of anger by the suggestion that they act as agents of social control, for such language conjures up images of coercion and constraint, if not the intentional infliction of hurt and harm. Such connotations are all very well in the overtly punitive realm of the criminal justice system, for retribution is an acknowledged and (within limits that vary in time and space), an acceptable face of punishment. But they consort uneasily with the pretensions of a profession that purports to be devoted solely to the interests of their nominal clients, the patients, and bent on curing them.

In the past decade or so, a new generation of scholars who cannot readily be seen as knee-jerk apologists for psychiatry have also increasingly abandoned the language of social control. To some extent, I think such a move reflects a weariness with an older set of debates on the subject. The positions of the combatants on each side of the question had tended to become fixed and somewhat predictable, and the arguments familiar. (On the one side, see Grob (1977, 1990); Quen (1974); Roth (1973); and on the other Rothman (1976; 1984).) There was a natural desire to open up new avenues of inquiry, and to push research in different directions, both topically and temporally. But that is not the whole story. In reaction against the earlier revisionist historiography, a younger generation of scholars has moved to embrace what the historian Joseph Melling has called a late-Whiggish position on the nineteenth-century asylum. Rather than viewing Victorian bins as mere warehouses, an array of hidden repositories for society's unhinged and unwanted, these historians have adopted a more benign role for these institutions.[1]

One element in this revised portrait has been the observation, well-established by now, that there was considerably more traffic across the boundary between asylum and community than the first generation of revisionist studies had allowed. (The pioneering study here was Ray 1981.) Even in the late nineteenth century, a substantial fraction of those who entered an asylum in any twelve-month period could expect to be discharged within a year, and a handful more over the next twelve months – perhaps a third or two-fifths of the intake. Adding to this the 10 to 18 percent of patients who died within a year of admission, and the repeated finding that the median length of stay for a new asylum inmate in the last third of the nineteenth century hovered between a year and a year and a half seems wholly unsurprising, if at odds with a previous insistence on the custodial character of the Victorian bins.

For some, this trafficking to and fro across the margins of the madhouse sector, the existence of patients who were "brought back" into society after being previously "cast out" (I echo here the title of John Walton's (1985) seminal paper on the subject.) was sufficient by itself to refute the image of the asylum as an instrument of social control, and to revive its credentials as a therapeutic institution. Such arguments, however, strike me as profoundly mistaken. First, to assert that mental hospitals serve vital social control functions is not by any means to assert that this is the *only* social role they play. Therapy and social control may be intertwined and were complementary aspects of the asylum system, not contradictory and binary opposites. Second, even temporary incarceration may serve important social control goals, whether viewed from the perspective of the patient's immediate family, of the local community, or of the larger society. And third, it will not do to replace a one-sided view of the late nineteenth-century asylum as a storage dump, a repository of dead souls, with an equally one-sided portrait of it as a benevolent and therapeutic institution.

For, notwithstanding the restoration of a significant fraction of its intake to the larger society, every year a very substantial fraction of asylum admissions remained behind to swell the population of chronic, long-stay patients, and as the size of public asylums grew relentlessly, annual admissions formed a smaller and smaller fraction of the whole. In the mammoth bins that were scattered across the fin-de-siècle landscape, a large and growing proportion of the asylum population quickly came to be composed of chronic, long-stay patients, for those who did not leave within twelve or twenty-four months seldom exited, save in a pine box. And it was this specter of chronicity, this horde of the hopeless, which was to haunt the popular imagination, to constitute the public identity of the asylums, and to dominate late nineteenth and early twentieth-century psychiatric theorizing and practice (see Scull 1993).

Central in other respects to the renewed attempt to reassert the humanitarian credentials of the asylum, and thus at least implicitly to contest both Foucault's broad-ranging assault on the Enlightenment project and the arguments put forward in the first generation of Anglo-American revisionist historiography, has been a growing move away from the macro-sociological level of analysis. As the more global analyses of the rise of the asylum have become unfashionable in recent years, so too there has been something of a retreat from efforts to connect the rise of asylumdom to the larger social and political context – to the dynamics of class society, for example, or to the growing commercialization of existence in the eighteenth and nineteenth centuries.[2] In an interesting rhetorical maneuver, those of us who insist on the relevance and importance of these factors find ourselves dismissed as "Marxists," a sufficiently damning epithet in the eyes of many, in the aftermath of the collapse of the Soviet empire, to discredit this whole line of argument, and "perhaps irrevocably," as one not unsympathetic critic would have it (Grob 1990; Dowbiggin 1997: 361). If more ammunition is needed to shoot down our claims, boiling down a complex argument to the crude claim that "asylum treatment was...an effort of the anxiety-ridden, capitalist, Victorian ruling class to incarcerate deviant paupers and subject them to managerial techniques of control" (Dowbiggin 1997: 361) has been mustered to provide it.

By no means, of course, does a shift in analytic focus from the macro- to the micro-social context *determine* a move away from a concern with the inter-relations of broader social, cultural, political, and economic forces with the psychiatric enterprise. For example, Jonathan Andrews' and my recent collaborative work on the eighteenth-century trade in lunacy, and the patrons and customers of its most famous mad-doctor, John Monro, places such concerns at the heart of its analysis (Andrews and Scull 2001, 2003). Yet an examination of a series of individual cases certainly encourages an emphasis on the particularities of person, institution and place, and in the celebration of what is idiosyncratic about a certain setting and the articulation of the complexities of an individual example, there is a natural tendency to criticize and shy away from global generalizations rather than refining and extending them.

The risk, of course, is the construction of meticulously detailed individual accounts that overlook or underweight larger structural and organizational imperatives, and lapse into telling stories of incremental change that retreat into a sort of neo-solipsism. That is not to deny the value of confronting general models with detailed empirical analyses. Only in this way can we hope to develop a more subtle and sophisticated understanding of the phenomena under study and expose the limitations of previous generalizations. But it is to emphasize that it is equally vital that we acknowledge that we can only achieve this larger aim if we consciously seek to show the more general significance of a given set of phenomena and to transcend the peculiarities of person and place. A mindless empiricism, a view of social reality as just one damn thing after another, is a stance that avoids the intellectual risks and inevitable pitfalls of a more vaunting ambition, but at the heavy price of embracing a constricted vision that flattens and distorts our sense of perspective, and leaves in obscurity aspects of historical reality that acquire meaning only when placed in a larger contextual frame.[3]

Regrettably, the division between those focusing on the micro-politics of insanity and those continuing to insist on the importance of a broader scholarly perspective corresponds to some considerable extent with disciplinary boundaries and loyalties. I say regrettably, because I have long argued that the distinction between sociology and history is an artificial and unfortunate one. To be sure, it is a distinction that has become entrenched over the years in institutional structures and professional organizations, but it is a foolish and distorting division, one that mirrors and reinforces the parochialism of much of contemporary academic life. That remains the case no matter how skillfully the separation is rationalized by the self-interests of academic guilds, and no matter how fiercely it is defended by the border guards who spend their days on the prowl, looking out for intellectual interlopers to shoot at.[4]

In what follows, I suggest some of the analytic gains that can flow from examining the evolution of psychiatry as an aspect of the changing structures of social control in modern societies. Before doing so (not that it will forestall criticism from some quarters), I would like to stipulate at the outset that some of the objections raised by the new generations of historians to an earlier historiography that stressed social control are well-taken. It should go without saying that it will not do to adopt an unduly reductionist view that treats psychiatry as *only* a form of social control and its interventions as nothing more than a relentless effort to control a particular class of deviants (the simplistic view promoted by Thomas Szasz and his followers). That bears repeating, even though one should emphasize that the Szaszian perspective had never drawn much support among the first generation of revisionist historians. More germane are recent critics' arguments that an earlier generation of scholarship, my own included, tended to focus too narrowly on a state-centered view of social control and to downplay issues of agency and resistance.

The emerging interest in recovering the perspectives of mental patients and their families forms part, of course, of a wider interest on the part of professional historians in constructing a "history from below." Rather than viewing those who ended up in asylums (and their nearest and dearest) as mere ciphers, passive victims whose fortunes and fates are wholly at the disposal of those funding and running the institutions, a sustained effort is now under way to give voice to the voiceless, and to provide a more nuanced, less one-sided account of the interaction of magistrates, Poor Law officials, alienists, families, and patients. Families, it is now fashionable to argue, were not just put-upon, submissive pawns pushed about by a Leviathan state and its minions, but actively used and manipulated the asylum system for their own ends (Forsythe *et al.* 1996; see also Wright 1998; Walsh 1999; Michael 2003).[5] Recent scholarship has suggested, for instance, that it was not so much the judgments of asylum superintendents, but rather the ability and willingness of patients' families to absorb particular individuals back into the household, regardless of continuing mental disturbances and infirmities, that must be seen as the central determinants of decisions over discharge or retention within the confines of the asylum (Wright 1999). On some accounts, too, patients are to be accorded a measure of agency. If not quite the masters or mistresses of their fates, neither the new orthodoxy would have it, nor were they wholly incapable of resistance and of influencing the terms of their confinement (Jackson 2000).

That is true, useful, and important to remember. Yet it is easy to push these arguments too far, and to fail to acknowledge that there are gross imbalances of power and resources at work here for families, and even more clearly for patients, for whom the problems of social subordination and economic powerlessness are compounded to an extraordinary degree by the impact of the label of insanity. For lunatics, the madmen, psychotics, schizophrenics – call them what you will – suffer a sort of social and moral death. Their wishes and will, their very status as moral actors, as agents capable of expressing valid preferences and exercising autonomous choice are deeply suspect in light of their presumed pathology, as the often dark history of their treatment under confinement abundantly shows. Erving Goffman's essays on the "moral career of the mental patient" and the "underlife" of the total institution (Goffman 1961) long ago pointed to acts of distancing and resistance employed by inmates. But the pathetic and self-defeating qualities of the "make-dos" he describes, which serve only to reinforce others' sense of them as pathologically different and inferior, are powerful reminders of the profound power imbalances that structure the over-matched inmates' lives, and of their moral and political insignificance in the larger equation. Uncomfortable as it may be for some to accept the obvious, I insist that issues of power and social control, broadly conceived, are indeed central, and necessarily so, to any balanced understanding of the psychiatric realm.

Over the course of the first half of the nineteenth century, in England, (Scull 1979) in Continental Europe (Doerner 1981; Castel 1988), and in North America (Rothman 1971; Grob 1973a) the typical response to the deranged underwent dramatic and radical changes. The metamorphosis occurred at the level of both ideas and social practices; and it made irrevocable the differentiation of the insane from the wider category of the merely indigent and troublesome. In a highly significant redefinition of the moral boundaries of Western society, insanity was transformed from a vague, culturally defined phenomenon afflicting an unknown, but probably small proportion of the population into a condition which could only be authoritatively diagnosed, certified, and treated by a group of legally recognized experts. Whereas in the eighteenth century only the most violent and destructive amongst those now labeled insane would have been segregated and confined apart from the rest of the community, with the achievement of what was widely portrayed as a major social reform, the asylum was endorsed as the sole officially approved response to the problems posed by mental illness. And, in the process, the boundaries of who was to be classified as mad, and thus was to be liable to incarceration, were themselves transformed.

The crystallization of this new ensemble of social practices and meanings; their striking and sinister embodiment of new physical forms that constitute such a notable example of the "moral architecture" of the nineteenth century;[6] the reciprocal constitution of new forms of expertise and knowledge alongside and in intimate relationships with this new institutional apparatus; the development of new theoretical codes and technologies of intervention; the redrawing of the boundaries between the normal and the pathological; and the shutting away of the mad in what was pronounced to be a therapeutic isolation – these mark the emergence for the first time of a relatively stable psychiatric complex, and the irruption of new modes and mechanisms of intervention and treatment, dominance, and control. Institutions and knowledge, theory and practice, and the constitution and the capture of particular sorts of problem populations do not develop in some linear, sequential fashion, with one side of these equations preceding and producing the other. They are, on the contrary, mutually reinforcing and deeply inter-dependent, the development of the one deriving from and simultaneously advancing the maturation of the other.

Pace Foucault (1965), the massive internment of the mad is essentially a nineteenth-century phenomenon; and notwithstanding the readily identifiable presence of medical accounts of madness as *one* strand – but only one strand[7] – in the complex of meanings attributed to Unreason in Western culture in the pre-industrial age, it is only from the Victorian era forward that one can speak without anachronism of psychiatry as a historical actor. It was on the basis of their control over the novel and rapidly expanding realm of asylumdom that alienists constituted themselves as a newly self-conscious profession, making use of their medical identity to attribute a particular status and meaning to the objects of their attention. Moreover, it is psychiatrists' supremacy over the asylum and its techniques of isolation, and the monopoly this gave them over the legitimate treatment of madness, which have subsequently formed the foundation from which the profession has sought to expand its jurisdictional reach, multiplying the range of behaviors and the classes of deviants subject to its intervention and dubiously therapeutic ministrations. To be sure, the emerging profession remained a hobbled and stigmatized enterprise, even well into the twentieth century, and one should be wary of exaggerating its role in the creation of asylumdom as well as properly cognizant of the limits of its professional powers. But the institutionalization of expertise in this sector of society is inextricably bound up with the rise of specialized institutional responses to the mad. It is thus with the origins of the asylum and its psychiatry that I shall begin my discussion.

Confinement was a not uncommon fate for some of the frenzied long before the age of the asylum. Those madmen whose loss of contact with or respect for consensually defined reality and whose wild and unpredictable behavior posed an obvious threat to social order were shut up with but little fuss or ceremony. They formed one element, for instance, of the heterogeneous population the French absolutist state crammed into its Hôpitaux Généraux; and they were freely consigned to jails or to a growing number of private madhouses by their families or by the English authorities, wherever domestic resources proved incapable of protecting the community from their imprecations and potential depredations. A still larger proportion of the melancholy or mopish, the disturbed and distracted – people who would certainly have been candidates for incarceration in the nineteenth century – were tolerated and provisionally left at large. But one should harbor no romantic illusions of a Golden Age of permissive madness, left untrammeled and untouched by the machinations of bourgeois Reason. In medieval and early modern Europe, folly did not flourish, free of pernicious social restraint. Where the mad proved troublesome, they could expect to be beaten or locked up; otherwise, they might roam or rot.

Physical restraint and coercion were scarcely hidden aspects of the traditional management of the mad. As I have demonstrated elsewhere (Scull 1989: ch. 3), the sense of madness as a condition that required taming, as one might domesticate and thus render predictable the behavior of a wild beast, runs through any number of eighteenth-century discussions of insanity. Widely viewed as a creature dragged down to a state of brutish insensibility and incapacity, the lunatic occupied a wholly unenviable ontological status, being seen as emblematic of the chaos and terror, of the dark, bestial possibilities that lurked within the human frame, waiting only on the loss of "that governing principle, reason" (Pargeter 1792: 2) to emerge in their full awfulness. Correspondingly, it was held that the madman's ferocity must be tamed by a mixture of discipline and depletion designed to put down "the raging of the Spirits and the lifting up of the Soul" (Willis 1684: 206). As Willis argued,

> To correct or allay the furies and exorbitancies of the Animal Spirits . . . requires threatenings, bonds, or strokes, as well as *Physick*. For the *Madman* being placed in a House convenient for the business, must be so handled both by the *Physician*, and also by the Servants that are prudent, that he may in some manner be kept in, either by warnings, chidings, or punishments inflicted on him, to his duty, or his behaviour, or manners. And indeed for the curing of Mad people, there is nothing more effectual or necessary than their reverence or standing in awe of such as they think their Tormentors. . . . Furious Madmen are sooner, and more certainly cured by punishment and hard usage, in a strait room, than by *Physick* or Medicines.
>
> (1684: 206)

(Which is not to say that madmen were spared the more conventional therapies of the Galenic medical practitioner – purges, bleedings, vomits, and the like – in those instances where they came under medical control.)

Whether confined in nominally medical establishments, in jails, in workhouses, or in lay run madhouses, the coercive, controlling aspects of the traditional treatment of the mad were in essence transparent and unadorned. The necessity for repression, the deliberate incitement of fear, and the infliction of physical suffering were openly acknowledged. Indeed, intimidation and forceful persuasion were viewed as essential techniques in the management of the mad and freely defended as such. Francis Willis, for instance, the Lincolnshire divine who was summoned to treat George III's madness, insisted as "the first principle of [his] practice" on the need "to make himself formidable – to inspire awe. In these terrible maladies," he boasted, "those who superintend the unhappy patients must so subjugate their will, that no idea of resistance to their commands can have place in their minds" (Anonymous 1794: 31–33). Notwithstanding the Queen's objections, and George's status as his king, Willis had him "sometimes chained to a stake. He was frequently beaten and starved, and at best kept in subjection by menacing and violent language" (The Countess Harcourt, quoted in Bynum 1974: 319).

Such practices were not without an underlying therapeutic logic (Scull 1989: chs 3 and 4), but their repressive, controlling aspects are scarcely ambiguous or hidden. It is quite otherwise with the approaches to madness which character-ized the nineteenth-century reforms. The founding myths of modern psychia-try are the picture of Philippe Pinel literally and metaphorically striking off the chains from the lunatics in the Bicêtre and (in the midst of the bloodiest excesses of the French Revolution) inaugurating the first rational and humane approach to the treatment of the mentally disordered;[8] and the companion por-trait of John Conolly completing this triumph of science and humanity by inaugurating an asylum regime that totally dispensed with even the remnants of the ancient reliance on "mechanical restraint" – whips and chains, manacles and muffs, stripes and straitjackets (Scull 1989: ch. 7). In the Manichean vision preferred by modern psychiatry and its apologists, the Dark Ages of the mad persists right up to the birth of alienism and of the asylum in the early nine-teenth century, when science and humanity united at last to produce a revolu-tion in the treatment of the mentally ill – a sequence of events which constituted, in the words of one of its least critical observers, "the most blessed manifestation of true civilization the world can present" (Paget 1866: 34–35).

Such is the official portrait drawn up by those our culture accords the status of experts in the treatment of mental disorder and by their scholarly allies.[9] And within such a vision talk of psychiatry as "social control" can find no place. Convinced of their own righteousness, they bridle at the very notion, emphasizing that the reformers (and the alienists who ran the new asylums) were "primarily concerned with uplifting the mass of suffering humanity…" (Grob 1973a: 109) not with restraining "deviant groups or largely lower class elements, thereby ensuring some measure of social control (if not hegemony)" (Grob 1978: 4–5). Psychiatrists were and are scientists and healers, devoted to providing humane care and cures for their patients. The language of repression and control is thus wholly misplaced, a positive anathema, and to make use of it is willfully to obstruct the relief of suffering (Roth 1973), virtually to commit blasphemy.

It would be difficult to imagine a more thorough-going assault on these orthodox triumphalist pieties than that launched by Michel Foucault almost three decades ago now. For Foucault, so far from the interventions of Pinel and Conolly marking the liberation of the insane from their fetters of iron and shackles of superstition, they constitute the imposition of an ever more thorough-going "moral uniformity and social denunciation" – the historical moment at which the medical gaze secured its domination over the mad, launching "that gigantic moral imprisonment which we are in the habit of calling, doubtless by antiphrasis, the liberation of the insane..." (Foucault 1965: 259, 278). The myth of progress is here turned upside down. For the mad, in Foucault's view, "[l]iberation from the racking of the body merely meant new tortures for the mind..., the imposition of more subtly terrifying 'mind forg'd manacles' of guilt and self-control" (Bynum *et al.* 1985a: 2).

My own view is that both these perspectives are too crude and one-sided. In its origins, at least, nineteenth-century lunacy reform was Janus-faced, simultaneously embodying (at least at the outset) "a humanitarian concern for the protection, against visible abuses, of people who were coming to be seen as curable sufferers whose condition was not their fault" (Walton 1985); while (to some degree unwittingly) fostering a concealed yet ever more systematic regulation of lunatics' lives. The new realm of asylumdom depended crucially upon the new technology of moral treatment developed independently by men like Pinel and Tuke (Pinel 1806; Tuke 1813); and embedded within moral treatment were structural tensions between repression and rehabilitation, between the imposition of moral discipline and the development of self-government and self-control. Only over time were these tensions systematically resolved in favor of an oppressive system of moral management, enforced conformity, and disciplined subordination.[10]

The central fact about moral treatment, and the reason for its immediate appeal, was the way it demonstrated that the most repellent features of existing responses to the mad were actually unnecessary cruelties. Tuke, for instance, was able to boast that "neither chains nor corporal punishment are tolerated, on any pretext, in this establishment." Instead, the patient's "desire for esteem" could generally be exploited to secure good behavior. Where this did not produce the desired result, "the general comfort of the patients ought to be considered; and those who are violent require to be separated from the more tranquil, and to be prevented, by some means, from offensive conduct towards their fellow-sufferers." This could be achieved when "the patients are arranged into classes, as much as may be, according to the degree to which they approach to rational or orderly conduct." Such a system had the crucial additional advantage of providing patients with a powerful incentive to exercise self-restraint for the insane "quickly perceive, or if not, they are informed on the first occasion, that their treatment depends, in great measure, on their conduct" (Tuke 1813: 141, 151).

To see in all this only the benevolent face of moral treatment – its break with the crude coercion of the past – is to ignore the latent power of these techniques as a mechanism for enforcing conformity. The pervasive authority of the alienist, and his ability to link classification with a system of rewards and punishments, constituted an extraordinarily powerful new form of "moral machinery" (Browne 1837), a superior mode of *managing* patients. The use of space in the form of the ward system to constitute and make salient moral boundaries, and the creation of an intimate tie between the patient's position in this classificatory system and his behavior, enabled alienists to use every aspect of the environment as "a more powerful lever in acting upon the intractable" (Browne 1837: 156). It was precisely the hidden strengths of moral treatment as a mechanism for the management and regulation of conduct and the production of docile bodies which made possible the abandonment of the brutal and harsh methods of management which had previously been inextricably connected with the concentration of large numbers of lunatics in an institutional environment. And in placing far more effective and thorough-going means of control in the hands of the custodians while simultaneously removing the necessity for the asylum's crudest features, the reality of that imprisonment and control simultaneously became far more difficult to perceive. It was the possession of this technology of domination which made it possible, in a very practical sense, for alienists to manage and clothe with a veil of legitimacy their expanding empire, the nineteenth and twentieth-century museums for the collection and confinement of the mad.

There were, however, clear limits to the power of these techniques. Alienists in the second quarter of the nineteenth century boasted of quite extravagant success in curing the crazy: 60, 70, 80, even 90 percent cures were allegedly within reach. Insanity, it was solemnly pronounced on both sides of the Atlantic, was one of the most readily cured of the afflictions to which human flesh was heir (Burrows 1828; Rothman 1971: 131–133; Grob 1973a: 182–185). And the high initial costs of a properly constituted asylum system thus would be rapidly offset by the production of a high proportion of cures and the return of the dependent to the ranks of the productive citizenry. But the claim that there existed what Ellen Dwyer has dubbed "an economics of compassion" (Dwyer 1987) foundered in the face of the recalcitrant reality of chronic mental disorder.

It was the utopian dream of the founding fathers of Victorian asylumdom that they possessed the untrammeled ability to impose their values and norms on the mad (Scull 1990), the capacity to inculcate a sufficient measure of moral discipline and self-control into the lunatic to allow their reabsorption into the social order as fully rehabilitated and re-programmed citizens. Possession of this sort of capacity "to domineer for good purposes over the minds of others" (Bucknill and Tuke 1858: 509) would have constituted the exercise of social control with a vengeance, the realization at once of the positive ambition to vanquish madness, but also of the insidious and worrying capacity to suppress non-conformity in the name of mental health. In reality, of course, the powers of psychiatry were far more modest and circumscribed, and with respect to its larger ambitions, fortunately or unfortunately, the profession "failed most abjectly" (Walton 1985: 143).

Within the closed universe of the asylum, however, moral management proved highly efficacious as a repressive instrument for controlling large numbers of people. I should emphasize "large," because publicly funded asylum systems underwent explosive growth throughout the nineteenth and well into the twentieth century. In England, for instance, the number of officially certified lunatics doubled between 1844 and 1860, while the general population grew by only 20 percent, and increase in their numbers continued to outstrip the growth of the population as a whole by a large margin for the remainder of the century, rising to over 100,000 by the early 1900s. Expansion was equally dramatic in France and in the United States (Grob 1973; Dowbiggin 1991), and not just the total number of patients, but the size of the receptacles within which they were confined grew remorselessly. Initially, the profession had demanded that asylums contain 200 or fewer, but already by mid-century, institutions containing a 1,000 and more were common. By the early twentieth century, Milledgeville in Georgia had grown to a vast series of barracks holding more than 10,000 inmates (Hurd 1916: 401), while the new London County Council was in the process of constructing no less than 5 utilitarian pauper asylums on a single, centrally serviced site, holding pens for more than 12,000 pauper lunatics (Cochrane 1988). Leading psychiatrists now claimed that "hospitals with 4,000 to 5,000 patients or more were not unreasonable" (Grob 1983: 236; for France, see Alexander 1976: 281).

Within these mammoth institutions, the reality of the patient's existence departed further and further from the conditions in the outside world, for his return to which the asylum was still ostensibly preparing him. Most institutions possessed a ward or two for show, where the better behaved patients were kept in an environment less immediately depressing. But the contrast with the rest of the asylum only emphasized more cruelly the bleak existence provided for the overwhelming majority of the patients who were left to languish on the back-wards, "subject to the rigid constraints of detention . . ., which [over time] became more and more degrading. Overcrowding, material misery, absence of therapeutic activities, daily violence" were everywhere the marks of "the asylum order, that immense cemetery that has swallowed up thousands of despairing lives" (Castel 1988: 218). The mechanical metaphor recurs again and again in contemporary descriptions of the asylum, with even the patients' diversions and recreations organized and bureaucratized, shaped to fit the asylum's timetable and routine.

Huge and impersonal, late nineteenth-century asylums were nonetheless proclaimed to be "marvels of order and regularity" resembling nothing so much as "a well-constructed piece of mechanism, which, once set in motion, needs but a certain amount of regular attention to keep it working smoothly and successfully" (Burdett 1891: 189–190). "Success" no longer meant cures. Indeed the proportion of their patients alienists claimed to cure fell steadily over the course of the nineteenth century, till ultimately more of their charges left the asylum in coffins each year than were restored to society in the possession of their senses. But if cures were beyond reach in all but a small minority of cases, the asylum regime at least provided the public with symbolic demonstrations that the disturbing and dangerous manifestations of madness were firmly under control; that the disorderly could be rendered tranquil and tractable.

In sustaining the whole operation, old, long-stay patients were vital "to give the newcomers the necessary example of industry, order, and obedience" (Yellowlees 1890: 488). Indeed, it was "the quiet, chronic patients who give stability to the asylum microcosm...the phalanx of failures, whose well-considered routine constitutes the *force majeure* of an ordinary asylum, into whose orderly ways the newcomer of ill-regulated brain drops by sheer force of numbers" (Dr Urquhart, superintendent of the Perth Asylum in Scotland, quoted in Burdett 1891: 189–190). Confinement year after year produced its own deadening effect, ensuring a sufficient measure of conformity so long as the patients remained safely within the walls of the institution:

> The effect of long continued discipline is to remove all salient parts of the character, all obtrusive and irregular propensities and peculiarities... [with the result that] the majority [of asylum inmates], enfeebled by monotony, by the absence of strong impulses and new impressions, tamed, and stilled, and frozen, by the very means to which they may owe life, and some remains of reason, exhibit a stolidity and torpor which are obviously superadded to their original malady.
>
> (Crichton Royal Asylum 1848: 35)

The failure of psychiatry to deliver on its original promise of cures produced, as might be expected, both an internal and an external "crisis of legitimacy" (Rosenberg 1975). In the 1860s and 1870s, in France (Dowbiggin 1985; Castel 1988: 220–293), in the United States (Pitts 1978; Blustein 1981), in Britain (Scull 1979: chs 5 and 6), both internal questioning and external attacks marked the upsurge of sharp challenges to psychiatric authority and the profession's pretensions to expertise. In beating back these threats, alienists were quick to re-emphasize the traditional notion that they were protecting the public and guaranteeing social order. Exemplary tales circulated to "prove" that the most apparently harmless lunatics were liable to commit totally unpredictable and often unprovoked acts of senseless violence. The public was informed, unfortunately,

> it is just those cases in which the signs of insanity seem slight to an ordinary observer [as opposed to the keener perceptions of the expert in mental medicine] that the greatest danger exists. The homicidal lunatic often shows scarcely a sign of the disease and the suicide may show nothing at all beyond a slight amount of depression. (Greene 1889: 498; for the employment of similar tactics by French alienists, see Nye 1984: 230–232)

But alienists increasingly articulated a broader and far more effective justification for the sequestration of the mad than the threat of random violence. As asylums silted up with the chronically crazy, "the waifs and strays, the weak and wayward of our race" (W.A.F. Browne, quoted in Anonymous 1857: 201), so late nineteenth-century psychiatry moved steadily toward a grim determinism, a view of madness as the irreversible product of a process of mental degeneration and decay. The rigid and pessimistic somaticism which increasingly pervaded psychiatric discourse provided a powerful rationalization for the profession's dismal therapeutic performance. More crucially still, as we shall see, it transformed (and broadened) the potential sites for psychiatric intervention.

The asylum remained at the heart of mental medicine, now and for almost a century more – albeit with its mission redefined as quarantining the incurable rather restoring the temporarily distracted to sanity. But psychiatry simultaneously sought to transform the failure to redeem its therapeutic promises into the basis for obtaining a wholly new importance in the battle to contain social pathology and to defend the social order. The march it now undertook into "the borderlands of insanity" (Wynter 1875; Cullere 1888), its embrace of the "demi-fous," the neurasthenic (Beard 1881; Levillain (1891), and the hysteric (Skey 1867; Charcot 1971) marked the opening shots of a campaign to secure "an awesome extension of the medical role" (Castel 1988: 232) in policing the boundaries of society, and in the regulation of asocial behaviors. That campaign has met with no more than a series of partial successes. It has been marked by a continuing parade of border skirmishes and uneasy compromises with proponents of a traditional and entrenched legal system of social regulation.[11] And it has heightened the controversial position occupied by psychiatry in modern systems of social control.

The essence of the new theoretical account of madness, a neo-Lamarkian explanation of the proliferation of organic pathologies, was laid out for the first time in B.A. Morel's *Traité des dégénérescences* (Morel 1857). Heredity had long been seen as a causal factor in the development of madness, but an inherited morbid constitutional defect now came to be viewed as the biological principle underlying all the protean forms of deviation from conventional morality. Linking together the physical, the environmental, and the social, alienists argued that dissolute and depraved conduct exacted a heavy biological price. It produced "a worsening physical and nervous disorder of a morbid type..." (Nye 1984: 121), a generalized degradation of all nervous tissue whose pernicious but entirely predictable sequel was an entrenched neuropathic hereditary "taint." This constitutional defect, in its turn, was transmitted without fail to succeeding generations, remorselessly bringing in its train alcoholism, criminality, madness, idiocy, sterility, and death.[12]

Borrowing freely from these formulations, English-speaking alienists soon advanced closely related views. The madman, as Henry Maudsley put it, "is the necessary organic consequent of certain organic antecedents: and it is impossible he should escape the tyranny of his organization" (Maudsley 1879: 88). Insanity constituted nothing less than a form of phylogenetic regression, which accounted, of course, for the lunatic's loss of civilized behavior, and regression to the status of a brute:

> Whence came the savage snarl, the destructive disposition, the obscene language, the wild howl, the offensive habits displayed by some of the insane? Why should a human being deprived of his reason ever become so brutal in character as some do, unless he has the brute nature within him?
>
> (Maudsley 1870: 53)

Employing ever harsher language, psychiatric discourse now exhibited a barely disguised contempt for the mad, those "tainted persons" (Strahan 1890: 337) whom it sequestered on society's behalf. They were, said Daniel Hack Tuke, the most unembarrassed apologist for asylumdom, "an infirm type of humanity ... on admission 'No good' is plainly inscribed on their fore-heads" (Tuke 1878: 152).

All this meant, of course, that psychiatry's dismal therapeutic performance was actually a blessing in disguise, a demonstration that Nature herself embraced Hegel's "cunning of reason." The public was warned that it must face up to the bitter truth that

> The subversion of reason involves not only present incompetency, but a prospective susceptibility of disease, a proclivity to relapse.... The mind does not pass out of the ordeal [of insanity] unchanged.... Recovery ... may be little more than the exercise of great cunning, or self-control, in concealing the signs of error and extravagance.
>
> (Crichton Royal Asylum 1857: 12–13)

But if "normality" is a mere facsimile of the genuine article, if, as Robert Castel puts it, "a cure risks being only 'apparent,' [then] the only good insane are those in the asylum" (Castel 1988: 182). The original justification for asy-lumdom, its potential as a new form of "moral machinery" for the manufac-ture of sanity from mad raw materials, was now turned on its head: "It is not probable," the new orthodoxy proclaimed, "that we can ever diminish the insane by any increase in recoveries; indeed, *the converse is more probable*" (Thompson 1890: 157, emphasis in the original). When all was said and done,

> No human power can eradicate from insanity its terrible hereditary nature, and every so-called "cure" in one generation will be liable to increase the tale of lunacy in the next ... it is evident that the higher the percentage of recoveries in the present, the greater will be the proportion of insanity in the future.
>
> (Greene 1889: 503)

The very defects in will-power and self-control which most characterized these "tainted persons" encouraged them to "attend upon the calls of their instincts and passions as does the unreasoning beast" (Strahan 1890: 337); and, in consequence, "every year thousands of children are born with pedigrees that would condemn puppies to the horsepond" (Strahan 1890: 334). Left to herself, Nature would set things right, since each of the several varieties of insanity "is but a stage in the descent towards sterile idiocy" (Maudsley 1867: 247). But misguided attempts to cure the mad and restore them to society

> prevent, so far as is possible, the operation of those laws which weed out and exterminate the diseased and otherwise unfit in every grade of natural life... [the insane] are not only permitted, but are aided by every device known to science to propagate their kind... [they are turned loose to act as parents to the next generation... centres of infection deliberately laid down, and yet we marvel that nervous disease increases.
>
> (Strahan 1890: 331, 332, 334)

Psychiatry could thus continue to point to the institutions which formed the core of its jurisdiction as vital elements in the maintenance of social order and tranquility. Asylums performed a social function of inestimable value, the "sequestration," even the "violent extrusion" of "morbid varieties or degenerates of the human kind" (Maudsley 1879: 115). They provided "in the cases of chronically insane persons, their detention for life" (Charles Lockhart Robertson, quoted in Burdett 1891: 263–264) – a convenient apparatus allowing for the collection of dead souls in a network of cemeteries for the still-breathing, "where they can be more easily visited and accounted for by the authorities" (Bucknill 1880: 122).

But if madness was almost wholly resistant to treatment once fully established, this did "not lead to pessimism and even less to abandoning the will to intervene." To the contrary, alienists sought rather "to shift the point at which this intervention was applied" (Castel 1988: 232) to an earlier period in the process, to promote prevention, programs of mental hygiene, (Sicherman 1967) and the treatment of the mildly disordered and still potentially salvageable (Rosenberg 1962; Blustein 1979; Showalter 1985: 121–164; Goldstein 1987: 322–377). Psychiatry now cast about for a place in those arenas where madness might emerge if not forestalled by expert intervention. The family, the school, the factory, the army – all were sites where it offered its services and advice, claiming to have at its disposal the means to secure, as Morel put it, the "moralization of the masses" through a "preservative prophylaxis" (Morel 1857: 687).

Its hereditarian emphasis brought psychiatry into close relationship with eugenic ideas, and not the least of the "services" it offered to clients beyond the confines of asylumdom was the provision of advice about who was, and was not, fit to marry. This effort to impose restraints on the profligate breeding of the unfit, and thus, within a generation, to trim the increase in the ranks of the mad was as successful at stemming the rising tide of insanity as the commands of King Canute on an earlier occasion. The emerging mental hygiene movement sought, with an equal lack of therapeutic success, to fore-stall mental illness, or to catch it in its incipient stages. But from another perspective, alienists' propaganda about the prevention of mental illness, the promotion of mental health, and the value of treating cases of incipient men-tal disorder both reflected and reinforced a new receptivity on the profession's part to the still-functioning, though symptom-bearing patient who could form the basis of an office-based practice. Such a development was vital if the profession was to transform the image of mental medicine as overwhelmingly concerned with the institutional custody of a chronically incapacitated and generally economically deprived clientele.

But this line of analysis requires both extension and qualification. In the regulation of madness, accredited experts, families, their soon-to-be excluded members, and the larger civil society all enter into the picture. We must acknowledge that the analytic model of the all-powerful state coercing entirely helpless individuals (patients and their families) has been shown to be hopelessly simplistic, however great its ideological appeal in some quar-ters. The same may be said, of course, about the way the concept of society has at times been applied to the study of punishment, where again there is a risk of narrowing one's focus too much. Two decades ago, writing of revisionist work on the prison and penitentiary, and including his own work in the crit-icism, Michael Ignatieff confessed that the new generation of scholarship had overstated the importance of the state. It had fostered, he suggested, the mis-conceptions "that the state enjoys a monopoly over punitive regulation of behaviour in society, that its moral authority and practical power are the binding sources of social order, and that all social relations can be described in the language of subordination" (Ignatieff 1983: 77).

But to acknowledge the importance of this broader array of actors, and to reject a simple reductionism that would equate the psychiatric (or the punitive) enterprise with nothing more than a relentless effort to control a particular class of deviants – one which adopts the Szaszian line, for instance, that psy-chiatrists are merely concentration camp guards in disguise (Szasz 1970) – is not at all the same thing as accepting the claim made by many in the profes-sion and their apologists that theirs is a purely therapeutic and humanitarian intervention. For as Goffman noted in an obscure and little-cited paper, men-tal illness is all about havoc and disarray, and efforts to contain and mitigate the problems that flow from that disorder and threat (Goffman 1971). Bringing family, community, profession, and patient back into the picture does not alter that reality, or in my judgment make the issue of social control any less central to a balanced assessment of the psychiatric enterprise.

Likewise, I remain as convinced as I was two decades ago of the centrality of psychiatry and of psychiatric ideologies and technologies to the study of social control in modern societies. Indeed, over the past century or so, their centrality has surely grown. Many astute analysts of the punitive sphere (Cohen 1985; Garland 1985, 2001) have been struck by the broadening and net-widening impact of "reforms" in this sector. One can readily observe a parallel extension and expansion of psychiatric forms of social control into new social settings and institutional domains.

For psychiatry in the twentieth century has clearly been operating in the context of a rapid proliferation of the sites and targets of intervention. Outpatient clinics and office-based practices developed quite rapidly in the early years of the century, as the profession defined and refined new syndromes requiring its services. Whole realms of "functional" nervous disorders were "discovered" and efforts made to invest them with a respectable status as genuine disease entities. With characteristic symptoms as varied as "sick headache, noises in the ear, atonic voice, deficient mental control, bad dreams, insomnia, nervous dyspepsia, heaviness of loin and limb, flushing and fidgetiness, palpitations, vague pains and flying neuralgia, spinal irritation, uterine irritability, impotence, hopelessness, and such morbid fears as claustrophobia and dread of contamination" (Sicherman 1977), the newly defined neuroses promised psychiatrists a large and varied clientele.

The invention of the neuroses was soon followed by a widening series of interventions in the psychiatric management of domestic life. The advent of psychoanalysis, at first merely one among several competing forms of psychotherapeutics with which the profession experimented (Scull 1981b: 21–23; Caplan 1998), greatly facilitated these developments.[13] Not without its drawbacks – the expense and time-consuming nature of the therapy in its fully elaborate, near interminable form; its lack of correspondence with what ordinarily passed for scientific medicine (and thus its tendency to exacerbate the divisions between psychiatry and the larger profession to whose coat-tails it so desperately clung); and its dubious efficacy (though given the gullibility and desperation of the clientele, and the difficulty of obtaining a clear-cut measure of success or failure, this was very likely the least of its problems) – psychoanalysis nonetheless offered a more than compensating set of advantages.

To begin with, it had the great merit of being non-testable, and hence non-refutable; and, like Marxism, it lent itself to simplification for the simple and sophistication for the sophisticated. Requiring prolonged and costly training, it developed in its devotees a presumptive expertise which readily justified the rejection of outside, non-professional interference – a dogma which even provided an "explanation" of why such "irrational" resistance to its method should arise in the first place (thus discrediting its critics while protecting itself from the dangerous task of actually having to supply answers to the objections they might raise). It provided an elaborate technology of treatment, "certain definite methods of procedure of a rational sort" (Hale 1971: 48), which could underpin and give substance to an office-based practice; a psychotherapeutics which its practitioners solemnly compared to "a surgical operation of the most delicate sort" (Putnam 1908: 411). ("[The analysis] of subconscious memories," James Jackson Putnam (1908: 411) proclaimed, was "the major surgery of neurological therapeutics.") Perhaps most important of all, psychoanalysis "made sense" of a whole range of phenomena previously left outside the realm of systematic observation, and in the process created "understandable order out of chaos" (Hale 1971: 48) – an ideological accomplishment of extraordinary significance and power. For madness is fundamentally behavior too unintelligible to be accorded the status of human action (Coulter 1973; Morgan 1975; Ingleby 1982, 1985); and psychoanalysis now provided plausible accounts, constructible only by experts, which replaced commonsense judgments that something was "irrational," literally did not make sense, with interpretations that were at once remarkably systematic, symbolically highly elaborated, and – once its premises were granted – both plausible and internally coherent.

Traditionally a profession structurally hamstrung by the extraordinary weakness of its claims to possess special knowledge and capacities, and thus compelled to hold on tightly to the reassuring social power that derived from its autocratic control over asylumdom, psychiatry in the second and third decades of the twentieth century now ventured forth to capture an ever wider sphere for its ministrations and interventions. The psychiatric casualties of war (Stone 1985a), the management of infancy and childhood (and particularly of delinquent childhood) (Ingleby 1973; Rose 1985: 197–209; Horn 1989), alcoholism and other forms of intemperance and excess (Conrad and Schneider (1980)), marital disharmony and divorce (Donzelot 1977; Lasch 1977), the alienation of the industrial workforce (Stone 1985b), the translation of these and other moral problems and disturbances not readily susceptible to legal sanctions and intervention into technical, medicalized conditions provided psychiatry with a greatly expanded territory within which to practice (Stone 1985b). A widening array of forms of deviance was thus systematized within an orderly framework, and in reducing them to a medical paradigm, an attempt was made to reconstitute them as conditions "completely emptied of moral significance" (Zola 1972; Ingleby 1983: 162).

Helpless, hopeless, and highly stigmatized, the institutionalized population that presumably remained at the core of psychiatry's claims to expertise proved an increasing embarrassment, one which the more "progressive" segments of the profession were anxious to leave behind. The suffocating constraints and frustrations of attempting to cope with the recalcitrant, increasingly senile occupants of the mental hospital (Goldhamer and Marshall 1953; Grob 1983: ch. 7) stood in ever starker contrast with the attractions of new worlds to conquer. A paroxysm of experimentation among institutional psychiatrists with various forms of physical therapy – surgical evisceration (Scull 1987, 2005) malaria and other forms of fever therapy, metrazol-induced seizures, insulin comas, electroshock treatment, and crude surgical assaults on the brain itself (Grob 1983: 291–308; Pressman 1986; Valenstein 1986) – provided no relief, indeed, may well have contributed its quota to the dilapidated denizens of the back-wards. And the upshot was the desertion of the professional elite, followed by a decisive shift in the profession's center of gravity away from the dismal, despised, and depressing institutional sector.[14]

The marginalization of the seriously deranged as targets of professional intervention and concern, and the attempted reconceptualization of a variety of other social problems as medical conditions in need of treatment, were thus symbiotic processes which marked a crucial transition in the development of the psychiatric profession (Abbott 1988: 280–314). What is generally termed the rise of the therapeutic state constituted a potentially massive expansion of psychiatry's role in the processes of social control, particularly since the

> thrust of the expansion of the application of medical labels has been toward addressing (and controlling) the *serious* forms of deviance, leaving to the other institutions [traditionally involved in social control, law and medicine,] a residue of essentially trivial and narrowly defined technical offenses.
>
> (Freidson 1970: 249, emphasis in the original)

Under the appealing banner of *parens patriae*, the profession laid claim to the right to intervene in an ever-widening range of spheres of social life, defining for others what was in their own best interests, and offering the benign reassurance that, like a good substitute parent, psychiatry always had benevolence and rationality on its side.

But the invention and embrace of psychotherapeutic treatment techniques and of psychodynamic accounts of functional "mental illness," vital as they were as weapons in the struggle for professional jurisdiction, were not unproblematic in their implications. Most seriously, of course, there was the question of why a branch of the medical profession was uniquely qualified (indeed, qualified at all) to diagnose and treat, if the etiology and therapeutics of these conditions were primarily *psychological*.[15] Unsurprisingly, a number of different professional disciplines – most notably clinical psychology and social work – now emerged to invade psychiatry's turf and, at least temporarily, to contest its dominance.[16]

The contest, however, rapidly proved to be one-sided. Psychologists and social workers largely lacked independent control of the institutions within which they worked. Their bureaucratic subordination to psychiatrists in such settings as outpatient and child guidance clinics (even though the psychiatrist-director often attended the clinic only part-time) (Abbott 1988: 307) limited their autonomy from one direction. Their aspirations to independence were further thwarted by medical monopolization of the psychoanalytical training institutes, an organizational source of domination which was of great strategic value given the insistence within psychoanalysis on the centrality of training analyses for the therapists themselves (Abbott 1988: 307–308). Social work, in particular, lacked any independent intellectual basis for its claims to jurisdiction and quickly surrendered any aspirations to autonomy, its subordination overtly acknowledged with the adoption of the term *psychiatric* social work.[17] Psychology gained somewhat more leeway from its independent control over the technology of mental testing (Stone 1985b), but despite the usefulness of these techniques to corporations and in schools, they provided the basis for only a limited degree of separate authority. Necessarily, therefore, psychologists for the most part also submitted to a submissive relationship with their medical rivals,[18] and, notwithstanding occasional outbreaks of "fratricidal strife . . . , a practical division of labour was established within the psychiatric units, hospitals and clinics" (Rose 1986: 79). (Jurisdictional settlements of this sort were made easier by the fact that psychiatry, lacking the manpower to service the expanding territory it laid claim to, had room to cede the marginal and less desirable portions to subordinate groups of specialists.) One suspects that one source of the relatively unproblematic subordination that ensued was the predominantly feminized character of both social work and clinical psychology, for notwithstanding ideological proclamations about gender equality, the fundamentally unequal place of the two sexes in the workplace remains, not totally impervious, yet still remarkably resistant to change.

In the years since the Second World War, psychiatry has thus been able to view with relative detachment the sharp curtailment (though not quite the total demise) of the institutional sector that formerly constituted its heartland. The rapid run-down of mental hospital populations, the de-institutionalization of even the chronically crazy, has simply marked a further step in the profession's retreat from socially contaminating contact with an impoverished and clinically hopeless clientele. (On the scope and sources of the mental hospital's demise, see Scull 1984b.) The "miracles" of modern psychopharmacology – the phenothiazines, lithium, and the burgeoning variety of anti-depressants – clearly played a subordinate role in bringing about these mass discharges (Lerman 1982; Scull 1984b; Gronfein 1984). But, notwithstanding their far from miraculous therapeutic properties, for the profession they have been a virtually unmitigated blessing. (For patients, however, given the serious and often irreversible iatrogenic "side effects" the treatments produce, the picture is distinctly more mixed.) Psychiatric involvement with the unrewarding cases which used to throng mental hospital wards can now be reduced to the occasional prescription of psychoactive drugs, preferably to be dispensed by others – a thin veneer of continuing medical attention in which profession and public can nonetheless take comfort. On a wider canvas, alongside the psychotherapeutic techniques that first allowed the spread of its jurisdiction beyond the asylum, psychiatry now can proffer a new treatment technology, adaptable without strain to the general hospital, the outpatient clinic, and the private consulting room. And psychopharmacology is a form of treatment which is unambiguously and indisputably the monopoly of the medically trained, thus furnishing a decisive means of re-cementing the profession's jurisdictional claims to the value-free realm of medical science.

Pills have therefore replaced talk as the dominant response to disturbances of emotion, cognition, and behavior. Pharmaceutical corporations have underwritten the revolution, and have rushed to create and exploit a burgeoning market for an ever broader array of drugs aimed at treating some of the hundreds of "diseases" psychiatrists claim to be able to identify (Healy 1997). And patients and their families have learned to attribute their travails to biochemical disturbances, to faulty neurotransmitters, and to genetic defects, and to look to their doctors for the magic potions that will produce better living through chemistry. Spurred on by the neo-Kraepelinean revolution embodied in Diagnostic and Statistical Manual (DSM III) and its revisions, psychiatry has embraced a conceptualization of mental illnesses as specific, identifiably different diseases, each allegedly amenable to treatment with different drugs or "magic bullets," though the whole conceptual edifice rests upon the shakiest of foundations, and the treatments themselves remain decidedly less efficacious than the public relations flacks for the industry would have us believe. Meanwhile, at the level of language, both the profession of psychiatry and popular culture have become saturated with biological talk, though, as David Healy has wisely remarked, "it can reasonably be asked whether biological language offers more in the line of marketing copy than it offers in terms of clinical meaning" (Healy 1997: 5). Most certainly, though, psychopharmacology has reinforced the notion that the behavioral and emotional problems its weapons are trained upon are purely intra-individual and biological in character. They thus provide a neutral "scientific" justification and technique for the control of the wayward, one their relations (and very often the deviants themselves) embrace with avidity. For pills and a biological etiology reduce or eliminate problems of morality, guilt, and blame, and suggest the existence of technical remedies for life's troubles.

Herein lies, perhaps, one of the most powerful attractions of psychiatry as a form of social control. In rationalizing the maintenance of social order, it can claim, more plausibly than potential competitors, to a foundation "laid firmly on the ground of the natural sciences" (Mayer-Gross *et al.* 1960). In reality a moral enterprise, actively engaged in the creation and application of social meanings to particular segments of everyday life, it masked (and masks) the necessarily evaluative dimension of its activities behind a screen of scientific objectivity and neutrality. Moreover, its explanatory schema locates the source of the pathology it identifies in intra-individual forces, and in principle can allow the redefinition of all protest and deviation from the dominant social order in individualistic and pathological terms. It was and is, therefore, of great potential value in legitimizing and de-politicizing efforts to regulate social life and to keep the socially disruptive in line, the more so since, so far from appearing as merely a repressive or negative force, psychiatry can often direct its interventions at willing subjects, "those who have come to identify their own distress in psychiatric terms, believe that psychiatric expertise will help them, and are thankful for the attention they receive" (Rose 1986: 83). Perhaps, when all is said and done, the power to exercise social control is most effectively exercised when it does not appear to constitute punishment.

One final point is that in stressing the substantial expansion that has taken place in psychiatry's jurisdiction, and the even greater potential for intervention in daily life that is implicit in the therapeutic approach, I do not want to minimize the countervailing forces which have to some extent held these tendencies in check. Clearly, one source of difficulty for psychiatry and its allied professions has been the continuing intellectual vulnerability of their cognitive claims, and the practical deficiencies of the "remedies" on offer to consumers of its services. The opposite concern – the persistent disquiet aroused in many quarters on contemplating the implications of an approach which threatens to equate any deviation from conventional moral and social standards with illness, and to impose compulsory treatment – has also placed significant constraints on psychiatric expansionism. (The polemical assaults of such figures as Thomas Szasz and Nicholas Kittrie (1972) on the dangers of the therapeutic state are only the most recent manifestations of a long history of spasms of public anxiety on this score). Finally, psychiatry operates within a larger matrix of contending professions, each jealous of any attempt to seize portions of its jurisdiction. Lawyers, in particular, have a highly developed sense of turf, and the social power and cultural authority to offer a vigorous defense of their territory. Psychiatrists, pushing their deterministic universe of discourse to its limits, have on occasion been rash enough to extend their imperial claims to encompass all forms of criminality, threatening to substitute pathology for sin, determinism for free will, and treatment for punishment. Such efforts have tended to provoke sharply adversarial responses from the legal profession, whose traditional mandate to control crime has the advantage of being rooted in a commonsense schema wherein will or intention and the voluntary basis of action assume a central place. Discretion being the better part of valor, and neither principle of social regulation being capable of fully vanquishing the other, both professions have more usually adopted a policy of conceding each other's heartland, with jurisdictional disputes only occurring at the margin – where they generally take on a ritualized, if symbolically charged character.[19]

10 Psychiatric therapeutics and the historian

> The physical therapies have emphasized the essential unity of mind and body. The fact that mental illnesses are in a degree amenable to procedures easily comprehended by all as "treatment" goes far to establish the attitude that these are really illnesses like all others, and not incomprehensible reactions which split the victim away from the rest of mankind and from ordinary concepts of sickness and treatment.
>
> ("Through the Years – Pilgrim [State Hospital]," [*New York State*]
> *Mental Hygiene News* January 18, 1948: 8)

Any comprehensive approach to the history of psychiatry, as to the history of medicine more generally, must surely find a central place for the study of therapeutics. The translation of abstract knowledge into socially acceptable recipes for intervention and practical action to combat disease and debility lies at the very heart of the medical enterprise, and psychiatry forms no exception to this generalization, despite the administrative origins and preoccupations of the specialty for much of the nineteenth century. Like other forms of illness, mental disorders produce pain and suffering, debility and distress, and psychiatry's claims to dominion over its territory necessarily rest in part on its claim to possess unique and valuable specialized knowledge: expertise that extends not just to the diagnosis of mental disturbance, but far more significantly, skills and understanding that allow members of the profession to intervene and treat those who fall victim to its depredations or benefit from its ministrations.

The analytic centrality of therapeutics emerges most obviously from certain central features of the market for professional services. A modern profession's claim to occupational closure and to the associated jurisdiction over a particular territory rests upon a successful prior assertion of the claim that it possesses specialized expertise and knowledge. Intellectual and organizational dominance of some significant segment of the social division of labor, the cultural authority to shape and regulate discourse about specific areas of social concern, the occupation of a privileged status in the social hierarchy, all these accoutrements of professional standing depend upon the ability of the members of a particular occupational group to secure general acceptance of their pretensions to control a body of unique and valuable skills and knowledge: their ownership, to put it another way, of those sorts of cognitive and practical talents which render human problems susceptible to expert intervention and servicing.

To be sure, in the struggle for professional turf, other cognitive elements besides therapeutics may play an important role. As Andrew Abbott has forcibly argued is the case for professions as a whole, stable medical control over their jurisdiction, and the constitution and defense of the boundaries of that jurisdiction require the development of abstract and intellectually powerful systems of knowledge. "Only a knowledge system governed by abstractions can redefine its problems and tasks, defend them from interlopers, and seize new problems.... Abstraction enables survival in the competitive system of professions" (Abbott 1988: 9). Technical skill, absent in any significant degree of formalization, is necessarily associated with the much weaker form of craft knowledge. It is context-bound, too easily routinized, obvious rather than esoteric. Here is one important source of the insistent pressure to systematize medical knowledge, and a powerful motive for orthodox practitioners to attempt to stigmatize their competitors as quacks and mere "empirics."

On other occasions, it may prove possible to erect viable jurisdictional claims on a foundation of diagnostic refinement and prognostic precision, even when the course of the diseases themselves remains largely beyond the reach of treatment. This was largely the situation of late nineteenth and early twentieth-century neurology, for example, a narrowly academic but high-status specialty for whose practitioners diagnostic refinement went hand in hand with therapeutic impotence – causing some dissident elements (who began to flirt with psychotherapy for the legions of patients with "functional" nervous afflictions) to complain that their role threatened to "sink into the narrow niche of curator of the scleroses or an appraiser of teratological defects" (Dana 1913: 755; see Abbott 1988: 285–290; Scull 1981b: 17–23). By and large, however, the problems of disease and debility with which the medical profession must wrestle are associated with much pain and suffering, and the stoicism requisite to ensure that these are endured with philosophical resignation remains in rather short supply. Consequently, the difficulty all professionals potentially confront – the fact that, "with no effective treatments, abstractions are simply generalities without legitimacy" (Abbott 1988: 103) – is here felt with particular force.

I shall suggest that opening up the changing character of psychiatric therapeutics to serious historical scrutiny presents real challenges to historians of psychiatry. But it also provides us with a fascinating range of intellectual puzzles to explore; it forces us to broaden the range of sources we examine; and it compels us to integrate our consideration of developments within the comparatively isolated specialty that psychiatry remained for much of its history with the history of the larger medical enterprise. I am going to concentrate, in what I have to say here, on the history of *somatic* treatments for mental illness. I do not mean to imply, in doing so, that the history of psychological accounts and treatments for mental disorders is not a worthy enterprise, every bit as challenging as the exploration of more conventionally medical approaches – or that the interaction and often the clashes between the somatic and the psychological are anything but a crucial part of the story we need to tell. But the history of the psychological and the psychodynamic approaches introduces new areas of complexity and sectarian squabbles; and besides, in my own view psychiatry's metaphysical embrace of the body has been central to the medical identity of the specialty for most of its history. From the humoral accounts of the origins of mania and melancholia which underpinned medical claims to understand and treat mental illness in the eighteenth century to the recent declaration by the paymaster of American academic psychiatry, NIMH, that the 1990s mark "the decade of the brain," we have witnessed repeated attempts to link madness to disorders of the body – and, in parallel fashion, to develop somatic treatments for the presumed underlying pathology.

For all its importance and potential, however, it must be said that the history of the introduction and utilization of somatic treatments in psychiatry is still in its infancy. Perhaps this is less surprising when one recalls that among medical historians more generally, until very recent years, there has been a surprising dearth of serious research into the history of what doctors have actually done to and for patients. Most historians, as Charles Rosenberg (1979: 3) recently put it, "have always found therapeutics an awkward piece of business. On the whole, they have responded by ignoring it." Alternatively, and scarcely more satisfactorily, they have confined themselves to taking up the most readily available materials, the theoretical pronouncements in the published professional literature, to construct a portrait of progressive therapeutic enlightenment and progress – themselves seen in turn as the product of an essentially intellectual process through which traditional routines and treatments were gradually replaced by scientifically based therapeutics.

There have been encouraging signs, over the past decade and a half, that this unsatisfactory situation has begun to change. Rosenberg (1979) himself has provided us with a wonderfully subtle analysis of the traditional humoral therapeutics that dominated Western medicine for millennia – illuminating the "conspiracy to believe" that subsisted between doctor and patient, the elaborate system of belief and behavior through which a painful and (in our eyes) useless set of remedies came to constitute a tenacious therapeutics which repeatedly "confirmed the physician's ability to understand and intervene in the on-going physiological processes which defined health and disease." John Harley Warner (1980, 1986) has developed equally remarkable accounts of the decline of blood-letting and the processes of therapeutic change in the late nineteenth century. Martin Pernick's (1985) meticulous examination of the introduction of anesthesia has similarly reminded us of the social and cultural complexities that we must attend to if we want to grasp the often tortuous pathways through which technical innovations become part of the medical mainstream. And for the early years of our own century, Joel Howell's (1995) examination of the beginnings of modern medicine's more broadly based love affair with technology have given us an invaluable perspective on the influence of the laboratory and the machine on the practice of clinical medicine – a body of work (forgive the pun) that I shall draw on in the latter stages of this paper.

One of the central messages of this emerging scholarship has surely been the foolishness of the old distinction between external and internal approaches to the history of medicine and, by extension, of psychiatry. The explosion of interest in our subject over the past quarter century has been marked, of course, by the invasion of the history of psychiatry by social historians, a development some have regarded as by no means an unmixed blessing. Relations between the historically trained and the clinically qualified have often been tense if not openly hostile, with both sides on occasion resorting to name-calling and demonization. (The tensions and the name-calling have both manifested themselves in the pages of the new specialist journal in the field, *History of Psychiatry*, whose editors and editorial board are divided between eminent representatives of both camps.) Initially, too, the research agenda of the new generation of social historians pointed them away from a concern with the content of psychiatric knowledge to a concern with providing a critical re-examination, for example, of the origins and character of nineteenth-century lunacy reform and of the emerging empire of asylumdom; or toward an interest in the social processes associated with the emergence of psychiatry as a professional specialty. In recent years, however, whether from a dawning recognition of the seemingly obvious point that a profession cannot be divorced from its work and from the *content* of the knowledge it lays claim to, or from the growth of a more focused interest in the psychiatric patient and his or her fate, therapeutics has begun to attract the same sort of sustained attention among historians of psychiatry as among medical historians more generally.

In my view, this is a wholly salutary development. In my more optimistic moments, I wonder whether it may not also create the occasion for a rapprochement between the two often hostile groups of scholars who work on the history of psychiatry. For if there is one thing I am convinced of it is that the intertwining of the scientific and the social, present throughout our discipline, is so central when one considers the history of therapeutics that the historian ignores at his or her peril. That means for the social historian that there must be a genuine commitment to paying serious attention to the content and development of psychiatric knowledge; and for the psychiatrist-turned-historian an understanding that therapeutic change and the continued employment of particular treatments are dependent upon much more than purely intellectual processes.

There have already been some signs that this is something more than a pious and utopian pipedream.

Joel Braslow, for example, a young scholar trained in both psychiatry and in the tradecraft of the professional historian, has recently produced a fascinating series of papers dealing with the use of therapeutic sterilization on a massive scale in my own home state in the early twentieth century (Braslow 1996a), and with the impact of malaria therapy for tertiary syphilis in California State Hospitals in the 1920s, 1930s, and 1940s (Braslow 1996b). At the end of 1997, his broader examination of the impact of a whole range of innovative physical therapies (insulin shock therapy, metrazol, ECT, lobotomy) on doctors and patients in the California asylums appeared in a book from the University of California Press (Braslow 1997).

Braslow's study of the use of deliberately induced "fever" as a remedy for general paresis provides perhaps the best example of the virtues of his approach. The differential diagnosis of paresis, or general paralysis of the insane, had been one of the psychiatric profession's few genuine achievements in the nineteenth century, and in the first decade or so of the twentieth century, the long-nurtured suspicion that the appalling neurological and psychiatric consequences of this condition had their roots in a prior infection with syphilis were finally confirmed. Quite apart from the singular misery such a diagnosis heralded, paresis was of major concern because it afflicted so substantial a portion of psychiatry's core patient population, perhaps as many as 15 or 20 percent of male asylum admissions in the early twentieth century. Symbolically and practically, anything that offered the hope of arresting the dismal downward spiral of its victims would naturally be of surpassing importance, and it is perhaps no surprise that the inventor of what came to be regarded as a sovereign remedy for the condition should be hailed as a savior, and become the only member of the psychiatric profession to ever win a Nobel Prize for Medicine (Wagner von Jauregg 1946).

Julius Wagner von Jauregg, professor of psychiatry at the University of Vienna, had long been intrigued by the therapeutic possibilities of induced fever. Before the First World War, he had tried such dangerous tactics as injecting his patients with erysipelas to raise their temperatures. (Erysipelas, or St Anthony's Fire, is a bacterial infection usually caused by streptococcus pyogenes. It consists of a rapidly developing skin disorder accompanied by pain, fever, chills, and shivering, and can cause lymphatic damage. In a pre-antibiotic era, there was no effective treatment for the disease.) In 1917, however, a more attractive febrile agent came to his attention, when he came across a soldier suffering from tertian malaria. Though he had earlier touted fever therapy as a remedy for "melancholy, manic states, and acute mania," he now focused his attentions on tertiary syphilis and the psychiatric and neurological catastrophes that accompanied it.

Within a few years of the war's end, Wagner von Jauregg's fever treatment for neurosyphilis spread rapidly in North America and elsewhere. For a uniformly fatal disease usually associated with a steep physical decline and a particularly nasty end,[1] even a therapy that promised marginal improvements had obvious attractions.[2] Soon, hospitals were using paretics with malaria as a source of infected blood,[3] and the precious liquid was passed among them in thermos flasks sent through the mail.[4] Others began experimenting with alternative means of inducing fever, and seeking to explore whether febrile reactions might not cure other varieties of mental disturbance. Injections of colloidal calcium[5] or rat bite fever organisms (Illinois Department of Welfare 1927–1928: 12, 23, 1928–1929: 23) were tried on occasion, but such exotica were generally discarded in favor of "diathermy machines," sweat cabinets that artificially broke down the body's homeostatic mechanisms.[6] But though fever therapy continued to be endorsed by many clinicians as a last-ditch treatment for tertiary syphilis, there was a broad consensus that other forms of psychosis did not respond to this approach.

Braslow goes to great lengths to understand these practices in the light of the science of the time. At the same time, he puts on display in a very sophisticated fashion the complex social, cultural, and individual consequences of these technical changes, showing how malaria therapy, for example, separate from the controversial and perhaps ultimately unresolvable issue of whether it "worked" by the standards of our time rather than theirs, transformed psychiatrists' attitudes towards and treatment of paretics in ways that extended far beyond the specifics of the therapeutic encounter; and the attitudes of these patients and their families toward not just their disease, but also toward the mental hospital and the psychiatrists who treated them. Case records are used in a remarkably creative way to tease out the social matrix within which intervention took place, and the complex reverberations of a "biological" intervention into the socio-cultural realm. Before the introduction of fever therapy, the case records show that psychiatrists viewed their neurosyphilitic patients as "hopeless," "immoral," and "stupid" paretics – objects to be acted upon and people who were sinful and depraved. The introduction of Jauregg's new therapy brought a marked change: psychiatrists wrote and presumably reacted far more empathically and positively toward their patients, who were allowed to become active participants in their treatment. Patients with GPI, reciprocally, voluntarily sought admission to asylums they had previously shunned, and began to see the asylum as a place of treatment rather than confinement. Therapeutic innovation thus led to powerful shifts in the perceptions and behaviors of doctors and patients, demonstrating emphatically that therapies do more than simply address disease processes.

The late Jack Pressman's (1998) long-awaited book on lobotomy, which sadly was destined to appear posthumously after his untimely demise, likewise refuses the easy route of treating psychosurgery as a paradigmatic example of science gone awry. He insists that lobotomy must be understood without benefit of hindsight, and that looked at by the standards of the time, it was both good clinical medicine and "worked." Indeed, one of his central chapters is subtitled "Why lobotomy worked in 1949, and not now." More than that, he accords lobotomy an honored place in the creation of a more scientific, methodologically sophisticated psychiatry. He claims that it forced re-evaluations of what constituted adequate experimental method in mental health research and even "in significant ways [laid] the foundation for the upcoming era of psychopharmacology, which is generally taken to be the beginning of 'scientific' psychiatry."

Many of these are claims I consider overblown or would dispute in their entirety. There is more evidence, for example, than Pressman allows of informed contemporary scientific opposition to and criticism of the scientific credentials of lobotomy – private objections by Jacobson, whose experiments with Becky the chimp launched the lopping of thousands of frontal lobes, that his work was being distorted when used to justify psychosurgery; vigorous criticism from psychiatrists like William Alanson White; and even threats by John Fulton to visit physical violence on Walter Freeman when the latter introduced and sought to publicize the transorbital approach to damaging the frontal lobes. White, for example, wrote to his friend and colleague Smith Ely Jelliffe of an approach by Walter Freeman, who sought to undertake lobotomies at St Elizabeth's Hospital in Washington, DC:

> I am asked to subject my patients to this operation as a legitimate experiment in therapy. I do not very often trouble you with the various propositions that are handed up to me, but here is one which I would like to have you tell me what you think of in as few words as possible. I could express the whole matter in one word, but I do not want to do that because it would be unmailable.
>
> (White 1936)

Nor was all of this opposition private and behind closed doors. Well-informed and responsible psychiatrists forcibly denounced lobotomy in print and in public as a disastrous failure, even as others continued to view brain surgery as a valid form of therapeutics. For example, Jay Hoffman (1949), chief of the Veterans' Affairs Neuropsychiatric Service, concluded in the *New England Journal of Medicine* that

> the evaluation of the results after prefrontal leukotomy will be greatly influenced by the frame of reference one uses. If the condition of the patient is compared with his condition prior to the onset of his psychosis, all the results must be considered failures...I think it should be re-emphasized that by psychosurgery an organic brain-defect syndrome has been substituted for the psychoses.

Later the same year, addressing the American Psychiatric Association, Nolan Lewis, the director of the New York State Psychiatric Institute, mounted an even blunter set of criticisms. Referring to the so-called successful cases, he suggested his colleagues needed to rethink what they were accomplishing:

> Is the quieting of the patient a cure? Perhaps all it accomplishes is to make things more convenient for the people who have to nurse them.... The patients become rather childlike.... They act like they have been hit over the head with a club and are as dull as blazes.... It disturbs me to see the number of zombies that these operations turn out. I would guess

that lobotomies going on all over the world have caused more mental invalids than they've cured...I think it should be stopped before we dement too large a section of the population.

(Anonymous 1949)

On the other side of the coin, however, other psychiatrists in the same period were willing to countenance a whole series of aggressive assaults on their patients in an effort to disrupt what they saw as the otherwise inexorable tendency of psychosis to eventuate in chronic illness and ultimately dementia. The inventor of one of the shock therapies that enjoyed a considerable vogue in the 1930s and 1940s, Ladislas von Meduna (1938), spoke without apology of the need to use "brutal force" in the treatment of the mentally ill. His own chosen method employed injections of a synthetic form of camphor to elicit grand malseizures, and he acknowledged that his technique, like its rival, the induction of comas via injections of insulin could seem disconcerting to outsiders:

we act with both [insulin and metrazol] as with dynamite, endeavoring to blow asunder the pathological sequences and restore the diseased organism to normal functioning...we are undertaking a violent onslaught with either method we choose, because at present nothing less than such a shock to the organism is powerful enough to break the chain of noxious processes that leads to schizophrenia.

Still another enthusiast for the somatic treatments of this era, Charles Burlingame, who was superintendent of the elite Institute for Living in Hartford, Connecticut acknowledged that

Certainly it is true that the human system takes a terrific battering during the process of insulin shock. If it were not for the amnesia concerning these episodes it would be difficult to get anyone to submit willingly to the treatment...one cannot help wondering...what damage is possibly being done to parts of that body. Sufficient information is not yet available to answer that question.

(Burlingame 1938)

But for Burlingame, as for many institutional psychiatrists of his generation, such lacuna in their knowledge did not serve to curb their enthusiasm or diminish their willingness to employ experimental therapies. For a profession and a public desperate for some therapeutic purchase on the major psychoses, radical interventions were perceived as acceptable risks, given the alternative of confessing therapeutic bankruptcy and administering a custodial holding operation.

Beyond these contextual arguments for reassessing lobotomy's place in the history of psychiatric therapeutics, Pressman argues that psychosurgery played an important role in transforming research methodology in psychiatry. Previously, he contends, anecdotal recitals of clinical case histories had sufficed as evidence of therapeutic efficacy. It was lobotomies, cingulotomies, and topectomies – the whole panoply of operations on the frontal lobes – that decisively ushered in an era which saw the "replacing of a system of clinical evaluation based upon personal judgment with one of uniform scientific criteria" (Pressman 1998: 384). It was through discussions of the difficulties of rationally assessing the results of brain surgery, he contends, that "psychiatrists became aware of the critical need to reassess their basic methodologies, to become more sophisticated in reporting research results" (Pressman 1998: 387). At least indirectly, therefore, he suggests that the transformation of modern psychiatry into a scientific enterprise can be attributed to the romance with lobotomy. For it was lobotomy that "in significant ways [laid] the foundation for the upcoming era of psychopharmacology, which is generally taken to be the beginning of 'scientific' psychiatry."[7] Ironic as it may seem, then, in view of many younger historians' determination to distance themselves from a Whig interpretation of the past, "revisionist" judgments about lobotomy's history are here deployed in a manner that allows the reassimilation of what many have seen as a paradigmatic example of science gone awry to a narrative of progressive change.

I have to confess that I find this final line of argument both strained and unconvincing. The growth of the medical-industrial complex, the rationalization of medical research more broadly, and the massive entry of the federal government into the research enterprise were transforming the whole medical enterprise in the years after the Second World War, just as the advent of the National Science Foundation and the Cold War were transforming the scientific enterprise more broadly. I would want to see far more evidence than Pressman provides before I could be convinced that such critical innovations as double-blind methods and better research designs would not have entered the psychiatric research enterprise anyway.

But these are issues that lend themselves to resolution by conducting further empirical research, rather than by ideological argument. And regardless of how the debate is ultimately resolved, studies like these have begun to open up a host of previously overlooked issues. The plethora of new therapies that emerged in the 1920s, 1930s, and 1940s demands that we explore the question of the origins and spread of particular new therapies, both within a single country and across national boundaries. As Pressman has attempted to do for lobotomy, we need to ask ourselves how treatments acquire (and in some cases lose) acceptance in professional circles as efficacious (and efficacious for what conditions). What did previous generations (and do we) mean by "efficacy," or "science," come to that? And what kinds of source materials can we look for as we seek to develop our understanding – the papers and correspondence of both leading psychiatrists and the rank and file, to the extent that these survive; oral histories and interviews with participants on both sides of the equation, doctor and patient alike (a particularly urgent task given the length of time that has now elapsed since many of these interventions fell into oblivion); case records, which for all their limitations can open up a remarkable window on an apparently lost world, as well as allowing us to explore the actual use and implementation of these approaches in clinical settings, rather than relying upon the claims and asseverations made in the published professional literature; and contemporary literary and pictorial representations of psychiatric treatments, including training films prepared to demonstrate the uses of particular techniques.

We must go beyond these explorations, however, and begin to break down some of the isolation of psychiatric history from the broader history of medicine. For a key question must surely be to what extent innovations in psychiatric therapeutics reflect and borrow from broader changes in medical understanding of disease processes and therapeutics – for example, the impact of the bacteriological revolution and the rise of laboratory-based approaches in the medical mainstream; or changing standards and methodologies for assessing the value of particular therapeutic interventions. (I am thinking here of Harry Marks' (1997) pioneering examination of the origins and spread of double-blind clinical trials as the "gold standard" for assessing therapeutic innovations.)

Once we are committed to raising these kinds of issues, writing teleological history becomes much harder. I recall that one of the first books I read in the history of psychiatry was Zilboorg's (1941) *A History of Medical Psychology*, an ideological tract that looked at the historical record as a combination of a series of serendipitous anticipations of Freud and more frequent blundering down biological blind alleys. Quite recently, I encountered an equally one-sided, equally teleological global history of the subject, Edward Shorter's (1997; see also Ch. 7 of this book) text published by the Free Press. But Shorter, of course, turns Zilboorg upside down (or as he would doubtless put it, right side up); treats Freud and his epigones as the deaf and deluded; and lavishes praise on everything that anticipates the acme of enlightenment, modern biological psychiatry. Most relevantly for my argument here, when examining the history of psychiatric therapeutics, Shorter proves himself incapable of avoiding anachronistic judgments or of appreciating the complexity of the processes of therapeutic change.

I have already stressed the need to grasp psychiatric innovations in relation to broader developments in medicine as a whole, and to understand therapeutics in its contemporary context. I want in the next to last section of this chapter to return to these suggestions, both to demonstrate the gains in understanding that flow from breaking down the artificial barriers between the two, and to point up the kinds of problems Shorter's approach inevitably brings in its train. And I want to do this by removing the discussion from the general plane on which I have pitched it so far and instead to consider one particular therapeutic intervention in more detail.

I have written elsewhere about the influence of the doctrine of focal infection in both British and American psychiatry in the 1913s–1930s (Scull 1987, 2005; and Ch. 12 of this book). As advocated particularly by Henry Cotton in the United States, and Thomas Chivers Graves in Britain, the notion that psychosis was the product of lingering, chronic, and largely overlooked infections that poisoned the brain and central nervous system seems at once somewhat bizarre, and easily dismissed as an aberration – albeit one that persisted for decades and that licensed dubious and even deadly interventions on the bodies of thousands of helpless patients. Indeed, dismissing the activities of those who embraced focal sepsis as having nothing to teach us, as simply malpractice on a grand scale by marginal men of no importance then or now, is precisely the approach Edward Shorter adopts (Shorter 1997; see also Shorter 1996). The reality, I would argue, is much grimmer and less comforting, and at the same time much more tightly linked to the central ideas and institutions of early twentieth-century medicine.

Cotton's and Graves' adoption of focal infection theory and their use of this doctrine to underwrite a surgical assault on the "perils of pus infection" (as they were termed by Senator Royal Copeland, the leading medical agony aunt of his generation), constitute but a single chapter in a much broader story of psychiatric experimentation on the vulnerable bodies of a literally captive patient population. The extraction of teeth, the extirpation of tonsils, the excision of appendixes, of colons, stomachs, and uteri constituted their effort to rescue psychiatry from the stigmatized margins of medicine, to bring it into the new world of X-Ray machines, blood tests, bacteriology, and aseptic surgery, and to anoint their activities with the holy oil of modern medical science.

Those enamored of focal infection theory advanced with increasing aggressiveness the thesis that mental disorder was the product of auto-toxicity, caused in its turn by the presence in a variety of organs of chronic untreated reservoirs of infection. The hypothesis was by no means a novel one among psychiatrists. Henry Maudsley's (1867) *Physiology & Pathology of Mind*, written more than half a century earlier had claimed that:

> There is no want of evidence that organic morbid poisons bred in the organism or in the blood itself may act in the most baneful manner upon the supreme nervous centers. The earliest and mildest mental effect by which a perverted state of blood declares itself is not in the production of positive delusion or incoherence of thought, but in a modification of mental tone. The further effect is to engender a chronic delusion of some kind. A third effect of its more acute action is to produce more or less active delirium and general incoherence of thought.
>
> (Quoted in Graves 1923: 465)

Both Cotton and Graves, however, could and did invoke a far wider range of medical authority in support of their basic contention that "clinically an important relationship can be demonstrated to exist between prolonged emotional disturbance and chronic septic processes, occurring in hard tissues, especially in connection with the jaws." (Graves 1923: 471). Indeed, in the context of the times their theories were anything but eccentric. The late nineteenth and early twentieth century was an era dominated by bacteriological models of disease. Though the medical profession had initially greeted the claims of Lister and Pasteur with skepticism and ridicule, its entrenched conservatism rapidly gave way in the face of the powerful practical advances that flowed from their work: gains in both etiological understanding and in therapeutic efficacy. In surgery, antisepsis (and the routine employment of anesthesia) prompted rapid advances in the technical capacities of surgeons, and equally striking therapeutic gains. For a variety of acute and life-threatening diseases, similarly remarkable breakthroughs occurred within a short time. Within a five-year period, the typhoid bacillus, the plasmodia parasites that cause malaria, the tubercle bacillus, cholera vibrio, and diphtheria bacillus were all identified in the laboratory, and with the development of antiserums for diphtheria and tetanus, the medical outlook seemed completely transformed. General medicine's prestige (and the prospects of its practitioners) soared, along with expectations that medical science would soon extend its dominion over yet wider realms of disease and debility.

Yet a number of chronic, debilitating disorders – and not just those that pre-occupied psychiatrists – remained frustratingly recalcitrant in the face of every attempt to unravel their secrets. Even effective palliative therapies were in short supply, while the etiology of these diseases remained speculative at best. Succumbing to the temptation to extend the reach of the bacteriological paradigm, however, a number of leading medical men on both sides of the Atlantic turned to the notion of focal sepsis for an explanation, suggesting that such chronic diseases as arthritis, rheumatic fever, nephritis, and degenerative diseases of the arteries "might be caused by bacteria disseminated through the lymph or blood-streams from a hidden primary focus of infection" (Billings 1914, 1916; Barker 1920).

Among the most prominent medical advocates of the wide-ranging significance of focal sepsis was Frank Billings, the dean of the School of Medicine from the amalgamation of Rush Medical College and the University of Chicago in 1901 through 1924, President of the AMA in 1902, and of the Association of American Physicians four years later. Throughout most of this period, with Billings' enthusiastic leadership, much of the research and clinical care at the school and its affiliated hospitals and institutes was devoted to the pursuit of focal sepsis.

Billings' own pronouncements sound no different from those of Cotton and Graves. In his Lane Lectures, delivered at Stanford Medical School in September 1915, he urged his listeners "to make sure that all sources of focal infection have been obliterated" (Billings 1916: 144). He warned darkly that "The existence of focal infection of the jaws . . . without the manifestation of much discomfort is remarkable . . . often not discoverable by inspection and escapes the attention of the physician and dentist. Properly made Röntgen ray films of the jaws will enable one to recognize the real morbid and anatomical condition" (Billings 1916: 130). Intervention must then be ruthless and thorough-going: "Deplorable as the loss of teeth may be, that misfortune is justified if it is necessary to obliterate the infectious focus which is a continued menace to the general health." (Billings 1916: 131) "Too often," he continued, "the tonsillar tissue in children and also in some adults is a culture medium of pathogenic bacteria and as such is a constant source of danger as a portal of entry of infectious bacteria through the lymph and blood streams to the tissues of the body" (Billings 1916: 128–129). Again, since "infected tonsils cannot be successfully sterilized by any known method of treatment...entire removal is the only safe procedure" (Billings 1916: 129). Moving down the digestive tract, intestinal stasis "should have proper medical management or, if necessary, surgical treatment...[and] the focal acute and chronic infections of the pelvic organs of woman...should be rationally managed and surgically treated when necessary to safeguard health and life" (Billings 1916: 132–133).

Nor were such beliefs the peculiar province of the medical elite of the Windy City. Similar views were held in the bastions of early twentieth century scientific medicine at the Mayo Clinic, for example, where Edward Rosenow had brought the doctrine with him from Chicago; and at Johns Hopkins, where the sainted Osler's successor as professor of medicine, Llewellys Barker, became a prominent and vocal proponent of focal infection theory. Across the Atlantic, too, leading figures in British medicine and surgery hastened to add their voices to the chorus, invoking Lord Lister and calling repeatedly for the development of a "surgical bacteriology." After Cotton and Graves had spoken at the 1923 meeting of the Medico-Psychological Association in Edinburgh, Sir Frederick Mott, the eminent pathologist of London's mental hospitals, rose to offer extravagant praise for their accomplishments, and Sir George Robertson, President of the MPA, lent his weight to the cause, terming Cotton's work on focal sepsis a scientific breakthrough that "should have served to draw members back from the alluring and tempting pastures of psychogenesis back to the narrower, steeper, more rugged and arduous, yet straighter paths, of general medicine" (Anonymous 1923). Again in 1927, after Cotton and Graves and many of their supporters had spoken at length at a joint meeting of the MPA and the mental diseases section of the BMA, Sir Berkeley Moynihan (1927) the then President of the Royal College of Surgeons, added his own fulsome endorsement of their work, which had "set us a new standard of inquiry in this branch of medicine." As for the connection between focal sepsis and disease more generally, he was convinced that the discovery of this link was "the most illuminating thing that had happened in medicine in the twentieth century."

Joel Howell's book on the impact of technology on early twentieth-century medicine suggests that these remarks by leading physicians and surgeons were not just idle theoretical pronouncements. I want to emphasize one very remarkable set of statistics that emerged from his study of the clinical records of the New York and Pennsylvania Hospitals: numbers that suggest the growing importance of surgery in making the hospital central to twentieth century medical practice; and that simultaneously reveal the penetration of the ideas associated with the doctrine of focal infection into the center of routine medical practice. At the Pennsylvania Hospital, the number of operations rose from 870 in 1900 to 4,180 twenty five years later, and the increase in surgery followed a similar pattern in New York. As for the nature of these operations, I would like to remind you of another remarkable finding that is, 0.52 percent of the surgery at the Pennsylvania Hospital in 1900 was for diseases of the tonsils, and 19.02 percent in 1920; 2.09 percent of surgery at the New York Hospital was performed on tonsils in 1900, and 25.51 percent in 1925 (Howell 1995: 60–65).

These statistics make clear that the ruthless pursuit and elimination of sepsis extended well beyond the bounds of psychiatry. Cotton's and Graves' activities were unusual in part because they persisted so long, and in part because the captive audience these doctors treated found themselves the beneficiaries of so remarkably broad and thorough-going assault on "the perils of pus infection." I hope I have said enough, however, to dispel the comforting illusion that Graves' and Cotton's work can be dismissed as some sort of weird aberration from the normal march of scientific progress, a gothic tale wholly disconnected from the medical mainstream; and to demonstrate the range of issues that surface when we turn our attention to what it is that psychiatrists and other doctors actually do to and for their patients.

For many people, patients and practitioners alike, such episodes can be explained away as part of the realm of pre-history, psychiatric dark ages that predates the emergence of modern biological psychiatry. Surely no one can doubt that we have moved far away from an era of surgical evisceration, of producing grand malconvulsions via injections of chemicals, or of deliberately damaging the brain's frontal lobes. Psychiatry, at least within the universe of the medical schools, has increasingly hitched its star to the high tech, high-status world of neuroscience, and clinically it has embraced an array of medications that allow its routine practices to approximate more closely those characteristic of mainstream medicine. In all sorts of ways and within the space of scarcely a half century, we seem to have decisively left behind the world of Victorian and post-Victorian loony bins and the therapeutics they produced.

And so, in some senses, we have. For the advent of the psychopharmacological age, conventionally dated from the introduction of Thorazine to the marketplace in 1954, has without question revolutionized psychiatric practice, transformed the profession itself, and underwritten a reassessment of the very categories through which we think about and approach mental illness – to say nothing of proving stunningly profitable for multinational pharmaceutical corporations. Many, both within and outside the ranks of organized psychiatry, have credited (or blamed) the phenothiazines for the emptying of mental hospitals and the advent of so-called community-based mental health services. Regardless of the accuracy of this assessment (and I shall suggest later that there are reasons to be skeptical of such claims), the historiography of psychiatric therapeutics must most certainly come to terms with this series of developments. And fortunately, it has begun to do so.

Early work on the pharmacological revolution, while moderately useful, suffered from some severe limitations. Judith Swazey's account of the introduction of the phenothiazines into American psychiatry, for instance, the first systematic attempt to survey the territory, blatantly embraced the "science as progress" motif (Swazey 1974). Read carefully, her account hints at the scientifically shoddy basis on which the "pharmacological revolution" in psychiatry was based, and the high pressure sales techniques by which pharmaceutical houses promoted its spread; but the book's primary intent is clearly a celebratory one. In the process, not only is the complexity of the process of therapeutic change slighted, but vitally important issues never receive the attention they deserve.[8]

Chlorpromazine (marketed in North America as Thorazine and in Europe as Largactil), originated from research seeking "an anesthetic potentiator" and much of the early testing of the drug was done with this use in mind (Swazey 1974: 9). By 1953, efforts to find a commercial use for this compound had been extended to include attempts to demonstrate its value as an anti-emetic, as a treatment for itching, as a general sedative, and as a help in dramatic and acute psychosis. An internal memorandum in the files of Smith, Kline and French (who were to market the drug in North America), dated April 8, 1953, indicates that "nausea and vomiting are still felt to be the most appropriate indications on which to conduct rapid clinical testing to try to get marketing clearance by the F.D.A. [Food and Drug Administration]" (Quoted in Swazey 1974: 179). Reflecting this emphasis, by the end of 1953, a mere 5 months before it was to be marketed, chlorpromazine had been tested on only 104 psychiatric patients in the North America (Swazey 1974: 195). Thirteen months later, it was being given to an estimated *two million* patients in the United States alone; and by 1970, US pharmaceutical manufacturers sold $500 million of "psychotropic agents" – of which the phenothiazines accounted for $116,500,000. A major proportion of Smith, Kline and French's growth, from net sales of $53 million in 1953 to $347 million in 1970, was directly or indirectly attributable to this enormously profitable product (Baiter and Levine 1969; Swazey 1974: 160–161, 202). The rapid commercial exploitation of this new drug by the medical-industrial complex thus ought to figure centrally in any serious examination of the pharmacological revolution in psychiatry (Healy 1990).

What of the science on which these massive early sales were based? Remarkably few of the early studies of chlorpromazine met even the minimal current criteria of a scientifically acceptable research design. To a limited extent, this reflected the underdevelopment of techniques for controlling experimental bias during the early 1950s, but many early studies failed to use what controls were available and used in other medical research; and long after a consensus emerged on "the double-blind, placebo-controlled method as virtually a *sine qua non* of clinical drug research," tests continued to be conducted, and claims of the drug's 'efficacy' supported, on the basis of nonblind and single-blind designs (Clarke 1957; Sainz *et al.* 1957; Leveton 1958; Glick and Margolis 1962). Lack of methodological rigor was apparent in all aspects of the testing program. Sample sizes were frequently very small – occasionally just a single patient – and sometimes the number of patients treated was not even noted. Reviewing 61 of these early studies, Bryant and his co-workers found that such potential sources of bias as "differential treatment of experimental subjects, previous and concomitant therapy experience, and duration of illness" were seldom considered or controlled, while long-term follow-up studies were entirely absent. "An adequate description of the method used to rate patients' improvement was lacking in many of the reports and reliability of the ratings was likewise neglected" (Byrant *et al.* 1956).[9] Subsequent careful reviews of the relevant literature have demonstrated, scarcely surprisingly, that "uncontrolled studies [of this type] gave a *systematically* more positive evaluation of drug effect than controlled studies" (Fox 1961; Glick and Margolis 1962; Gittleman *et al.* 1964; Davis 1965, who note "the prevalence of generally faulty research designs").

The relationship between the introduction of the phenothiazines and the decline in mental hospital populations is a very complex matter, and the connections are far more intricate and surprising than the conventional wisdom would suggest. I first attempted to examine this matter systematically, in a broad-ranging critique of the failures of deinstitutionalization that appeared as long ago as 1976 (Scull 1976, 1977). Based upon my review of the historical record, I advanced the then-controversial position that the drugs' role in the run-down of hospital census was secondary, indirect, and far less significant than was generally assumed to be the case; and that deinstitutionalization was more importantly the result of other changes in governmental policy. A series of other studies since that time have confirmed the essential correctness of that assessment. (For an early psychiatric skeptic, see Lewis 1959; see more generally Aviram and Cohen 1976; Aviram *et al.* 1976; Segal and Aviram 1978; Smith and Hanham 1981; Lerman 1982; Gronfein 1985a,b; Grob 1991: 264–272.)

Nor have the anti-psychotic drugs proved an unmixed blessing for those taking them. The first published reports of serious side-effects, oro-buccal dyskinesia, appeared in the scientific literature in 1957,[10] but drew little attention for more than a decade. The profession's defenders have suggested that delays of this sort reflected the fact that it took approximately that "length of time for enough clear-cut cases of tardive dyskinesia to develop" (Merskey 1994: 391). It is hard to take such suggestions seriously.

In the first place, it is not at all clear that it took anything like a decade for a sufficient number of cases to develop (as opposed to be recognized by the profession for what they were). Clinicians in the 1960s and early 1970s reported that the time lapse between the administration of neuroleptics and the appearance of symptoms of tardive dyskinesia could be as brief as three months in a handful of cases, although in a large fraction of the patient population, the disorder took between one and three years to surface (Crane 1968, 1973b).[11] Given the massive numbers of patients being treated long-term on neuroleptics, the severity of the symptoms in many cases,[12] and a prevalence of tardive dyskinesia among chronic neuroleptic users estimated as falling between 13 percent and 56 percent (e.g. Tepper and Haas 1979, who found a range of 24–56 percent; and Woerner *et al.* 1991, who found a range of 13.3–36.1 percent), Merskey's claim that there simply weren't enough cases surfacing to alert the profession about the problem until a decade had passed strikes me as grossly implausible.

In any event, such counter-arguments founder on a far more serious obstacle. For the available evidence suggests that a very large proportion of the profession ignored these side-effects, or minimized them, not for 10 years, but for more than 20. (There are obvious parallels here with the recent allegations that the pharmaceutical companies have suppressed evidence of the dangers of antidepressants and – outside psychiatry – such drugs as Vioxx and other Cox-2 selective inhibitors.) In an authoritative review of the status of "clinical psychopharmacology in its twentieth year," published in *Science* the director of research at a Maryland State Hospital, attributed part of the problem to the difficulties psychiatrists faced in the wake of state-sponsored programs of deinstitutionalization:

> Inadequate programs for the management of [patients released from hospitals] have created new and unexpected problems, and, in an effort to solve them, the psychiatric community has become more and more dependent on the use of neuroleptic agents. One of the consequences of this reliance on psychopharmacology has been the tendency to minimize the potential danger of long-term exposure to powerful chemical agents. Thus permanent neurological disorders have become very common among patients treated with neuroleptics, but little effort has been made to come to grips with this problem.[13]

Remarkably, despite the publication of "more than 100 papers reporting 2000 cases of 'tardive dyskinesia' in the scientific literature, and despite the fact that diagnosis offers no major difficulties...[in 1973] the majority of clinicians continue to ignore the existence of this problem...or seem to be completely unconcerned about it." Equally strikingly, "So far little effort has been made to carry out the necessary long-term studies on the onset and evolution of neurological and other cumulative effects of drugs." What we had observed during the first twenty years that phenothiazines had been used, Crane concludes, was "the neglect of a serious health problem by practising psychiatrists – a neglect which 'has deeper roots than mere ignorance of facts'."

None of these drawbacks has seriously slowed the shift back to a biologically reductionist model of mental illness over the past three decades, or diminished the growing influence of the pharmaceutical industry. For better or worse, we now live in a psychopharmacological age. Prozac and Valium. Thorazine and

Zoloft, and a host of other psychoactive substances are daily ingested by millions, and have made fortunes for those creating and peddling them to an ever expanding market of eager (and sometimes not-so-eager) consumers. Since 1980, when the American Psychiatric Association promulgated the third edition of its DSM III, American psychiatry has achieved worldwide hegemony, and pills have replaced talk as the dominant response to disturbances of emotion, cognition, and behavior. Pharmaceutical corporations have underwritten the revolution, and have rushed to create and exploit a burgeoning market for an ever broader array of drugs aimed at treating some of the hundreds of "diseases" psychiatrists claim to be able to identify.[14] And patients and their families have learned to attribute their travails to biochemical disturbances, to faulty neurotransmitters, and to genetic defects, and to look to their doctors for the magic potions that will produce better living through chemistry.

Here is a vast territory that as yet has only begun to attract serious scholarly attention. Once again, the best of that recent work refuses to accept the traditional divide between social historians and clinician historians, or to examine the social and the scientific in isolation from one another. The work of David Healy, in particular, has provided us with a wide-ranging and searching examination of large portions of the terrain, a provocative synthesis that should and undoubtedly will serve as an example and a stimulus for others. His book on *The Antidepressant Era* provides a wide-ranging assessment of developments in the field since the first application of chlorpromazine to the treatment of psychosis in 1951, though, as his title suggests, focusing most centrally on the emergence of drug treatments for depression. He brings to the task a background as secretary of the British Association for Psychopharmacology, but also as a researcher into cognitive therapy. He has, besides, read widely in the relevant historical and sociological literature, and approaches the subject with a skeptical and sophisticated eye. Naïve cheerleaders for a biologically reductionist view of mental disorder may read Healy's history as an endorsement of their blinkered viewpoint (and indeed, one of their number, Edward Shorter, provides a remarkably enthusiastic encomium on the book's dust-jacket); but in reality, Healy's subtle and probing examination provides as little comfort for such a position as for those who dismiss the drugs as universally useless or actively harmful weapons of a "toxic psychiatry" now loosed upon the land (cf. Breggin 1991).

Healy is, as he confesses at the outset of his book, "by nature...an enthusiast." His book, however, is a skeptical one, "skeptical of the motives of clinicians as well as the pharmaceutical industry, skeptical of both pharmacotherapists and psychotherapists" (Healy 1997: 3). He remains uncertain of whether the drugs work as well as they are supposed to do, and insists that "in many respects the discovery of the antidepressants has been the invention of and marketing of depression" – a once rare condition that has now been transformed by their entrepreneurial efforts into "the common cold of psychiatry" (Healy 1997: 5, 58). Spurred on by the neo-Kraepelinean revolution embodied in DSM III and its revisions, psychiatry has embraced a conceptualization of mental illnesses as specific, identifiably different diseases, each allegedly amenable to treatment with different drugs or "magic bullets," though the whole conceptual edifice rests upon the shakiest of foundations, and the treatments themselves are decidedly less efficacious than the public relations flacks for the industry would have us believe. Meanwhile, at the level of language, both the profession of psychiatry and popular culture have become saturated with biological talk, though "it can reasonably be asked whether biological language offers more in the line of marketing copy than it offers in terms of clinical meaning" (Healy 1997: 5).

Yet skepticism, as Healy insists, is not the same as cynicism, and though he resists a simple narrative of magic potions and medical breakthroughs, he is not blind to the way these drugs modify behavior, cognition, and emotion, often in ways that both sufferers and healers interpret as beneficial. *The Antidepressant Era*, in other words, is neither the work of an antipsychiatric ideologue, nor a celebratory tome. The very complexity of the argument it makes, and the nuances its author insists upon, are at once the book's great strength, and the elements that sometimes make it heavy going.

Healy attempts repeatedly to place developments in psychiatry within a broader historical and socio-political framework. He reviews, for example, the development in medicine as a whole of the notion of specific illnesses and specific remedies from being a perspective associated with quackery to the status of orthodoxy in the aftermath of the bacteriological revolution. Such a view of psychiatric troubles was advanced by Kraepelin in fin-de-siècle Germany, and then essentially submerged, especially in North America, where the growing dominance of psychoanalysis brought with it an increasing emphasis on mental health and illness as a continuum and an associated adherence to what he refers to as a dimensional view of mental disorder. One of Healy's most successful and interesting passages analyses the revival of neo-Kraepelinian ideas in the last quarter of the twentieth century, and their close ties to both the psychopharmacological revolution and the revision of psychiatric nosology and nomenclature over that same period. He has penetrating things to say about the intra-professional maneuvering and conflicts that marked this process, and its connections to the interests of the pharmaceutical industry and particular sectors of the profession, noting, for example, that these revolutionary changes emerged outside elite departments of psychiatry such as those at Yale and Harvard, where psychoanalysis was (temporarily) firmly in the saddle, and then transformed the entire field, with the emphasis on large, multi-site clinical trials tied to the exploration of the possible efficacy of novel drug therapies for individual disorders helping in turn to bring psychiatry everywhere under the hegemony of the Americans.

Equally impressive is Healy's dissection of the advent of random controlled trials (RCT) in the psychiatric arena. Again, local developments are firmly anchored in the larger context, but at the same time, the particular importance of this technology for psychiatry is emphasized, as are the conflicts and controversies that divided the profession, with both the personalities of those involved in the disputes, and the roots of the divisions in the structural location of the disputants nicely brought into the equation. Healy uses the fight over the now-discredited insulin coma therapy in 1953 to illustrate some of his central themes, pointing out how many heavyweights within the field reacted with outrage and venom to the suggestion that the treatment might be useless. The whole episode, he points out, should serve to remind us "just how open to bias the evaluation of psychiatric treatments is." Precisely because "in psychiatry more than in any branch of medicine, many of the end-points are either unclear or the subject of intense ideological division" (Healy 1997: 93) and because of the powerful role of the placebo in treatment (another topic treated with great insight), randomized, placebo-controlled, double-blind trials assume a particular importance in this context, as a control on the profession's repeatedly demonstrated susceptibility to often dangerous fads and enthusiasms. The convoluted path through which each element of the RTC entered the field is carefully anatomized, and the consequences, negative *and* positive, neatly laid bare.

Two crucial events lie at the heart of Healy's discussion: the central role of the Food and Drug Administration (FDA); and the radical restructuring of the epistemological world-view of American, and subsequently international, psychiatry that is embodied in DSM III and its revisions. The FDA's prominence, as he shows, dates back to the 1962 passage through Congress of the Kefauver–Harris drug amendments, in the aftermath of the Thalidomide tragedy. In the years since, "the FDA has come to occupy something of a magisterial role on the world stage" (Healy 1997: 100). The need to sell in the American market has ensured that its writ runs everywhere, and what has nominally been an institution charged with regulating an industry has in practice become the arbiter of what passes for scientific knowledge. The power of the FDA as gatekeeper has ensured the hegemony of the RCT. In turn, that methodology has encouraged a view of psychiatric illnesses as an array of specific, delimited diseases (as though depression, for instance, were akin to a bacterial infection), to be treated with individually targeted drugs.

The pressures thus created to adopt a division of mental illness into discrete disorders whose core symptoms reflected aberrant brain functioning were decisively reinforced with the promulgation of a new diagnostic classification in 1980, the product of work that had begun in 1973. Healy shows just how political the process of arriving at this new classificatory system was, and argues that "The creation of DSM-III was the Trojan horse by which [the neo-Kraepelinians] effected entry into the citadel of psychoanalysis"(Healy 1997: 233) – and the result, a document "whose concepts have yielded rich pickings for the pharmaceutical industry" (Healy 1997: 213). Subsequent revisions, growing to elephantine proportions, ironically show that "it is clearly a mistake to think that mental illnesses are something that have an established reality and that the role of a drug company is to find the key that fits a predetermined lock or the bullet that will hit an objective target"

(Healy 1997: 212). But this illusion is precisely what has been manufactured, and much of it by "astute marketing that extends right into the heart of academe itself" (Healy 1997: 213). Healy is not disposed to dispute that "there are clearly psychobiological inputs to many psychiatric disorders" (Healy 1997: 212), but he certainly *is* skeptical (and rightly so) of the notion that psychiatric science is now cutting Nature at the joints. In crucial respects, commerce rules:

> knowledge in psychopharmacology doesn't become knowledge unless it has a certain commercial value...[On a broader scale], it has become more and more difficult to distinguish between the marketing of scientific ideas and the marketing of psychotropic compounds. The selection of scientific ideas according to their coincidence with commercial interests is becoming an increasingly important factor in shaping the academic marketplace. Put another way, drug companies obviously make drugs, but less obviously they make views of illness.
>
> (Healy 1997: 176, 180–181)

Curiously, as Healy points out, pharmaceutical houses were slow to recognize the commercial possibilities of the market for mood-altering drugs. Through the 1970s, they were convinced, for example, that "the antihypertensive market was much larger and more important than the antidepressant market" (Healy 1997: 168). Once they realized their mistake, however, they reoriented their efforts with a vengeance, selling both profession and public on the seductive idea that defects in neurotransmission were at fault when people became depressed. Such perceptions have fueled an immense expansion of neuroscientific research, and a vast expansion of our knowledge of the basic functioning of the brain. Perversely, however, while "there has been astonishing progress in the neurosciences" there has, on the other hand, been "little or no progress in understanding depression" (Healy 1997: 174). Successive hypotheses about why antidepressive drugs might work have been undermined, and current evidence "points strongly to the fact that [depression] is simply not a single neurotransmitter disorder" (Healy 1997: 174), but "a complex disorder, whose management might require specifically non-specific treatments" (Healy 1997: 169). Wedded to the idea of specific treatments, and to targeting designer drugs at particular receptors or proteins, however, researchers have proclaimed an era of "rational drug development". Yet, "If anything the efficacy of psychotropic compounds stemming from this process seems to be falling off" (Healy 1997: 135).

Healy's book is replete with ambiguities and ironies of this sort. His text fizzes with provocative ideas, and reading it is calculated to unsettle the prejudices of both critics of and enthusiasts for contemporary psychiatry. As with the work of Pressman and Braslow, Healy's research reminds us of much we can learn from paying serious attention to the practical interventions psychiatrists make. We are all better off now that the traditional neglect of the history of psychiatric therapeutics has begun to be remedied.

11 "A Chance to Cut is a Chance to Cure"

Sexual surgery for psychosis in three nineteenth-century societies*

> In the sexual processes, we have the indispensable "organic foundation" without which a medical man can only feel ill at ease in the life of the psyche.
>
> > (Sigmund Freud to C.G. Jung, April 19, 1908.
> > Reprinted in *Freud-Jung Letters: The Correspondence
> > Between Sigmund Freud and C.G. Jung* (1974))

> Cures, like fish, do not grow any smaller by being talked about, and many wonderful stories shrink immensely when traced back to their original sources.
>
> > (Robert T. Edes, *Points in the Diagnosis and Treatment
> > of Some Obscure Common Neuroses* (1896))

> It is not our business, it is not in our power, to explain psychologically the origin and nature of any of [the] depraved instincts [manifested in typical cases of insanity]...it is sufficient to establish their existence as facts of observation, and to set forth the pathological conditions under which they are produced; they are facts of pathology, which should be observed and classified like other phenomena of disease.
>
> The explanation, when it comes, will come not from the mental, but from the physical side – from the study of the neurosis, not from the analysis of the psychosis.
>
> > (Henry Maudsley, *Responsibility in Mental Disease* (1874))

The medical therapeutics of mental disorder seem peculiarly susceptible to fads and fashions. Over the course of the past two centuries, new forms of treatment have emerged at regular intervals and their curative potential has been trumpeted loud and long, only for subsequent experience to demonstrate that the initial estimates of their value were wildly over-optimistic. At the same time, these treatments (particularly the somatic therapies) have been the subject of debate and controversy among laymen to an extent that is without parallel in almost all other areas of medicine.[1] Those who are inclined to defer meekly to medical expertise over the treatment of pneumonia, hepatitis, or measles, are far less likely to do so over the administration of electroshock

---

* Written with the assistance of Diane Favreau.

or the employment of brain surgery in the treatment of the psychotic. Nor is this in any sense a recent development. In what follows, we examine two earlier episodes in the history of somatic treatments for mental disorder. Both involve treatments directed exclusively at women. And both were originated not by psychiatrists (or to use the historically more correct term, alienists), but by other medical men, in this case gynecologists.

For nineteenth-century physicians, few facts were more incontestably established than that the female of the species was "the product and prisoner of her reproductive system" (Smith-Rosenberg and Rosenberg 1973: 334). Woman's place in society – her capacities, her roles, her behavior – was ineluctably linked to and controlled by the existence and functions of her uterus and ovaries. To the crises and periodicities of her reproductive organs could be traced all the peculiarities of her nature such as the predominance of the emotional over the rational, her capacity for affection and aptitude for child-rearing, her preference for the domestic sphere and her "natural" purity and moral sensibility. Her status as "a moral, a sexual, a germiferous, gestative, and parturient creature" (Meigs 1847: 5 quoted in Smith-Rosenberg and Rosenberg 1973: 334) thus rested firmly upon the findings of science, which repeatedly demonstrated that "the functions of the brain are so intimately connected with the uterine system, that the interruption of any one process which the latter has to perform in the human economy may implicate the former" (Burrows 1828: 146). Such "interruptions," of course, profoundly threatened women's health, and formed the physiological foundation of her greater delicacy and fragility. And given that the central mediating role between brain and generative organs was played by the nervous system, it was no wonder that perhaps the most fearsome threats that were thus presented were to the feminine hold on sanity. Not surprisingly, then "Victorian psychiatry defined its task with respect to women as the preservation of brain stability in the face of almost overwhelming physical odds" (Elaine Showalter 1985: 64).

Medical theorizing about the source of the "sympathetic connection existing between the brain and the uterus" (which was, so it was blithely asserted, to be "plainly seen by the most casual observer" (Blandford 1871: 69)) became more self-confident from the mid-century onwards. Through the researches of Marshall Hall, Thomas Laycock, and Johannes Müller, the largely circumstantial and inferential claims about the involvement of the sympathetic nervous system were replaced by more elaborate conceptions of reflex physiology grounded in experimental evidence (Hall 1837; Müller 1839–1842; Laycock 1840; Laycock 1876).[2] Presenting their findings in the more sophisticated vocabulary of "reflex irritability," medical men offered fresh confirmation of the heightened susceptibility to emotional disorder and mental disease produced by the unsettled character of the female reproductive economy. Puberty, pregnancy, parturition, lactation, menstruation, and the menopause, each added to the constant shock and strain on the bodily system, prompting in all too many cases, the shipwreck of the intellect, the collapse of the will, and the dissolution of all semblance of self-control.

While women were thus "the victim[s] of periodicity" which produced a variety of mental defects with "neither homologue nor analogue in man...." (Storer 1871: 78), they were not the only psychiatric casualties for whom anatomy was destiny. Obsessed by ideas of Morelian degeneracy and hereditary taint (Nye 1984; Dowbiggin 1985), Victorian alienists in the last third of the century adhered to an ever more pessimistic and rigidly somatic view of mental disorder. In the words of Henry Maudsley, the dominant English psychiatrist of the period "There is a destiny made for each one by his inheritance, he is the necessary organic consequent of certain organic antecedents; and it is impossible he should escape the tyranny of his organization" (Maudsley 1879: 88).

This rigid somaticism appeared to provide the bleakest prospects for therapeutic intervention, and the institutional treatment of the insane generally reflected the prevailing climate of hopelessness and despair. Supervising their "museums for the collection of insanity" (Scott 1879: 138), asylum superintendents subsided into a torpor barely distinguishable from that exhibited by their patients, "cursed," in Weir Mitchell's words, "by that slow atrophy of the energizing faculties which is the very malaria of asylum life" (Mitchell 1894: 430).[3] Increasingly, they redefined their task in more limited terms such as comfort, cleanliness, and freedom from the more obvious forms of physical mistreatment, rather than the elusive and often unattainable goal of cure.

Their sense of impotence in the face of the biological laws of degeneration makes comprehensible the pronounced therapeutic conservatism that characterized late nineteenth-century alienism. At the same time, it accentuated their vulnerability to criticism – which was not slow in coming from both within and beyond the medical profession. In particular, members of the newly emerging specialty of neurology, whose varied clientele included many a hysteric or neurasthene on the borderlands of insanity, were at once more willing to experiment with such therapies as electricity, massage, and the rest cure; and all too eager to portray asylum superintendents as bumbling incompetents, "experts at everything except the diagnosis, pathology, and treatment of insanity" (Spitzka 1878: 209).

Aggressive therapeutic intervention as part of a planned assault on insanity came not only from neurology, but from another new group of specialists, gynecologists. The doctrine of reflex insanity had found some of its earliest and most energetic advocates in their ranks.[4] And such advocacy was not confined to the theoretical realm when on two separate occasions, eminent gynecologists on both sides of the Atlantic played major roles in devising and implementing surgical treatments for mental disorder.

A surgical remedy for madness

The advance of gynecology as a medical specialty simultaneously produced and was dependent upon the increasing role of technology in the birth process and in approaches to the diseases of women's reproductive organs. At a period in which the bankruptcy of traditional heroic therapeutics was becoming increasingly visible, prompting many physicians to embrace therapeutic nihilism and many patients to desert allopathic medicine for homeopathy, Thomsonianism, and a variety of other sectarian competitors, it was on advances in surgical technique and practice that orthodox medicine's continued hold on the public perhaps most crucially rested. In gynecology, as in surgery more generally, these advances derived, in the last analysis, from two crucial developments: the use of anesthesia, beginning in the 1840s; and the acceptance in the last third of the century (though not without a struggle) of Lister's emphasis on anti-sepsis. Anesthesia and anti-sepsis, particularly in combination, made the routine employment[5] of invasive surgery possible for the first time, and allowed refinements of skills and capacities that constituted spectacular confirmation of medicine's claims to scientific legitimacy.

Among the gynecological operators of the 1850s, few were more enthusiastic and audacious than Isaac Baker Brown, whose technical skills (and willingness to risk his patients' lives) soon placed him in the forefront of the London medical elite. Elected a fellow of the Royal College of Surgeons in 1848, his operating theater soon became "one of the most attractive to the professional visitor in all London – admiration being invariably evoked by his brilliant dexterity and the power he displayed in the use of his left hand when operating on the female perineum" (*Lancet* 1873b: 223). The publication of *Surgical Diseases of Women* in 1854, and his major role in the foundation of St Mary's Hospital, marked further steps on his path to professional prominence, culminating in his election, in 1865, as President of the Medical Society of London.

In the early 1850s, Baker Brown became one of the first to use chloroform in midwifery and in obstetrical operations. He pioneered new techniques for repairing vaginal and rectal fistulae, and for dealing with the prolapsed uterus. And notwithstanding the deaths of his first three patients, he experimented enthusiastically with ovariotomy as a cure for "ovarian dropsy."[6] The predictable result of "his celebrity as an operator at once bold, ingenious, and successful" (*Lancet* 1873b: 223) was to bring him a steady influx of affluent and aristocratic patients, so that by 1858, he felt secure enough to withdraw from his association with St Mary's and to establish his own proprietary hospital, The London Home for Surgical Diseases of Women.

Like many of his colleagues "engaged in the treatment of the female genitals," Baker Brown had been repeatedly frustrated and foiled in those cases in which physical pathology was complicated "with hysterical and other nervous affections.... [Such women] defied my most carefully conceived efforts at relief" (Brown 1866: vi). Brown-Sequard's lectures on "The Physiology and Pathology of the Central Nervous System," published in the *Lancet* the same year the London House opened its doors, at last suggested a line of attack on these recalcitrant cases. In keeping with the contemporary doctrine of reflex irritability, the French physiologist had argued that damage to the central nervous system might be caused by over-excitement of the peripheral nerves. Baker Brown immediately saw the relevance to his own practice for the source of his patients' hysteria and nervous complaints must surely lie in a pernicious and all-but-unmentionable habit, "peripheral excitement of the pubic nerve" – or, to put it bluntly, female masturbation.[7]

In invoking masturbation as a cause of insanity, Baker Brown was scarcely advancing a novel hypothesis. Masturbatory insanity had been a staple of early nineteenth-century psychiatric texts,[8] and had acquired new credibility in many quarters through the growing emphasis on the importance of the conservation of energy. In other hands, this theory had already been invoked to justify a number of painful, or more accurately sadistic "remedies." Particularly popular was the "continual application of the strongest caustics to the seat of the irritation," in an effort to dissuade the patient from the filthy habit (Brown 1866: 10). Characteristically, however, Baker Brown scorned these sorts of half measures as wholly inadequate to "destroy such deep-seated nerve irritation" and proceeded at once to "a surgical test, by removing the cause of excitement," the woman's clitoris (Brown 1866: 10, vi).

This desperate remedy was justified, in Baker Brown's eyes, by the danger that nervous exhaustion posed to the whole system. Loss of nerve power as a result of masturbation was, he assured his readers, followed successively by hysteria, spinal irritation, hysterical epilepsy, cataleptic fits, epileptic fits, idiotcy [*sic*], mania, and finally death. And the record of his operative results between 1858 and 1866 proved that "the treatment must be the same whether we wish to cure functional disturbance, arrest organic *disease*, or, finally, if we have only a chance of averting death itself" (Brown 1866: 7–9).

Patients deemed suitable cases for treatment were operated upon immediately, pausing only to ensure that they had "been placed completely under the influence of chloroform" before "the clitoris is freely excised either by scissors or knife" (Brown 1866: 17, emphasis in the original). The results, according to Brown himself, were enormously gratifying, and within a month, "it is difficult for the uniformed, or nonmedical, to discover any trace of an operation" (Brown 1866: 18). Idiots, epileptics, hysterics, paralytics, the young and the old, all proved readily curable through surgical intervention. Even in cases of nymphomania, where "under medical treatment, of how short duration is but too frequently the benefit," success was all but guaranteed indeed, "in no case am I so certain of a permanent cure ... for I have never after my treatment seen a recurrence of the disease" (Brown 1866: 70). Yet others of his cases were women who sought to take advantage of new Divorce Act of 1857, usually diagnosed as suffering from "incipient mania." Case 48, for example, Mrs SM, had developed "a great distaste for her husband ... and [for] cohabitation with him. I pursued the usual surgical treatment, which was followed by uninterrupted success; and after two months' treatment, she returned to her husband, resumed cohabitation, and stated that all her distaste had disappeared; soon became pregnant, resumed her place at the head of her table, and became a happy and healthy wife and mother." The conclusion, he thought was obvious: that marital disharmony might typically be cured in such a fashion, obviating the need for "a judicial separation of husband and wife, with all the attendant domestic miseries" (Brown 1866: 84).

Despite, or perhaps because of, these vaunted successes, and notwithstanding its apparent conformity with some of the central assumptions of mid-Victorian medical theory, Baker Brown's work brought him opprobrium rather than the hoped for fame; and within a year of his book's appearance, both clitoridectomy and its author had been consigned to the outer darkness. Why was this?

Not, for all appearances, because of the cruelty or failures of the treatment. As Elaine Showalter (1985: 66) points out, "The mutilation, sedation, and psychological intimidation ... seems to have been an efficient, if brutal, form of reprogramming ..." and in any event, the issue of inefficacy was never seriously pursued in the storm of criticism Brown's work raised.[9] The treatment was certainly brutal, as is made clear in the description given by one of Brown's former assistants, "Two instruments were used: the pair of hooked forceps which Mr. Brown always uses in clitoridectomy, and a cautery iron. ... The clitoris was seized by the forceps in the usual manner. The thin edge of the red hot iron was then passed around its base until the origin was severed from its attachments, being partly cut or sawn, and partly torn away. After the clitoris was removed, the nymphae on each side were severed in a similar way by a sawing motion of the hot iron. After the clitoris and nymphae were got rid of, the operation was brought to a close by taking the back of the iron and sawing the surfaces of the labia and the other parts of the vulva which had escaped the cautery, and the instrument was rubbed down backwards and forwards till the parts were more effectually destroyed than when Mr. Brown uses the scissors to effect the same result" (*British Medical Journal* 1867g: 407–408).

But the brutality of the surgery was likewise not the central issue, and scarcely could be, since some of Brown's fiercest critics themselves used treatments that were every bit as unpleasant with their own female patients.[10] Instead, it was the "ethics" of Brown's behavior that drew down on his head the almost universal wrath of his colleagues. In fact, close attention to the record reveals that even before the appearance of his book, Brown's activities had drawn unfavorable comment from influential segments of the medical press. Mid-nineteenth-century medical practitioners could lay only a precarious claim to gentlemanly status (Peterson 1978; Scull 1984a), and medical elites were thus extraordinarily sensitive about behavior that threatened the profession's social standing. Brown's activities raised this vital issue in multiple and mutually reinforcing ways.

In the first place, he had aggressively sought public attention for and approval of his activities. In early 1866, for example, before his book on clitoridectomy appeared in print, he had arranged with a friendly reporter for the *Standard* for a hyperbolic article on "An Admirable Institute – The London Surgical Home." This immediately drew sharp criticism from the editor of the *British Medical Journal*, who commented tartly "We doubt whether the profession will approve of the way in which this particular institution is brought before the public. . . . A superfluous amount of self-laudation is not always a real recommendation" (*British Medical Journal* 1866a: 77). Baker Brown failed to take the hint. A few issues later, the *British Medical Journal* (1866c: 440) returned to the attack: the recent annual report of the London Surgical Home was permeated by "a regrettable spirit of exaggeration. . . ." And his new book on clitoridectomy, while demonstrating that "the operation may be of value in certain forms of nervous disease," made similarly wild and unsupported claims. Equally unforgivable was the presentation of subject matter fit only for the eyes of fellow medical men in a binding more suited "to a class of works which lie upon drawing room tables." The impression that Brown was seeking lay instead of professional approval was only accentuated by the appearance in the *Church Times* of an article which endorsed his operation and which urged clergymen to recommend it to practitioners;[11] and by the claim that Brown had sent the annual report of the London Surgical Home "to half the nobility in the kingdom" (*British Medical Journal* 1866d: 456, 1867e: 478)." And when Brown again resorted to barely disguised advertising in the public press, planting another laudatory story touting his unique remedy in cases of insanity (on this occasion in the *Times* [London] December 15, 1866), the editors finally lost all patience, and referred his activities to the Commissioners in Lunacy (*British Medical Journal* 1866h: 702).[12]

Brown thus proved fatally unwilling to abandon a line of conduct that deeply offended professional norms. His relentless pursuit of publicity smacked of the tradesman, an association medical men (especially surgeons) were desperately anxious to live down. Moreover, in the fiercely competitive medical world of mid-century London, advertising – direct or thinly disguised – was doubly threatening: to one's economic interests, since it deprived fellow practitioners of patients; and to social status, since it testified to the presence of mercenary concerns unworthy of a gentleman. Accordingly, few behaviors were so predictably stigmatized and anathematized. At least equally serious was Brown's preference for lay approval over the opinion of his professional peers. For this raised the specter of quackery, an association rendered the more plausible by the extraordinary array of hitherto untreatable conditions that Brown claimed to cure.

By the close of 1866, the London medical elite was all but unanimously turning on someone who had, till recently, been one of its leading lights. Between November 24, 1866 and March 16, 1867, the correspondence columns of the *British Medical Journal* were filled with attacks on Brown's activities. Letters came from fellow gynecologists, like Charles West; from former visiting surgeons at the London Surgical Home, like Robert Greenhalgh and John Locking; and from two of the most eminent alienists of the period, Henry Maudsley and Forbes Winslow. In the flurry of criticism, new charges now emerged, some of them prompted by Brown's own attempts to disarm his critics.

Though Maudsley claimed that masturbation was a consequence, not a cause of insanity, and West complained that Brown's work was "based on erroneous physiology" and the operation "completely unjustifiable when done for the alleged relief of...painful defaecation, for the cure of amenorrhoea, or for the mitigation of the symptoms of uterine misplacement or disease" (West 1866: 585) it was "the moral and professional aspects of the charges" (*British Medical Journal* 1867b: 61) that remained central to the case. Masturbation was "a dirty subject, and one with which only a strong sense of duty can induce professional men to meddle; and then it needs to be handled with an absolute purity of speech, thought and expression, and, as far as possible, in strictly 'technical' language." Yet Brown had deliberately trespassed over the boundary that kept knowledge of such subjects strictly within the ranks of professional men. Even worse, he had initiated "the public discussion, before mixed audiences, of sexual abuses" (*British Medical Journal* 1866g: 664). Such "public attempts to excite the attention of nonmedical persons, and especially of women, to the subject of self abuse in the female sex" threatened "to injure society," violating the weaker sex's natural purity and perhaps spreading the reprehensible habit; and they were, into the bargain, likely "to bring discredit on the medical profession" (West 1866: 585).

As other details of Brown's activities now began to emerge, it became even more apparent that his conduct represented a serious threat to the credibility and authority of a still precarious profession. Allegations repeatedly surfaced that he operated "upon married women without the consent of their husbands, and upon unmarried women without the consent of their friends and of the patients themselves..." (*British Medical Journal* 1867g: 407);[13] and that "terrorism," in the form of threats to commit the patient to an asylum, had "been used to frighten patients into submission, where need for operation there was none" (*British Medical Journal* 1867b: 61). Brown's disingenuous attempt to circumvent the charge that he had illegally admitted insane patients to the London Surgical Home only added fuel to the flames. Pressed by the Lunacy Commissioners unequivocally to confirm or deny the allegation, he first tried to dismiss the whole affair as a misunderstanding; then, when the Commissioners pressed for "a plain and direct contradiction of its being open for the reception of females of unsound mind," he resorted to a legalistic quibble stating he had never advertised the Home as an asylum and "the institution is not open for the reception of females of unsound mind."[14] Yet, as his critics promptly and gleefully pointed out, his own publications on clitoridectomy claimed to be "taken from the records of the London Surgical Home," and included at least five cases of insanity "cured" by his operation (*British Medical Journal* 1867c: 94, February 2, 1867d: 119, 1867e: 144). Caught on the horns of a dilemma of his own making, Brown's "explanation" was of a sort "which I can hardly venture to characterise among a society of gentlemen" (Dr Robert Barnes in *British Medical Journal* 1867g: 400).[15]

His reputation as a "gentleman" in tatters, Brown now seems to have become increasingly frantic. Seeking to shift the focus of attention away from issues of ethics and honor, he instructed the Secretary of the London Surgical Home to write to the editor of his chief tormentor, the *British Medical Journal* promising a moratorium on further clitoridectomies pending an impartial investigation into "its validity as a scientific and justifiable operation" (*British Medical Journal* 1867f: 154). But he could not keep his word, for less than two weeks later, he operated yet again, only to find his "decided breach of faith with the profession" exposed by another physician on the Home's staff who promptly resigned and then notified the medical press.

Events now moved rapidly to a conclusion. Urged on by the *Lancet* and the *British Medical Journal*, the Council of the Obstetrical Society announced an emergency meeting to consider Baker Brown's expulsion. The Society convened on April 3 with more than 200 members in attendance. From the outset, the hostility to Brown was palpable. The Council had threatened to resign if he were not expelled, and the meeting was run in a blatantly partisan fashion. An hour after the meeting began, only two speakers had been heard from, both excoriating Brown, when the President announced that the ballot box was now open. The wretched man protested that he had as yet had no opportunity to answer the charges, but his protests were over-ruled and he had to make do with the assurance that the balloting would not actually be *closed* until after he had had a chance to speak.

When he did finally obtain the floor, he was interrupted and heckled unmercifully. Rounding on his accusers, he did his own cause no good by impugning their character and motives and claiming that he had written evidence (which unfortunately he had neglected to bring with him) demonstrating the falsity of the central allegations against him. From a man whose veracity was already damaged beyond repair, the performance could scarcely have been more ill judged.[16] Appeals for mercy from one of his few supporters fell on deaf ears, and just after midnight, an overwhelming vote for his expulsion was announced.[17]

Though Baker Brown was not erased from the register of the recently established General Medical Council, his career was effectively ruined. A few weeks later, the London Medical Society announced the forced resignation of its former president, and in the tightly controlled, hierarchical world of metropolitan medicine. Brown was rapidly reduced to penury. His health failed, and for the last two years of his life he was supported only by the charity of the profession that had ostracized him (*Lancet* 1873a: 151–152).

As Michael Clark has rightly argued, the physician's moral and pastoral responsibilities were an essential – perhaps the essential foundation of the Victorian medical man's claims to authority and prestige. Anything which cast even a shadow upon the appearance of moral rectitude and strict probity simultaneously threatened the profession's paramount concern with safeguarding the basis of its social standing and mandate. It was his violation of this "first principle of the physician's professional conduct" (Clark 1981: 293) that destroyed Baker Brown. For the injunction to uphold the basis of professional honor was always likely to be enforced with particular force and fury in the case of gynecology, a specialty whose practitioners, "beyond other [medical] men, are not only the guardians of life, but, by force of circumstance, often also the guardians of female honour and purity" (*British Medical Journal* 1867g: 388).

The very precariousness of their position, having only just "emerged from the difficulties and clouds under which we lay during previous centuries," made it essential that the Obstetrical Society demonstrate to "the public that their health in our hands, as men of honour and gentlemen, is safe" (*British Medical Journal* 1867g: 409, speech of Dr T.H. Tanner). As men, and more particularly, as medical men, gynecologists possessed extraordinary power over the weaker sex; yet their social mandate to exercise that power would rapidly evaporate were they to use their authority irresponsibly and "unethically." In the words of Seymour Haden, proposing the notion to expel Baker Brown,

> we have constituted ourselves, as it were, the guardians of [women's] interests, and in many cases . . . the custodians of their honour. We are, in fact, the stronger, and they the weaker. They are obliged to believe all that we tell them. They are not in a position to dispute anything we say to them, and we therefore may be said to have them at our mercy . . . . Under these circumstances, if we should depart from the strictest principles of honour, if we should cheat or victimize them in any shape or way, we would be unworthy of the profession of which we are members.
>
> (*British Medical Journal* 1867g: 396)

Quite unambiguously, then, Baker Brown's conduct constituted "a breach of faith with every individual member of the profession . . ." (*British Medical Journal* 1867g: 407); a betrayal of trust that, without a forceful response from the guardians of professional morality, might have delivered a body blow to the reputation for moral rectitude and probity upon which the profession's privileged place in the division of labor ultimately rested. Hence the harsh and unforgiving treatment by his peers.

The normal ovariotomy

The first attempt to introduce gynecological surgery as a cure for insanity thus ended abruptly and ignominiously, with such catastrophic effects on the career of its originator that others were effectively deterred from adopting his technique.[18] (Not that some weren't tempted to do so. Some years later, for example, the prominent English gynecologist, Lawson Tait, lamented the ostracization of Baker Brown and the barrier to his employment of so useful a remedy.)[19] A substantial portion of most gynecologists' practices, however, continued to consist of functional disorders of apparently "nervous" origin, and within a few years, an even more radical form of surgical treatment for mental disturbance was proposed.

The new operation, "normal ovariotomy," was designed to produce an artificial menopause. Its originator, an American surgeon from Rome,

Georgia with the rather apt name of Battey, announced his breakthrough in suitably apocalyptic tones:

> I have felt it to be my duty to...carve [*sic*] out for myself a new pathway through consecrated ground. ... I have invaded the hidden recesses of the female organism and snatched from its appointed set a glandular body, whose mysterious and wonderful functions are of the highest interest to the human race.[20]
>
> (Battey 1873: 1; see also Battey 1872: 321–333)

Others, of course, had previously "snatched" ovaries from their appointed seat. Battey's originality consisted in deliberately extending the operation to the extirpation of *healthy* organs. Hence the term "normal" ovariotomy, a choice of language he later came to regret.

Although Battey offered his operation as an effective treatment for a variety of pathological conditions that were held to depend upon the periodicities that plagued menstruating women, its allegedly marvelous curative properties were soon concentrated upon the treatment and cure of nervous ailments. As an operation on the external genitalia, Baker Brown's clitoridectomy could be undertaken even in the pre-anti-sepsis era, with only occasionally fatal complications from fulminating infections. But ovariotomy, or as it was also called, oophorectomy, only became technically feasible on a major scale once the importance of anti-sepsis had been grasped and generally accepted. Even then, during the first decade of the operation, mortality rates averaged one-third of all cases treated (see, for example, Peaslee 1872), so that those experimenting with the treatment found themselves "generally condemned, and at times even ostracized" (Marcy 1887: 6).

By the 1880s, however, death rates had declined quite markedly, to what were regarded as more acceptable levels (Battey himself, for example, reported a series of 70 cases with only 2 deaths and 68 "recoveries") (Battey 1886), and with the technical feasibility of the operation now established, a veritable mania for ovariotomy swept the United Stales and (to a lesser extent) Britain.[21] The precise number of operations performed during the 1880s and 1890s can never be established, since they were, "with a few exceptions, confined to private practice, or to general hospitals" (*Journal of the American Medical Association* 1893: 135); but by himself, the English surgeon Lawson Tait performed several hundred, and judging from the published cases alone, several thousand and quite possibly tens of thousands of women must have submitted themselves to the surgeon's knife. With only slight hyperbole, one critic waspishly commented:

> Pelvic operations on women has [*sic*] become a fad. It is fashionable, and the woman who cannot show an abdominotomy line is looked upon as not in style, nor belonging to the correct set. It is a mark of favor and considered "as pretty as the dimple on the cheek of sweet sixteen."[22]
>
> (Maclean 1894: 382)

There was no great mystery about the operation's popularity among gynecologists for the treatment of mental disorders. If the remedy was safe enough to use on *sane* women for the treatment of physical disorders, there surely could be no objection to its use on the mad – carriers of an otherwise hopeless hereditary disorder:

> For, in the first place, an insane woman is no more a member of the body-politic than a criminal; second, her death is always a relief to her dearest friends; third, even in the case of her recovery from her mental disease, she is liable to transmit the taint of insanity to her children, and to her children's children for many generations.[23]
>
> (Goodell 1881a: 639)

Within such a world view, normal ovariotomy would by definition be accounted a success, whether the outcome were mental recovery, sterilization, or death.

Despite this, throughout the 1880s, gynecologists made remarkably little progress in persuading asylum superintendents to allow them to operate on the mad. A.J.C. Skene was briefly affiliated with the Kings County Asylum in Flatbush, New York, and W.P. Manton, a Detroit gynecologist, was appointed to the staff of the Eastern and Northern Michigan Lunatic Asylums, but otherwise those running the state asylums proved all but immune to their colleagues' blandishments.[24]

In many ways, this refusal to give credence to a new form of treatment developed outside their own ranks was entirely typical of late nineteenth-century American alienism. An isolated, poorly regarded, and embattled group of men on the margins of medicine, asylum superintendents in the 1870s and 1880s characteristically responded with barely concealed hostility and scorn to attempts by others to trespass on "their" field of expertise, charging those who criticized their work with being animated by a deadly combination of "ignorance and malevolence" (Callender 1883–1884: 29). Critics "sermonizing and drooling" on the subject of insanity found themselves accused by alienists of being people "who live and move upon the borderland of insanity" (Chapin 1883–1884: 29, 37). And attempts by "medical societies and prominent physicians...to discuss and accomplish the best methods of treatment of the insane" were dismissed by the alienists' leaders as ill-founded meddling which served primarily "to excite distrust and destroy public confidence" in the only group with real expertise in the management of the mad, themselves (Chapin 1883–1884: 42, quoted in Caplan 1969: 210).[25]

In rejecting the claims of gynecologists to have discovered more efficacious forms of treatment for mental disorder (just as they were simultaneously attempting to discredit another group of potential rivals, the neurologists), alienists were fortified by their growing conviction that the prognosis of insanity was almost uniformly grim. Asylum superintendents had been notable a generation earlier for the extreme optimism of their claims about the curability of insanity (Bockoven 1963; Rothman 1971; Grob 1973a; Scull 1981a, 1991). However, in the face of the awkward situation created by the massive accumulation of chronic cases and the steady decline in official cure rates in their asylums, they had recently reversed themselves and begun to emphasize the essential hopelessness of the condition.[26] To do otherwise, of course, was to call into question the appropriateness of their treatment of their charges, and to undermine their own vulnerable claims to expertise.

In view of the difficulties for their position and status created by the uncertainties of their account of the biological mechanisms underlying insanity and by their now patently obvious therapeutic impotence, alienists thus possessed powerful reasons to reject the surgical remedy proffered by their medical colleagues. Having just engaged in massive "ideological work" (Berger 1981) designed to discredit the extravagant claims of an earlier generation of their own specialty to be able to cure the insane – a defense which rested upon a strong emphasis on the intractability of madness – asylum superintendents possessed little incentive to embrace a new panacea offered by a group of rivals to their therapeutic hegemony. Moreover, the retreat to a far more modest estimate of the efficacy of psychiatric interventions had come at a considerable cost to the alienists' public standing and to the legitimacy of the institutions they headed. In such a context, as the more astute leaders of the profession realized, to embark on a novel, potentially controversial, and highly experimental therapeutics was to court unnecessary peril. In the words of John Chapin, the President of the Association of Superintendents of American Hospitals for the Insane, "Hospitals for the insane might easily lose a portion of the slender hold they now have upon the public and friends of patients, if it were understood that the patients were subjected to experimental operations of a hazardous nature" (Quoted in *Journal of the American Medical Association* 1893: 136).[27]

With the gates of the asylum at least temporarily barred, the bulk of the insane thus remained beyond the reach of the gynecologists's scalpels, and if one may judge by the cases reported in print, most of their patients were not unambiguously mad, but rather "hovered on the narrow borderland which separates hysteria from insanity" (Goodell 1881a: 640).[28] Typically, that is, those subjected to Battey's operation were not the poor, but middle and upper-class women who suffered from mysterious and chronic "nervous" complaints.[29] Hysteria was the bane of the late nineteenth-century physicians and the profession's desperation when confronted by this pernicious malady at least equaled that of its patients and their families.[30] Consequently, doctor, patient, and family could agree with few qualms that, as a way station on the road to chronic insanity, hysteria and related conditions called for drastic measures designed to provide "a ray of hope," perhaps an "only chance" (Goodell 1890: 395) of staving off a life of permanent invalidism or – worse yet – the stigma of confinement in an asylum.

If such arguments persuaded many gynecologists of the merits of the normal ovariotomy, their clientele appear to have required little urging from their doctors. Physicians repeatedly claimed that husbands, families, and friends, to say nothing of the women themselves, pleaded for Battey's operation, since "it might offer a reasonable chance of recovery" (Hamilton 1893: 181, 182; Bloch 1894: 5). Women were described as insistent, "morbidly importunate and so unreasonable on the subject" (Goodell 1890: 394) that their medical attendants feel pressured into performing operations they might otherwise have hesitated to undertake.[31]

To some extent, this stress on the volunteerism of these women may have been intended to head off any possible criticism from the rest of the medical profession or from the public at large about the wisdom of persuading women to submit to such an irreversible operation, one which blighted forever any prospect that their patients could contribute to that most vital and sacred of feminine tasks, the propagation of the species. Hence, perhaps some of the ritualistic quality of the emphasis on how patient importunities forced them to wield the knife. The attitude gynecologists sought to convey appeared to be that since these women were so desperate and had indeed begged for this drastic treatment, the physician's professional duty was to oblige them.

But to argue that gynecologists may have had ulterior motives for emphasizing the willingness of their clientele is not to question the honesty of their reports. In many ways, it would have been surprising had this phenomenon *not* existed. After all, the connection between menstruation and women's emotional liability has deep-seated roots in folk "wisdom." Moreover, from the mid-century on, medical men had provided scientific support for this venerable belief through an emphasis on the reflex sympathy between women's brains and their reproductive organs. In the words of Howard Kelly, America's leading gynecologist at the turn of the century, "it is difficult even for a healthy girl to rid her mind of constant impending evil from the uterus and ovaries, so prevalent is the idea that women's ills are mainly 'reflexes' from the pelvic organs" (Kelly 1908: 73).

It should come as no surprise, therefore, that nervous patients were "fully convinced that, directly or indirectly, all their grief emanates from the pelvis" (Cokenower 1904: 293). Moreover, whatever secondary gains female hysterics may have derived from their condition (Smith-Rosenberg 1972), the reality of their primary suffering must not be minimized. Battey's early patient who declared "with emphasis that 'her life was but a living death': that to her the bare hope of cure – full and final cure – was of infinitely greater value than the realization of life coupled with her suffering..." (Battey 1872: 325) had many counterparts, who "were willing to accept anything that might offer a reasonable chance of recovery" (Bloch 1894: 5). "The result," as one critic of ovariotomy was later to note, "is that we have an overwilling surgeon and a pliant patient" (Van de Warker 1906: 372).

For the most part, any doubts most medical men may have felt about the value of ovariotomy as a treatment for mental disorder were suppressed during the 1880s. There were, however, a handful of exceptions to this generalization, most notably the famous English surgeon, Sir Thomas Spencer Wells.

Wells had made a substantial part of his reputation by being one of pioneering ovariotomists in England. By 1880 he had personally performed more than a 1,000 such operations, gaining renown by publishing his unsuccessful as well as his successful cases (Gwillim 1962: 87–88). But he was convinced that "in nearly all cases of nervous excitement and madness, [the operation] is inadmissible:" and he denounced "the fanaticism in America," as well as the depredations of his provincial rival, Lawson Tait. "Gynecologists," he insisted, "will never empty the lunatic asylums." To the contrary, "he who cuts mad people must himself be mad." Nor, in his judgment, could this remain a purely intra-professional squabble. To the contrary, those who succumbed to "this contagion of folly" were increasingly provoking jeers from "men in clubs" and fury on the part of the husbands of those they mutilated, so that their "personal degradation" was also, and far more seriously, "a crime against society and a dishonor to the profession" (Wells 1886: 455–471).[32]

As he recognized, such violations of the profession's "sacred trust" posed a serious threat to their craft. The claimed cures were in all probability the product of suggestion, or the "physical shock" associated with any operative interference, so that "many women have been doomed to sterility that would have been equally relieved by a farce or a failure." Moreover, it was only because its victims were women that such a state of affairs was allowed to persist, as was immediately obvious if one held "the mirror up to nature, only changing the sex of the actors" (Wells 1886: 470–471).

Suppose, he suggested, we lived in a world where women were the doctors and men the patients.

> Fancy [then] the reflected picture of a coterie of the Marthas of the profession in conclave, promulgating the doctrine that the most unmanageable maladies of men were to be traced to some morbid change in their genitals, founding societies for the discussion of them and hospitals for the cure of them, one of them sitting in her consultation chair, with her little stove by her side and her irons all hot, searing every man as he passed before her: another gravely proposing to bring on the millennium by snuffing out the reproductive powers of all fools, lunatics, and criminals; a third getting up and declaring that she found, at least, seven or eight of every ten men in her wards with some condition of his appendages which would prove incurable without surgical treatment, and a bevy of the younger disciples crowding around the confabulatory table with oblations of soup-platefuls of the said appendages; if, too, we saw, in this magic mirror, ignorant boys being castrated almost impromptu, hundreds of emasculated beings moping about and bemoaning their doltish credulity... should we not, to our shame, see ourselves as others see us?
>
> (Wells 1886: 470–471)[33]

As Wells knew, there were good reasons why such scenes were confined to the realm of fantasy. In general, the late nineteenth-century medical construction of the female, with its emphasis on their physical and mental inferiority, provided ample theoretical justification for their differential treatment. For many physicians, it was a truism that woman's

> mental characteristics...offer a marked contrast with that of a male. Her physical organization is not fully developed, and...she is...more like a child in disposition and also anatomically...in a general way...women are less intellectual than man, less original in thought, less capable of continuity and logic of thought, and hence they have been called more childlike in their mental characteristics, and in this respect resemble rather the primitive races.
>
> (Skene 1895: 80)

More directly relevant to the question of operating on the reproductive system, and another possible motive for the lack of attention to the testicles, as James Russell sarcastically suggested a few years later, was the absence of technical difficulty and challenge in operating on the male:

> Happy, thrice happy should man be because of the simplicity of his genital outfit and its meagre attraction for the operations of surgical science. Had Nature decreed him to wear his genitals within the abdominal cavity, he too might have been compelled to suffer surgical martyrdom for the sake of restoring his reason.
>
> (1898: 580)

More seriously still, as Thomas Morton (1893: 399) noted, there were the likely consequences of castrating the male: "The medical superintendent who would advocate or practice such mutilating operations upon men would be promptly denounced, if not legally prosecuted."

But if the selective attention to women was not necessarily scandalous and could to some degree be accommodated within the domain assumptions of late nineteenth-century medicine, it was also not without its hazards. A lively sense of these potential difficulties was, of course, implicit in Wells' remarks, which embraced both a formidable critique of the scientific basis of the whole craze, and a realistic fear of what the long-term effects of the episode might be on the reputation of the profession. Within a few years, other members of the medical elite on both sides of the Atlantic clearly began to share Wells' concerns, and through the 1890s controversy raged in the medical journals over the value of Battey's operation. Fearful of "[t]he increasing frequency of these experimental mutilations and their doubtful ultimate success" (*Journal of the American Medical Association* 1893: 135) a number of major figures in the profession called, in steadily more strident terms, for a re-evaluation of the whole approach. Significantly, these critics included not only eminent physicians from the leading segments of other medical specialties, but also many of the most prominent gynecologists.[34]

Neurologists, who had long been harshly critical of asylum superintendents for being out of touch with the cutting edge of medical advances, were even more contemptuous of the claims of the advocates of sexual surgery. Wharton Sinkler, an eminent Philadelphia neurologist, commented sardonically that

> A first successful abdominal section seems to have the same effect upon an operator as the taste of blood upon the Indian tiger. A thirst insatiable is aroused, and life is spent in looking for new victims. Cases running into double and triple figures are cited, where all the worst features of the most stubborn nature have disappeared, as though the surgeon's knife were gifted with the power of an enchanter's wand.
>
> (Sinkler 1891: 173)

Re-asserting that insanity and related conditions were the product of "nerve exhaustion" or disease, and hence belonged securely within the neurologist's province, they accused their colleagues of having fallen into a trap: "We are liable to be misled by what we see" particularly in cases of hysteria, "which very much simulate organic disease" (Maclean 1894: 38). But such cases merely counterfeited organic mischief, while the true causes of the disorder resided in the nervous system.

In consequence, leading neurologists denounced ovariotomy as a treatment for mental disturbance as simply a mutilation, a variety of "heroic surgery, of...the most flagrant and pernicious form," whose "evil and uselessness can not be too strongly condemned" (Hamilton 1893: 181; Edes 1896: 1080). Even were one to assume that the procedure had some therapeutic value, it was far too drastic and dangerous to be employed against "a comparatively hopeful malady [like hysteria]" (Church 1893: 495). In fact, however, despite all the exaggerated claims, "the relief is either none at all or only such as may be temporarily obtained from any strong impression whose effect is hopefully awaited" (Edes 1898: 1135).[35]

All of these objections were substantially shared by the leaders of the gynecological specialty, who added some further criticisms of their own. Their comments make clear the double and mutually reinforcing basis for the growing opposition to sexual surgery for mental disorders: discomfort about the increasingly shaky scientific basis for these operations; and anxieties about the long term effects of "exsective and amputative gynecology" (Kelly 1896: 249) on the profession's reputation and public standing.

Technique, they feared, was outrunning judgment and knowledge. Careful attempts to assess therapeutic results were "relatively scanty, compared with the large numbers of operations performed" (*Journal of the American Medical Association* 1893: 135) but accumulating experience suggested that, notwithstanding frequent claims to the contrary, the actual "results are not so gratifying and wonderful." Worse yet, even apparent successes were, as likely as not, the accidental by-product of post-operative shock or of taking "as a cause what is simply a synchronous occurrence" (Skene 1895: 335).

Others pointed out the difficulty of defining "the limits of health and disease in an ovary" (Ross 1897: 229). After all, "The ovaries in any woman who has menstruated twelve or more years are battered, wrinkled-appearing organs and it needs some experience to enable one to say that they are normal" (Van de Warker 1906: 368; see also Edes 1896: 1077). Moreover, wider experience with abdominal surgery had demonstrated that so-called pathology of the ovaries commonly existed without producing either mental or physical symptoms, raising legitimate doubts about whether ovarian pathology was any more common among the mad than among their sane sisters.[36]

A yet more serious objection to the operation now loomed. One of the major developments in late nineteenth-century physiology was an increasing recognition of the importance of internal secretions. Prompted in the first place by Brown-Sequard's experiments in 1889 with testicular extract, endocrinology rapidly established chemical regulation as at least as important as nervous regulation of the body (on these developments, see Brooks 1962; Borrell 1976; Hughes 1977). While many rank and file gynecologists remained strikingly ignorant of these advances,[37] the leading cadres were not slow to grasp their significance. Given the "vital importance" of the ovaries, one must now question the casual assumption of an earlier generation that their removal was of slight import, serving only to hasten the onset of menopause. The multiple contributions of the glandular system to the economy of the body meant there must be grave doubts about the wisdom of extirpating the ovaries, doubts that were reinforced as reports began to appear of protean varieties of side-effects following upon double oophorectomy.[38]

At least as important as these medical objections were a series of "ethical" qualms about the operation (see especially Kelly 1893). Throughout the nineteenth century, the medical profession sought to persuade the public of its status as guardian of the patient's interests.[39] Yet the claim to be proceeding in the patient's best interests was in this instance hard to square with the general belief that ovariotomy "ruins a woman in all the essentials of womanhood," preventing her from fulfilling her divinely ordained duties – to serve as wife and mother. Operative interference created equally powerful *practical* difficulties for its female clientele: "Economically, as the world is constructed, many women have no other prospect in life than marriage. Besides, unless a woman has means, or education, or unusual strength of character, a single life is insupportable." Yet for moral reasons, "a mutilated woman" could not hope to marry: "there is no hope and no happiness in such a union; there is no end to look forward to; there is nothing which makes marriage perfect and holy." Absent the possibility of procreation, a woman who engaged in sexual relations was little better than a whore and the gynecologist who brought about this condition could thus count himself "the destroyer of everything that makes a woman's life worth living."[40]

Small wonder, then, the elite physicians, who felt most keenly the need to protect their reputations, worried that "such operations bring surgery into bad repute" (Carstens 1897: 210). Ill-trained and inexperienced men, anxious "to carve [*sic*] their way to fame and distinction" (Haughton 1896: 256), were threatening the public's trust in the profession as a whole. And all too often they were actuated by mercenary motives, realizing that "ovariotomies are a source of income; [and that] many have grown rich on them." It was thus the duty of the leaders of the profession "to do something to stem the torrent of mutilation" ("the leading practitioner in one of our large cities," quoted in Kelly 1896: 251).

Such fierce criticism drew an equally strong response from some quarters. Supporters of the conservative position were accused of embracing a "fashionable craze" preaching "that it is better for one hundred suffering women to die unrelieved than that one should be relieved at the expense of the organs which are not only useless but a source of danger" (Praeger 1895: 322); and reports continued to appear of the wonderful cures that could be attributed to gynecological surgery (see, for example, Meyer 1894: 503–504). But those who continued to advocate operative interference in print were almost without exception provincial physicians who at best acquired some small measure of local fame.[41] Each knew that all his arguments could only "bring down on my head a storm of disapprobation" (Gilliam 1896: 315) from the profession at large. And none succeeded in reversing the operation's steady decline in popularity.

Curiously enough, it was only as normal ovariotomy became controversial, and then acquired the status of a fringe therapy, that some public asylums began to experiment with gynecological surgery as a treatment for mental disorder. The number of institutions involved was never large, and in only 3 or 4 were more than a handful of operations performed. Still, in a strange historical irony, this ill-conceived episode reflected psychiatry's belated attempt to break out of its self-imposed professional isolation and to acquire some of the trappings of modern medicine.

By the early 1890s, in a somewhat delayed reaction to the criticisms by neurologists and others of their scientific failings and detachment from the medical mainstream, asylum superintendents at last began an internal reform movement, granting membership in their professional association to their assistant physicians, and seeking to ensure that the latter brought into the asylum some of the recent advances in medical knowledge.[42] It was precisely through this route that a few institutions began to experiment with ovariotomy and other forms of gynecological surgery. Gynecologists were hired by some superintendents, and in a handful of cases persuaded their superiors of the value of surgical treatment of the female insane. At the Iowa Hospital for the Insane in Mount Pleasant, and at the Minnesota State Hospital, the superintendent was quickly disillusioned with the results, and operative treatment was quietly abandoned. In three other instances, however, at state hospitals in Pennsylvania, Maryland, and Ontario, Canada, the experiment drew greater attention and publicity.

At the Norristown State Hospital in 1892 and early 1893, a half-dozen ovariotomies were performed, and plans allegedly devised to set aside a special 50-bed ward to continue the experiment. Almost certainly urged on by the alienists' conservative leadership, the Pennsylvania Board of Charities, formally charged with the supervision of state hospitals, stepped in to forbid the scheme. Suggesting that "The zeal of the gynecologist is being carried to an unusual extent when it proposed to use a State Hospital for the Insane as an experimental station where lunatic women are to be subjected to doubtful operations for supposed cures" they denounced these "experimental mutilations" as "unwarrantable and indefensible" – "not only illegal, but... brutal and inhuman and not excusable on any reasonable ground" (Morton 1893: 397–401).[43] And in the face of their opposition, further experiments along these lines were quietly abandoned.

Meanwhile, in neighboring Maryland, George Henry Rohé, a former professor of obstetrics at the Baltimore College of Physicians and Surgeons, was installed in 1891, not as an assistant physician, but rather as superintendent of the Maryland State Hospital at Catonsville. This was in many respects a curious appointment, since nothing in Rohé's earlier career had evidently fitted him to run an asylum. Having originally practised as a dermatologist and syphilologist for a number of years, he had suddenly switched to obstetrics in 1890, and then, only a year later, to an interest in mental diseases.[44]

Author of a text on the medical uses of electricity, Rohé was clearly willing to experiment with novel therapeutics. Along with many of his professional brethren, he was convinced from the outset that "bodily conditions influenced mental states," and soon concluded that it was "not irrational to suppose... that diseases of the female sexual apparatus would have a not inconsiderable influence in the production or perpetuation of mental disorders." Within a few weeks, he had diagnosed a variety of gynecological ailments among his female patients and had begun to operate. His results were scarcely spectacular – 3 of his first 16 cases recovered, while 2 died – but somehow they sufficed to convince him that "there is a fruitful field for gynecological work among the insane" (Rohé 1892: 327).

Over the next several years, as general medical opinion was moving more and more decisively in the opposite direction, Rohé became a vociferous advocate of sexual surgery as a remedy for mental diseases (see, for example, Rohé 1893). His own efforts in this direction were abruptly terminated by his premature death in New Orleans in 1899 at the age of 48, but in the interim, at least one other asylum superintendent, Richard Bucke of the London Asylum in Ontario, Canada, had announced his conviction of the value of sexual surgery as a treatment for psychosis.[45]

Initially skeptical of the value of gynecological intervention when Rohé brought the topic before the superintendents' association in 1892, Bucke began to change his mind some three years later. The catalyst in this process was the appointment of a new assistant physician, A.T. Hobbs, to the staff of the London Asylum. Hobbs had little prior surgical experience, but, anxious to keep up with recent medical advances, he seized upon Rohé's claims and moved to implement a Canadian program of gynecological surgery.[46]

The earliest operations at the London Asylum involved improvised facilities – "a crude, wooden operating table, a couple of gas stoves, some granite basins and surgical instruments" – and an unskilled operator (Hobbs 1898: 514). But, Hobbs and his superior convinced themselves that the results were so promising that the former promptly left for New York for an intensive six-week course in gynecological surgery (Mitchinson 1982: 469). On his return, the number of operations expanded rapidly. An extraordinary proportion of the women the asylum staff examined were diagnosed as suffering from operable pathologies (122 of the first 132 cases), and as they employed surgery on a larger and larger scale, Hobbs and Bucke began to make sweeping claims for the value of the "eradication of pelvic disease" as a remedy for female insanity (Bucke 1898: 78; Hobbs 1898: 516–517).[47] In their view, "The almost instantaneous resolution of the mental faculties in some, and the steady evolution of the normal cerebral functions in others [following gynecological surgery], cannot but afford incontrovertible evidence in support of the relation of physical cause and mental effect" (Hobbs 1898: 523).

Such was hardly the general conclusion. Even among those who might have been expected to respond positively to Bucke's and Hobbs' claims, reactions were instead quite skeptical. Walter Manton, called upon to serve as discussant for Bucke's paper given at the 1900 American Medico-Psychological Association Meeting, noted his own pioneering role in introducing gynecological treatment into the lunatic asylum, and then proceeded to cast public doubt on the "large recovery rate" claimed by his Canadian colleagues, adding that he had "never yet ... seen a case of insanity, other than puerperal, that could be attributed to pelvic disorder alone. And I ... have never yet seen a mental cure of insanity through purely surgical procedures" (Manton 1900: 102–103).[48] Bucke's fellow alienists were much less restrained. His Canadian colleagues, in particular, denounced his work as "criminal," "wholesale mutilation of helpless lunatics," "a crying evil" inflicted upon the mad by someone who "always finds what he searches for" (all quoted in Hobbs 1899: 380; see, for example, Clark 1899; Russell 1898).

Led by the superintendent of another Ontario asylum, Dr James Russell of Hamilton, the critics succeeded in choking off all financial support for surgical treatment from the provincial government. Hobbs and Bucke at first sought to fight back against their opponents, denouncing them for "a deliberate attempt to strangulate a scientific advance upon the obsolete methods still so largely vogue in many asylums of today. ... The ridiculous sentimental cry of 'mutilation' should not prevent true surgeons from doing their whole duty towards their patients ... and scientific surgery will, in spite of the Rip van Winkles, supersede ancient and crude modes of treatment" (Hobbs 1899: 381–382). But it soon became apparent that such rhetorical attempts to appropriate the mantle of science and progress were falling on deaf ears, not least among those who held the asylum's purse strings. In December 1900, Hobbs retired to enter private practice, and with Bucke's accidental death a few months later, the last concerted attempt to attack madness through the "extirpation of diseased sections of the [female] reproductive system" (Hobbs 1898: 523) came to an abrupt halt.[49]

Conclusion

In the last third of the nineteenth century, lay and medical stereotypes of femininity and its connections with madness, coupled with the largely powerless status "enjoyed" by women of all social classes created among those of their number defined as mentally unbalanced a persistent vulnerability to radical, useless, and often dangerous interventions with allegedly marvelous curative properties. At any given point in the evolution of medical "knowledge," medical theories and models of the interaction of body and mind provided a rich source of speculations about ways to attack women's penchant for irrationality. Gynecological surgeons repeatedly drew upon this reservoir of ideology to generate novel, therapeutic interventions and to lend a scientific gloss to their depredations.

Paradoxically, however, the overwhelmingly male medical profession's need to preserve its social mandate, and to retain and extend the measure of public confidence essential to its social standing, meant that physicians had themselves to take very seriously their claims to act in their patients' interests and to serve as women's paternalistic protectors. The very centrality of certain aspects of sexuality, and especially of reproductive capacity, to the cultural construction of the female repeatedly created grave divisions and dissensions within the ranks of the profession over the wisdom of sexual surgery – concerns that were the more marked as the grandiosity of the surgeons' claims, and the latter's tendency to appeal directly to a lay audience desperate for remedies for so intractable a condition, raised in many minds the disquieting specter of quackery. Furthermore, for complex reasons of their own, alienists on this occasion proved peculiarly resistant to the siren songs of colleagues offering panaceas for the psychotic (or even the merely hysterical). Ultimately, the construction of a more elaborate and sophisticated picture of the workings of the body associated with the rise of endocrinology and the recognition of the importance of internal secretions became the occasion for orthodox medicine to turn its back on claims to provide a gynecological cure for madness.[50] In England, where control over the profession was relatively tight and hierarchical, sexual surgery was simply suppressed; in North America, where this degree of professional control was not yet established, these forms of gynecological intervention rapidly lost all semblance of respectability and became the province of a collection of crackpots and cranks.

12 Focal sepsis and psychosis

The career of Thomas Chivers Graves (1883–1964)

Thomas Chivers Graves, like most of his contemporaries in the psychiatric profession, has now fallen into obscurity. For more than a quarter of a century, though, he was one of the major figures in British psychiatry, his standing among his peers being recognized by his election in 1940 as President of the Royal Medico-Psychological Association (RMPA). Because of the war, he was to continue in that office until November, 1944, making his tenure as its head the longest in the organization's history. Of more direct moment from a practical point of view, his position as Chief Medical Officer to the Birmingham Mental Hospitals Committee (even as he simultaneously served as superintendent of two of them, Rubery Hill and Hollymoor Mental Hospitals) "gave him supervisory powers over all the other mental hospitals controlled by the City of Birmingham" (Anonymous 1964a: 1711) and placed him in charge of many thousands of patients, thereby ensuring that his views on psychiatric therapeutics were implemented on a broad scale.

Graves was born on May 11, 1883, in Histon, Cambridgeshire. His father was a veterinary surgeon, and an itinerant preacher for the Plymouth Brethren (V. Graves 1986). Thomas absorbed his father's sectarian religious beliefs (including a lifelong and very passionate prejudice against Roman Catholics) (F. Graves 1986).[1] At least initially, he also chose to follow in his father's footsteps when choosing his career. Educated at the Perse School in Cambridge, he proceeded from there to the Royal Veterinary College, from which he graduated in 1904, at the age of 21. Graves had proved an exceptionally talented and adept student, however, and his mentor, Professor Shave, whose assistant he now became, urged him to consider applying his talents to humans rather than animals.

Though related to the well-to-do Chivers family (whose wealth derived from its jams and preserves business), Thomas came from an impecunious household, and could not ordinarily have endured the additional expense of obtaining a medical qualification. His obvious abilities, however, allowed him to secure the Bucknill Scholarship at University College Hospital Medical School,[2] and together with income from some part-time work as an anatomy demonstrator and from giving veterinary instruction in his spare time, these funds allowed him to complete his medical education. By any measure, his student career was a glittering one. Almost incidentally, he obtained a BSc in Anatomy and Physiology as he proceeded, and by the time he took his MBBS with honors in Forensic Medicine and Hygiene in 1912, and qualified as MRCS and LRCP, he had won gold medals in Anatomy, Physiology, Pharmacology, Hygiene, and Public Health, as well as the Liston Gold Medal in surgery.

Of all these sub-specialties, it was surgery to which he was most attracted, and in which he sought to make his name. After a period as house-surgeon to Bilton Pollard at University College Hospital, he secured an obstetric residency there, and in 1914, at the age of 31, became a Fellow of the Royal College of Surgeons. At once, however, his career plans, like those of all men of his generation, were interrupted by the outbreak of war. He promptly joined the Royal Army Medical Corps, and by the time he was demobilized at the end of the war, he had elected to abandon his previous plans, turning instead to psychiatry as the means to secure his livelihood.

There is every indication that this radical change of plans was primarily motivated by economics rather than any alteration in Graves' intellectual horizons. Building a surgical practice in London in this period was a drawn-out and uncertain business, and even the most talented could look forward to several years of fluctuating and inadequate income before success might materialize. By the end of the war, though, Graves was not only approaching 40, but he had acquired a wife, Evelyn Dorothy Lang, the daughter of a colonel and a member of Queen Alexandra's Royal Army Nursing Service. Under the circumstances, a surgical career must have seemed out of the question.

In turning from surgery to psychiatry, however, Graves was moving from one of the most to one of the least prestigious branches of medicine. To be sure, appointment as an asylum superintendent brought with it a measure of economic security, and a large measure of authority over the self-contained world over which one presided – some measure of compensation for the personal and professional sacrifice the career change cost him. Still, the choice was undoubtedly an unusual one, and both directly and indirectly, it probably reflected the influence of the war, not just on his personal circumstances, but in bringing him into sustained contact with psychiatric casualties. Perhaps the encounter with victims of shell-shock prompted him to take an intellectual interest in the problem of mental disorders (though, as we shall see, virtually from the outset of his asylum career, Graves sought to counter the distinction between mental and physical disease). Certainly, however, it was these wartime experiences that provided him with relevant experience on the basis of which he could plausibly become a candidate for an asylum post.

A glance at the status of psychiatry in the first decades of the new century serves to make clear the magnitude of the career change which a move into the mental hospital sector represented. As early as the 1880s, as advances in basic science began to have demonstrable relevance for the understanding and then the treatment of disease, leading psychiatrists had responded by publicly expressing anxiety about being left behind the rest of medicine. The profession, in W.T. Gairdner's words, saw itself as being at risk of becoming "wholly divorced from the progress of medical science" (Gairdner 1882: 321–322; see also Newington 1889) – and such fears had proved to be well founded. By 1911, the Medico-Psychological Association (MPA), mindful of their increasing marginality and of the disparaging attitudes of their medical brethren, set up a committee under the chairmanship of Bedford Pierce, the superintendent of the York Retreat, to examine the status of the profession and to suggest ways of improving its standing. Both the committee's interim report, presented in 1913, and the final version brought to the Association's annual meeting a year later, must have made sobering reading for the membership at large. "The lunacy service," the committee acknowledged, existed in a twilight world "divorced from ordinary medical education and practice" – and the committee found itself forced "to consider what means could be devised to remedy the grave defects in the present position of psychiatry" (Anonymous 1914: 667–669).

It was far easier, however, to enumerate the difficulties which confronted the profession than to suggest effective means with which to "wipe out the reproach at present attached to our specialty" (Anonymous 1914: 675).[3] In the first place, "Psychiatry as a branch of medicine is in a decidedly inferior position to practically every other branch in the lack of educational facilities, and in the absence of any career for those who desire to undertake scientific work in it" (Anonymous 1914: 670). At best, a third of those serving as assistant medical officers in asylums could aspire to obtain an asylum superintendency, even after decades of service, "while short of this there are few attractive posts" (Anonymous 1914: 671). Isolation from the world at large was all but complete; "in many asylums no organised research work is carried on, and clinical and pathological investigations are often ill-directed, haphazard, consequently fruitless"; in other respects, "the work assigned to Junior Medical Officers is in the majority of cases monotonous, uninteresting, and without adequate responsibility [which] leads to the stunting of ambition and a gradual loss of interest in scientific medicine"; the routine and desultory qualities of asylum life tended "to kill enthusiasm and destroy medical interests [as well as] to produce a deteriorating effect upon those who remain long in the service"; and in return for enduring such miserable working conditions, and serving at the sole whim and discretion of the asylum superintendent, most medical men in the specialty could look forward to salaries so pitifully inadequate as to force them to remain celibate (if, indeed – as was often the case – the regulations of the asylum itself did not directly forbid them to marry) (Anonymous 1914: 667; see also Anonymous 1913).

These myriad disabilities and discouragements, together with the widespread perception that lunacy was a congenital and all-but-incurable condition, had predictable effects on the quantity and quality of the recruits to the profession. The war years, however, precipitated a still more serious crisis for psychiatry, since a veritable epidemic of disabling nervous breakdowns at the front brought into question the intellectual consensus that had developed within asylumdom about the etiology of mental disorder, and cast grave doubt upon the practical value of its conventional therapeutics. Shell-shock, as it came to be known, became an ever more threatening problem as the war proceeded, accounting for as many as "40 percent of the casualties from heavy fighting zones," afflicting the officer corps twice as often as the other ranks, and producing devastating effects on army morale (Stone 1985a: 249).

As Martin Stone (1985: 245) has noted, "The psychiatric establishment lost a great deal of credibility over shell-shock." Not only was there an epidemic of "a new war disease before which doctors seemed well nigh helpless" (Mitchell and Smith 1930: 9), and in the face of which their therapeutics seemed especially useless; but of perhaps still greater moment, the status of its victims – the manly heroes who had volunteered for the front – made it all but impossible to assimilate these cases of mental disorder to the ubiquitous explanation pre-war psychiatry had proffered to account for the legions of chronically insane pauper lunatics – the notion that insanity was predominantly a symptom of hereditary degeneration.[4] Marginalized as a source of ideas about etiology or therapeutics, asylum doctors also found that in practice, other branches of the medical profession – neurologists, but also general practitioners and even surgeons – were stepping into the breach and involving themselves in the treatment of the disorder.

Indeed, it is precisely in this context that Graves had his first contact with psychiatric patients. Joining the Royal Army Medical Corps at the outset of the war, he soon found himself working in a unit dealing with shell-shock cases (F. Graves 1986), and as early as 1915, somewhat surprisingly (for he had shown no prior interest in psychiatry), he became a member of the MPA. Though a sizeable minority of the medical men called upon to cope with the epidemic came to attribute the disorder to psychodynamic factors (and indeed some scholars have forcibly argued that shell-shock played an indispensable role in the emergence of psychodynamic psychiatry in Britain) (Showalter 1985; Stone 1985a) such views remained "anathema" (Culpin 1931: 24) to most of their colleagues in the RAMC, who strongly preferred an organic explanation of shell-shock's pathology. Here, at least, the army doctors were at one with what had long been the orthodox British psychiatric view of the origins of all varieties of mental disorder. Unfortunately, we have no direct knowledge of Graves' position on the matter, but there seems little doubt, given his prior medical background and his subsequent views on the etiology of mental disorder of all sorts, that his own sympathies must have lain with the somatic viewpoint.

At all events, by war's end, Graves had decided to pursue a career in psychiatry, and on demobilization, he promptly obtained qualification in Psychological and Nervous Diseases from the University of London, and equally rapidly secured the superintendency of the Hereford County Asylum. Less than a year later, he had moved to a more powerful and visible position, taking up on January 1, 1920 the post of Medical Superintendent of Rubery Hill and Hollymoor Hospitals in Birmingham, and by 1926, his empire had expanded still further, with his appointment as Chief Medical Officer to the City of Birmingham Mental Hospitals Committee. The retirement in 1926 of Cecil Roscrow, the superintendent of the third Birmingham mental hospital, made it possible to join all the hospitals together administratively as the City Mental Hospital. Graves' authority was further strengthened when the Committee then proceeded to appoint Dr Forsyth, who had served seven years as Graves' Deputy Superintendent at Hollymoor, as the new superintendent at Winson Green (Ogden 1983: 5).[5]

Despite the paucity of his prior experience in psychiatry, Graves' stellar medical credentials coupled with his wartime clinical duties had enabled him to move into the psychiatric service at its highest levels, avoiding entirely the years of drudgery and subservience as an assistant medical officer which were ordinarily the precondition for a superintendency.[6] He brought with him reservoirs of energy and enthusiasm, and "a determination to bring the study of pathology and the basic principles of medicine into the practice of psychiatry" (Anonymous 1964a: 1711). And he entered upon a position in which he had, like other superintendents of the period, considerable latitude to implement his ideas and enthusiasms. If not quite the monarch of all he surveyed, a superintendent nonetheless possessed near autocratic powers over all aspects of the artificially closed community over which he presided; and Graves' imposing physical stature (he stood over 6' 1" tall) and his domineering and charismatic personality[7] allowed him to exercise his nominal authority to its full extent.

His early months at Rubery Hill were occupied with the task of retransforming the institution back from the war hospital it had been to the mental hospital it was once again to become, and renovation and expansion of the physical plant were to occupy a substantial part of his time through the mid-1920s. The almost uninhabitable set of buildings he had inherited, bereft of any residents, had by early 1921 been refitted to house 560 patients, and by 1925, he had added new day-rooms and a number of bungalow-wards at both Hollymoor and Rubery Hill (Ogden 1983: 3). A larger than life figure who possessed considerable talents as an administrator, Graves reveled in his position, dominating both his colleagues and his patients, and seizing opportunities to secure the spotlight – whether in lectures to fellow psychiatrists illustrated with copious slides and statistics; or in taking the leading role in asylum productions of Gilbert & Sullivan and annually in "the part of Pooh-Ba at the hospitals' Christmas show, where the applause stopped the performance at several points" (Anonymous 1964a: 1711). He even had the opportunity to play the gentleman-farmer where like most hospitals of its era, his had a farm attached, whose milk, butter, meat, and eggs were worth more than £7,500 in 1922. Indirectly, therefore, Graves' veterinary training was thus eminently useful on a regular basis.

It was, however, his background as a surgeon that was to place a more distinctive mark on his psychiatric practice during the next three decades. Though a psychodynamically orientated psychiatry had made notable advances during and immediately after the war, and was rather less often the target of open hostility and intemperate criticism than it had once been, the long-standing disdain and distrust felt by the mainstream of the profession still lingered only barely beneath the surface (Clark 1981; Pines 1991). Graves' refusal to place much stock in a "childhood history of frustration" as the source of mental disorder (Anonymous 1964b: 4) thus made him very much a part of mainstream professional opinion. In opposition to psychodynamic explanations, beginning in 1922 he was advancing, both in print and in person, a very different account of the sources of mental illness, one which from the outset found a sympathetic audience among leading figures in the medical profession at large, as well as among many of his fellow specialists.

First articulating his views in a short paper published in the *Lancet* in 1922 (Graves 1922), Graves advanced with increasing aggressiveness the thesis that mental disorder was the product of auto-toxicity, caused in its turn by the presence in a variety of organs of chronic untreated reservoirs of infection. The hypothesis, as he was quick to acknowledge, was by no means a novel one. A more substantial paper delivered the following year to the MPA's Annual Meeting in London opened with a quotation from Maudsley's *Physiology & Pathology of Mind*, written more than half a century earlier:

> There is no want of evidence that organic morbid poisons bred in the organism or in the blood itself may act in the most baneful manner upon the supreme nervous centres. The earliest and mildest mental effect by which a perverted state of blood declares itself is not in the production of positive delusion or incoherence of thought, but in a modification of mental tone. The further effect is to engender a chronic delusion of some kind. A third effect of its more acute action is to produce more or less active delirium and general incoherence of thought.
>
> (Quoted in Graves 1923: 465)

Graves then proceeded to invoke a variety of authorities in support of his basic contention that "clinically an important relationship can be demonstrated to exist between prolonged emotional disturbance and chronic septic processes, occurring in hard tissues, especially in connection with the jaws" (Graves 1923: 471).

However odd these and later extensions of Graves' views may now seem, in the context of the times they were seen as anything but eccentric. The late nineteenth and early twentieth century was an era dominated by bacteriological models of disease. Though the medical profession had initially greeted the claims of Lister and Pasteur with skepticism and ridicule, its entrenched conservatism rapidly gave way in the face of the powerful practical advances that flowed from their work such as gains in both etiological understanding and in therapeutic efficacy. In surgery, antisepsis (and the routine employment of anesthesia) prompted rapid advances in the technical capacities of surgeons, and equally striking therapeutic gains. For a variety of acute and life-threatening diseases, similarly remarkable breakthroughs occurred within a short time. Within a five-year period, the typhoid bacillus, the plasmodia parasites that cause malaria, the tubercle bacillus, cholera vibrio, and diphtheria bacillus were all identified in the laboratory, and with the development of antiserums for diphtheria and tetanus, the medical outlook seemed completely transformed. General medicine's prestige (and the prospects of its practitioners) soared, along with expectations that medical science would soon extend its dominion over yet wider realms of disease and debility.

Yet a number of chronic, debilitating disorders – and not just those that pre-occupied psychiatrists – remained frustratingly recalcitrant in the face of every attempt to unravel their secrets. Even effective palliative therapies were in short supply, while the etiology of these diseases remained speculative at best. Succumbing to the temptation to extend the reach of the bacteriological paradigm, however, a number of leading medical men on both sides of the Atlantic turned to the notion of focal sepsis for an explanation, suggesting that such chronic diseases as arthritis, rheumatic fever, nephritis, and degenerative diseases of the arteries "might be caused by bacteria disseminated through the lymph or blood-streams from a hidden primary focus of infection" (Billings 1916).[8] In view of the wide currency and scientific respectability of these views among the medical and surgical elite in the first decades of the twentieth century,[9] both Graves' embrace of the idea of focal infection as a cause of mental disorder and his ability to secure a sympathetic hearing for his theories among his colleagues are anything but surprising.

Nor was he the first to suggest a connection between infection and mental illness. As early as 1900, the British surgeon, William Hunter, seeking to apply the principles of "Listerism" to general medicine, had suggested a role for focal infection in the causation of a wide variety of diseases (Hunter 1900: 215–216).[10] Six years later, the Scottish psychiatrist, Lewis Bruce, extended the array of troubles rotting teeth could cause, implicating them in the causation of insanity (Bruce 1906),[11] and similar suggestions began to surface in psychiatric circles in the United States at around the same time (Upson 1907, 1909, 1910).

A year before Graves made his first presentation on focal sepsis to his colleagues in the MPA, these and other adumbrations of the importance of bacterial poisoning of the brain in the genesis of mental disorder had been forcibly brought to their attention at their 1922 meeting in Edinburgh, by Chalmers Watson, physician at the Royal Infirmary (Watson 1923). In his own remarks on the subject, Watson had placed at least as much emphasis on "excessive putrefaction in the bowel" as on decay in the mouth, and had invoked the sainted Lister in urging his audience to recognize

> the urgent need at the present time to all cases of mental disorder being studied by alienists more from the standpoint of the general physician, full use being made of the routine modern methods of investigation as carried out by physicians with a modern outlook and knowledge.
>
> (Watson 1923: 63, 75)

Few in his audience were likely to be more receptive to such an appeal than Graves, essentially an outsider to the psychiatric profession in any event, and someone whose own primary "ambition was to bring the study of pathology and the basic principles of medicine [as he understood them] into the practice of psychiatry" (Anonymous 1964a: 1711).

In the event, Graves' own advocacy of the treatment of focal infection was far overshadowed at the Association's 1923 annual meeting by the performance of a visitor from across the Atlantic, a man with whom he would afterwards enjoy the closest professional relations, Henry Aloysius Cotton (Scull 1987). For while Graves presented a handful of cases to illustrate his claim that "clinically an important relationship can be demonstrated to exist between prolonged emotional disturbance and chronic septic processes occurring in hard tissues, especially in connection with the jaws" (Graves 1923: 471), Cotton advanced a much more far-reaching and revolutionary set of claims. From 1919 onwards, Cotton had been publishing a series of papers based on his work as superintendent at the Trenton State Hospital in New Jersey, in which he proclaimed with growing certainty to have found the key to understanding and treating mental disorders. His claims were the focus of increasing controversy in American psychiatric circles (Anonymous 1922), but here, given the chance to address a new and receptive audience, Cotton's self-confidence knew no bounds.

Flattering his listeners by first stressing the British origins of the doctrine of focal infection, he then launched upon a panegyric to the effects of mounting a full-blooded assault on its presence in the mentally ill, urging them to join in "the fight against sepsis in medicine" and for "antiseptic medicine" – a term he credited to William Hunter. Like Graves, he had begun by extracting infected teeth, but in his case the battle had soon extended to a variety of other fronts in what amounted to a thorough-going assault designed "to literally 'clean up' our patients of all foci of chronic sepsis" (Cotton 1923). Sinuses, tonsils, stomachs, gall bladders, colons, cervixes, and seminal vesicles, all these and more might be potential sites of silent chronic infections leaching toxins into the lymphatic system and the bloodstream and poisoning the brain; and any or all might require excision by the surgeon's knife.

Such ruthless pursuit and elimination of sepsis, however, was blessed with the happiest of outcomes, that is, an increase in "our recoveries in this group from 37 percent to 85 percent" (Cotton 1923: 438).[12] All of these efforts, Cotton insisted, were dependent upon the most recent scientific advances of modern medicine such as gastric analyses and serology, bacteriological work and X-rays, serums and vaccines, and above all, the miracles of modern aseptic surgery – for only the surgeon's knife and the dentist's forceps could in the last analysis ensure successful "detoxification." His audience were perhaps made somewhat uncomfortable by the scorn he poured upon what had long been British psychiatry's preferred explanation of mental disorder, defective heredity ("This doctrine was more or less fatalistic, and simply served as a cloak to hide our ignorance of other factors" and it "has had the most unhappy result of stifling investigation, and retarding constructive work.")

(Cotton 1923: 439);[13] but most found themselves nodding in agreement when he turned to a far more savage assault on psychoanalysis ("The extravagant claims made by its advocates are without foundation or justification. Freudism has proven to be a tremendous handicap to psychiatry.") (Cotton 1923: 440). Making the obligatory bow towards a multi-factorial origin of "the so-called functional psychoses," Cotton insisted that instead

> the most constant [cause], and, from the standpoint of treatment, the most important one, is the intra-cerebral, bio-chemical cellular disturbance arising from circulating toxins originating from chronic foci of infection.... Instead of considering the psychosis as a disease entity, it should be considered a *symptom*, and often a *terminal symptom* of a long-continued chronic sepsis or masked infection, the accumulating toxaemia of which acts directly or indirectly on the brain-cells.
>
> (443, 444)

Such findings were, the more significant in that they applied to the overwhelming majority of patients who ended up in mental hospitals. Praising his British audience for not swallowing Kraepelin's classification *in toto*, Cotton truculently asserted that

> as a result of our work, I do not believe there is any fundamental difference in the functional psychoses. The more we study our cases, we are forced to conclude that distinct disease entities in the functional group ... do not exist. The aetiological factors are the same ... [in] the whole so-called functional group, such as manic-depressive insanity, dementia praecox, paranoid conditions, the psychoneuroses, etc.
>
> (1923: 444–445)

The attentive listener would have heard Cotton confess to certain unfortunate side-effects that sadly were the inevitable accompaniment of this massive advance. There were, for example, the patients whose "serious lesions of the colon" necessitated remedial action – amounting to "about 20 percent of the 'functional' group." As with other kinds of sepsis, the only remedy in his view was "elimination," a term which here turned out to have an unfortunate double meaning:

> In our early operations the caecum and ascending colon were resected only.... Further examination of the unsuccessful cases proved that the splenic fixture and descending colon were also involved. Consequently, in the last two years total colectomy has been performed in practically every case. This operation was done in 133 cases, with 33 recoveries and 44 deaths. Partial resection at the right side was done in 148 cases, with 44 recoveries and 59 deaths.
>
> (1923: 454, 457)

Mortality statistics which, he explained, could be tolerated since they were "largely due to the very poor physical condition of most of the patients."

But it was the extraordinary therapeutic success that Cotton claimed, and the degree to which his approach seemed to call up the most "scientific" features of modern medicine, that his audience chose to focus upon. A series of prominent figures took advantage of the discussion session which followed to lavish praise on their American visitor. Chalmers Watson pronounced his work "wholly admirable," while Sir Frederick Mott, the pathologist to the London County Council Mental Hospitals, offered extravagant praise for Cotton's accomplishments. And William Hunter, the surgeon to whom Cotton attributed the original hypothesis connecting mental illness and focal infection, declared they had just listened to "one of the greatest accomplishments connected with the subject of mental disease" – an "utterly sound" piece of scientific work that in the words of George Robertson, the President of the MPA, "should have served to draw members from the alluring and tempting pastures of psychogenesis back to the narrower, steeper, more rugged and arduous, yet straighter paths, of general medicine. [For after all,] here were results which no one could deny" (Anonymous 1923a).

In a separate editorial on "Chronic Sepsis and Mental Disease," the editors of the *Journal of Mental Science* complimented Cotton on his "remarkable courage and tenacity" and expressed the hope that his work "will herald the dawn of a brighter day for those afflicted with mental disease and for the practice of psychiatry." Certainly, they added, "the idea that there may be one basic morbid condition underlying all these psychoses will not come as a matter of surprise to many psychiatrists." The prospects were simply revolutionary: "If, by eliminating chronic sepsis in cases of manic-depressive insanity, dementia praecox, paranoid conditions, the psychoneuroses, and toxic psychoses, between 80 and 90 percent recover, what a jettisoning of cherished theories, beliefs, and writings there will be!" [*If*, indeed!] The editors recognized that the breakthrough, Dr Cotton's kind gestures towards British antecedents notwithstanding, was essentially American, but thanks to Dr Graves, "a beginning has been made in Birmingham. It is now up to London and other great cities... not to lag behind" (Anonymous 1923b).

Graves certainly had no intention of leaving it to others to prove the truth of his contentions. Nor was he content, like some of his colleagues, simply to lament the fact that "psychiatry has failed to keep pace with progress to the same extent as other branches of medicine" or to bemoan a fate which left the specialty in "regrettable isolation... occupying a position in relation to medicine as a whole analogous to that of a certified patient to the life of the community." Encouraged by the reception accorded to his and Cotton's ideas, he moved promptly and aggressively to implement a broader assault on focal sepsis than had previously been possible. A visiting gynecologist and ear, nose, and throat (ENT) specialist were added to the hospital staff (a full-time dentist, Yaxall, had already been appointed); and Neville Chamberlain, MP arrived to open a newly established research laboratory at Hollymoor, before the year's end. By 1926, Graves had at his disposal a whole new set of buildings at Rubery Hill to which patients could be brought for the most advanced forms of treatment such as operating theatres, as well as rooms for hydrotherapy, ultraviolet light treatment, and colonic lavage. With a full-time pathologist (F.A. Pickworth),[14] bacteriological laboratories, X-ray facilities, etc. he could boast that he had moved decisively to break down the barriers between psychiatry and general medicine, and to introduce the latest scientific advances into the treatment of mental disorder.

The following July, Graves received a visit at Rubery Hill from Henry Cotton, who was *en route* to the joint meeting of the British Medical Association and the RMPA (as it had become in 1926) in Edinburgh, and took the occasion to compare notes. Cotton's extravagant claims of therapeutic success had in the interim prompted his hospital managers to sponsor an external review of his work, a report they intended to use to document his successes, but one whose findings in the event threatened to discredit his whole approach, and with it the general enthusiasm for the focal sepsis theory. He seems, however, to have given no hint of his troubles to Graves, let alone to the profession at large when he addressed them a few weeks later, and when his mentor, Adolf Meyer, suppressed the negative findings, the crisis passed and Cotton's work could continue unchecked.[15]

Unquestionably, though, Cotton was relieved to find himself in more sympathetic surroundings and in the company of another true believer. At Birmingham, he discovered that Graves had developed the treatment of focal sepsis in a number of directions that had not yet occurred to him using injections with anti-typhoid vaccine, for instance ("It produces a chill and a sharp rise in temperature, 103 to 105, which in an hour subsides .... The results were remarkably satisfactory."); and a superior method for diagnosing and treating sinus infections ("pushing a cannula through the nose, puncturing the sinus, withdrawing the contents, and actually seeing the pus").[16] On another front, "The treatment was rather similar to ours as far as teeth and tonsils were concerned [though] it was rather astonishing to see them extract teeth without any local or general anesthetic ... the patients did not seem to object to this method of extraction" (Cotton 1927).[17]

From Birmingham, the two men traveled north together to Edinburgh, where they took starring roles together at the joint meeting of the RMPA and the mental diseases section of the BMA, virtually all of which was devoted to a series of papers promoting the idea of focal infection as the common cause in the functional psychoses – a constellation of diseases William Hunter (1927) suggested should now be renamed "septic psychoses."[18] Graves himself spoke forcibly about "the possibilities of thorough disinfection"; and Cotton once more reviewed his astonishing achievements at Trenton, modestly adding in the informal discussion that followed that "The work at Birmingham under Dr Graves went beyond anything that had been done in the United States" (Anonymous 1927: 807). Both men then basked in the praise of the assembled luminaries, with Sir Berkeley Moynihan, the incumbent President of the Royal College of Surgeons, providing a particularly lengthy and fulsome endorsement of their work. Emphasizing the pioneering role of his fellow-surgeon, William Hunter in demonstrating "the part played by slight and continuously overlooked forms of sepsis in causing distant and apparently unconnected disorders" (it was "the most illuminating thing that had happened in medicine in the twentieth century [and] of the truth of his teaching there is not the slightest doubt"), Sir Berkeley concluded his speech with a bow towards the two alienists:

> The work of Cotton...in New York,...and of Graves in this country seems to set us a new standard of inquiry in this branch of medicine, and to show that no mental hospital will in future be considered as adequately equipped unless it has an x-ray laboratory, a skilled bacteriologist, and can command the services of an enlightened surgeon.
>
> (Moynihan 1927: 815, 817)[19]

Only D.K. Henderson, superintendent of the Gartnavel Royal Hospital in Glasgow, ventured any serious dissent from the prevailing atmosphere of mutual self-congratulation. His attempt to draw attention to the work of some of Cotton's American critics, Kopeloff and Kirby, was roundly dismissed by William Hunter (the Americans had failed because they had made only token efforts to remove the sources of sepsis, generally extracting only a handful of teeth at a time; and besides "Kopeloff was not even a doctor; he was a bacteriologist. He did not think psychiatrists need worry about Kopeloff's work") (Anonymous 1927: 726; Hunter 1927: 464–466). And Henderson's objection that "it was a great mistake to lay down dogmatic generalisations regarding cures founded on an individual case," coupled with a suggestion that "the cure of the woman cited by Dr. Hunter who had eleven bad teeth extracted might be due to the building up of her strength during two years in the hospital ward" was greeted by derisive laughter.[20]

Graves, as it happens, characteristically adopted precisely the style of reasoning Henderson complained about in his reports on the successes associated with his work (see Graves 1929, 1932a, 1938), and was convinced beyond any shadow of a doubt that his clinical experience was sufficient to prove the validity of his theory. In demonstrating the value of his treatment methods, he routinely added sections to his papers illustrating a variety of cases "cured" as a result of his interventions. He also showed how, where the disease proved resistant to one or another means of "detoxication," it could be overcome by yet further interventions directed at "daughter infections" or designed to stimulate the body's defenses on a more global level. Henderson's appeal for controlled studies, with patients "divided into two groups as nearly identical as possible...one group...treated surgically, while the other group had no surgical treatment" (Anonymous 1927: 817) evidently fell on deaf ears so far as Graves was concerned.

At the Edinburgh conference, Henry Cotton had announced (not entirely accurately) that "he no longer recommended colectomy, but used copious colonic douches instead," and added that "the results of this irrigation in 600 cases had been very satisfactory" (Cotton 1927: 817).[21] Following Cotton's return to Trenton in 1927, Graves wrote for advice about this new approach, and subsequently devised an elaborate new apparatus of his own to permit "continuous colonic irrigation," with different solutions used to wash out the bowel and treat "intestinal toxaemia" – a technological breakthrough he subsequently shared with his colleagues (Graves and Turner 1930).[22] Nasal washouts became an equally routine part of the therapeutic regime, as the sinuses came to be seen as a site of dangerous infections rivaled only by the teeth and gums. Meanwhile, alongside surgical intervention to drain or eliminate sources of infection, simultaneous efforts were made "to stimulate a focal reaction" of the body's own defenses through what was termed "non-specific therapy": injections of colloidal calcium oleate, of colloidal sulphur, or TAB – with the latter often inducing nausea and fever, reactions Graves saw as "an indicator of the activity of the agent" as well as a measure of "the severity of the general toxaemia" (Graves 1931, 1932a,b).

The death of Graves' first wife in 1932 was followed a year later by his marriage to one of his assistant doctors at Rubery Hill, Kathleen Sykes, an anesthesiologist-turned-psychiatrist. Sykes' published account of the hospital routine makes clear what a newly admitted patient could look forward to in these years. First, all new patients would be confined to bed for a week or more, rest being obviously essential to gathering one's internal resources for the fight against infection. A complete physical examination and a series of blood tests followed, and then the visiting specialists were mobilized: "dental and ear, nose and throat...gynaecologist...opthamologist [and] the X-ray Department." All of this activity allowed the formation of a rational and individualized treatment plan. Active therapeutic efforts generally began with attention to the teeth, whose extraction permitted "an obvious source of infection [to be] removed with little shock to the patient." Further bed rest was generally followed by operations by the ENT specialist to remove the tonsils and explore the state of the sinuses while the patient was under general anaesthetic. After a further period of bed rest to recuperate, next there was an attempt at "stimulating his resistance with some form of non-specific therapy" (injections of colloidal sulphur or Burroughs Wellcome's TAB vaccine), interventions aimed at inducing "a pyrexial response of between 103 and 105." Meanwhile, the "large proportion of female patients...found to have uterine endocervitis" could expect treatment by "cauterization followed by antiseptic douches." Male and female alike, if they were among the "many patients found to have infected colons," were then taken into special treatment rooms where "muco-pus or pus in quantities is washed away and the condition greatly improved by a course of continuous colonic lavage administered on one of the special tables in use here." Now "relieved of their sources of gross toxaemia," the convalescing finished up with "a course of ultra-violet light treatment" (Sykes 1933).[23]

Though Graves was to remain a forcible advocate for the position that "psychotics are physically infirm" and that there existed "a common cause for the mental and physical illness" (Graves 1940: 608), it is not clear how many converts he managed to win and retain for his views among his psychiatric colleagues. At the outset, as we have seen, a number of leading figures, not just in psychiatry but in general medicine and in surgery, were enthusiastic converts to the focal sepsis hypothesis. Wagner von Jauregg's discovery of the malarial treatment for general paresis had both stimulated a certain degree of therapeutic optimism, and had brought renewed attention to the realm of somatic treatments. With little else of comparable promise or appeal on offer, with extraordinary results reported from its practical implementation in the United States, and presenting an etiological account of insanity that corresponded to the dominant contemporary model of disease and was linked rationally in its turn to a set of straightforward therapeutic interventions, the doctrine of focal sepsis had some obvious attractions. For psychiatrists, such an explanation of mental illness offered a way back into the medical mainstream, and since the treatment of focal sepsis required the use of the most advanced forms of medical technology as well as the services of a variety of medical specialists (surgeons, gynecologists, oto-laryngologists, and pathologists, not to mention dentists) it was likely to appeal to a broader medical constituency as well. Even patients and their families, desperate for some glimmer of hope and anxious to distance themselves from the stigma that had hitherto attached itself to mental disorder, were likely to find an explanation of their troubles couched in such familiar terms almost irresistible.

Who, after all, could argue against the need to eradicate infection? The most skeptical of Graves' and Cotton's claims – Henderson in the United Kingdom, Kopeloff and Kirby in the United States – were nonetheless hard-put to assert that the physical ailments now targeted for attack could be safely left untreated, inhibiting the force of at least some of their criticism.[24] Disinfecting the body, washing out or excising pus, infection, and decay – these were approaches and a terminology with a powerful appeal, symbolic, and otherwise, to both professional and lay audiences. Nor, particularly among working class patients, was there any shortage of troublesome chronic infections in evident need of treatment such as malnutrition (an increasing problem in these years of growing unemployment), inadequate (or non-existent) medical care, and poor (and often infected) teeth were endemic problems among the lower orders, providing a demonstrable array of somatic pathologies to which attention could be directed once patients were admitted to the mental hospital.

Even in the 1920s and early 1930s, however, Graves hardly won everyone over to his cause, and many who voiced some degree of support were nonetheless some considerable distance from fully embracing his approach. In the immediate vicinity, both Rampton Hospital and the Worcester County Mental Hospital at Powick[25] enthusiastically adopted Graves' techniques, and other evidence suggests his ideas were being implemented at the Chester County Mental Hospital, at the East Sussex County Mental Hospital, at the Cardiff City Mental Hospital, and at the Hallam Hospital in Sheffield

(Shera 1930; Anonymous 1931; Goodall 1932; Potts 1935). The unprecedented turnout when the Northern and Midland Division of the RMPA held its autumn 1932 meeting at Rubery Hill likewise indicates at the very least a high degree of interest in Graves' ideas (see Anonymous 1933).

Whether because he was more honest or less deluded than Cotton, however, or perhaps because of the relatively strict oversight exercised by the Board of Control, Graves never laid claim to the kinds of extraordinary cure rates his American counterpart insisted he had achieved. Since vague claims that "His figures for discharges proved that his methods were more successful than those generally employed in other mental hospitals" (F.A. Pickworth, quoted in Anonymous 1964b: 1400) were scarcely borne out in the statistics appearing in the hospitals' annual reports, spectacular therapeutic success could not be invoked to convert the doubtful. As for other means of winning converts, the very force of Graves' personality could repel as well as attract, and his insistence that focal sepsis was the common cause of the functional insanities scarcely endeared him to his more eclectic colleagues. More seriously still, published reports began to cast doubt on just how widespread sepsis was among the mentally ill, to query whether the rate of focal infection differed as between the sane and the insane, and to call into question the methods Graves and his colleagues used to assess the presence of focal sepsis (see Rumbaut 1934; Jowett 1936).[26] When coupled with spreading doubts about the therapeutic efficacy of such measures as sinus irrigation, autogenous vaccines, and so forth, these developments gradually weakened his influence on the profession.

The appeal of the doctrine of focal sepsis to most psychiatrists suffered a further series of blows in the late 1930s and early 1940s, as a number of other somatic treatments, generally resting upon a very different logic, came to the fore. At the time such innovations as insulin coma therapy, cardiazol, and electrically induced convulsions (the only treatment of this sort still in widespread use today), together with various forms of leucotomy, were widely hailed, and represented an obvious rival for the profession's intellectual loyalties. Though inclined to experiment with insulin (and subsequently in a more limited way with cardiazol), as still another method of stimulating the body's own defenses (V. Graves 1986), Graves was sharply critical of alternative somatic approaches, even as other psychiatrists hastened to adopt them.[27]

Graves' marginalization in his own profession grew more marked as his own views became more and more eccentric.[28] Ironically, this process must have accelerated once he was elected President of the RMPA (a development that owed much to the outbreak of the Second World War, and the departure into military psychiatry of men who might otherwise have been his rivals for the honor). His "Presidential Address," issued under the long-winded title of "Diphasic Vascular Variation in the Treatment of Mental Inefficiency Arising From a Common Somatic Cause" (Graves 1940), reiterated his prior views about focal sepsis with a new and peculiar twist, couched in prose which verged upon (and at times lapsed into) incoherence. (For a similar assessment of this speech, see Ogden 1983: 5–6.)[29] Graves now insisted that sepsis could be either "open" or "closed" (i.e. draining or encapsulated), requiring different therapeutic responses and imposing different risks on the organism. Therapies which increased vascularity in the presence of open sepsis would allow more toxins to be expelled from the body, thus promoting healing, but increased vascularity in the presence of closed lesions would have counter-productive effects, promoting the production and absorption of the poisons thrown off by the hidden focal infections. Quite explicitly, he invoked a homeostatic vision of the bodily economy deriving from Hippocrates, and, arguing that "an abscess, an excretory disease if its discharges are drainable, can be an excellent development," drew the parallel with "the use in the past of setons and blisters in order to induce what was hoped would be such excretory conditions" (Graves 1940: 757, 760).

The following year, he organized a symposium for the one hundredth meeting of the RMPA, held in London on July 17, 1941. Significantly, while a whole series of ENT specialists[30] appeared to testify to the crucial significance of sinusitis in the genesis of mental disorder, only his long-time supporter H.F. Fenton of Worcester joined Graves in whole-heartedly endorsing their claims. Several psychiatrists, indeed, voiced the heretical view that

> in most of these cases one was not dealing with sinus infection as a cause of mental disorder at all. What was being done . . . was to introduce a very radical method of suggestion into the minds of patients and it was not remarkable if they showed the same "improvement" as was apparently to be found in all the recently introduced "successful" treatments of schizophrenia.
>
> (Anonymous 1941)

Since "medicine in general had rather abandoned focal sepsis," it was surely "rather a pity" for their President to insist that "they should have to examine all their patients for nasal sepsis," particularly when their own "ear, nose, and throat surgeons told them it was not as common as all that" (Anonymous 1941: 526–527).

Graves would have none of such skepticism. He insisted that "he was quite satisfied that the essential point was to get at the portal of entrance" (Anonymous 1941: 527). With the outbreak of the war, Hollymoor had been transformed into a military hospital, with its existing patients redistributed to the other mental hospitals in the Birmingham region and Graves installed as its commandant (alongside his continuing role as superintendent at Rubery Hill). Many of the soldiers now arriving for treatment had suffered head injuries, and, given Graves' convictions, these patients, too, soon found themselves being treated vigorously and thoroughly for hidden foci of infection (Graves 1941a,b: 10–14; F. Graves 1986).

One of the most remarkable therapeutic changes of the era, of course, was the advent of penicillin, which opened up new vistas for the assault on bacterial infections. By the closing year of the war, Graves had recognized the significance of the new antibiotic and was anxious to incorporate it into his treatment of sepsis. Supplies, however, remained short, and the authorities proved reluctant to divert some of the precious drug to a mental hospital. Accordingly, Graves began culturing his own crude "penicillin filtrate" in jam jars all over the hospital, giving the resulting solution orally (V. Graves 1986).[31] Subsequently, when he obtained "a small supply of 'pure' penicillin" it was "given to a few cases by intramuscular injection," with what Graves reported were uniformly favorable results (Graves 1946). By this time, however, the doctrine of focal infection had lost whatever credibility it had once possessed, and his psychiatric colleagues appear to have greeted his assertions with indifference.[32]

Still supported by the Birmingham Mental Hospitals Committee, and aided by the uncertainties attending the end of the war, Graves nonetheless continued as superintendent at Rubery Hill and Hollymoor until 1948, and with the advent of the National Health Service, he was retained as a consultant psychiatrist until his retirement in 1950. Convinced till the end of the correctness of his own theories, he planned to devote his retirement to writing up his case materials and to producing a monograph which would decisively demonstrate the crucial importance of treating focal sepsis. But the world was now passing him by. With the advent of the psychopharmaceutical era in the mid 1950s, the biological treatment of mental disorder, for which he had tirelessly campaigned, acquired a wholly new focus and meaning. Publishers displayed no interest in the results of his labors, and as his own mental condition deteriorated, he labored endlessly over his elephantine manuscript (now grown to several thousand pages, much of it scribbled on the backs of old envelopes) (V. Graves 1986).

In the end, Graves' declining condition led to his admission into a nursing home. Here, on June 6, 1964, aged 81, his life came to a close. He was buried in the grounds of the Baptist chapel at Histon, what began as a promising career having come to what must have been a bitter and depressing conclusion.

Notes

1 Musings about madness

1 "The ordinary and efficient means by which the aberrations of the human mind are detected, are minute observations of the individual's conduct, inspection of his written documents, and protracted conversations to develop his delusions: and these examinations, on many occasions, require to be frequently repeated, before the insanity of the person can be exposed. For these tedious processes Dr. Burrows has a remedy, which must be considered a peculiar endowment, the operation of which constitutes the greatest of modern improvements, and may be viewed as a short cut to the discovery of madness.... The maniacal odour is not noticed by every writer on the signs of insanity; nor as I have said, is it always present; but I consider it a pathognomonic symptom so unerring, that if I detected it in any person, I should not hesitate to pronounce him insane, every though I had no other proof of it."

2 The insanity of place

1 A slightly different version of this paper was originally presented as the plenary address to the conference on "Space and Psyche," held at Oxford Brookes University in December 2002. I am grateful to German Berrios for his comments on the original text.

2 Compare on this point W.A.F. Browne's panegyric to the asylum for its value "in establishing tranquility, and in suggesting a deportment which closely resembles, if it do [sic] not entirely realize, that of sanity and serenity" Crichton Royal Lunatic Asylum (1851: 28).

3 A half century earlier, John Charles Bucknill (1860: 7) had lamented that "he who efficiently discharges the arduous functions attendant on the care and treatment of the insane, dwells in a morbid atmosphere of thought and feeling, a perpetual 'Walpurgis Night' of lurid delusion, the perils of which he, who walks though even the most difficult paths of sane human effort, can little appreciate.... The number of mental physicians who have suffered more or less from the seeming contagion of mental disease, would form, perhaps, if enquired into, a proportion of those who really fight in this warfare which might bear some comparison even with that of men who fall in the strife of the sword." Note that the effects of this morbid atmosphere on the vastly greater number of patients were passed over in silence.

4 Humanity and economics (the so-called economics of compassion) were, of course, precisely the major arguments nineteenth-century lunacy reformers had advanced for building the asylums in the first place.

5 Ben Silcock, a schizophrenic, made headlines when he climbed into the lions' cage at the London Zoo and was mauled by the animals.

3   A failure to communicate? On the reception of Foucault's *Histoire de la folie* by Anglo-American historians

1   Stone reprints Foucault's reply, as well as his own ill-judged attempt to have the last word, in Stone (1987). See my discussion of this episode in Scull (1988). As I shall demonstrate in what follows, several of Stone's criticisms (e.g. that Foucault is careless with historical detail, neglects elementary conventions of historiography, and ignores the cross-societal *differences* in European responses to madness), though clumsily made and poorly documented, turn out to contain a substantial kernel of truth. Perhaps this explains the interesting publication history (or non-history) in France. Lawrence Stone has informed me that, before his exchange with Foucault was published in the *New York Review of Books* (and before he had seen Stone's reply), Foucault insisted that the exchange should also appear simultaneously in the French journal *Le Débat*. Stone and Robert Silvers, the editor of the *New York Review*, agreed to these terms, subject to the proviso that the debate was to be reprinted in its entirety, and that Stone would be allowed to respond to any further comments by Foucault. To meet an urgent deadline at the French end, the galleys containing the exchange were rushed to Paris. But the planned French translation never appeared, because Foucault intervened at the last moment to prevent its appearance. (The key elements in Lawrence Stone's account of these events have been confirmed separately by Robert Silvers and by Pierre Nora, editor of *Le Débat*, in letters to me dated July 13, 1990 and October 25, 1990 respectively.) In acknowledging that the non-publication was at Foucault's insistence ("Il m'a demandé ensuite de ne pas le faire"), M. Nora hastens to add that this was "non par censure mais parce qu'il [Foucault] pensait que ce échange n'avait pas beaucoup d'intérêt et ne méritait pas...'le voyage transatlantique'." Bien sûr. Its "triviality" and lack of intrinsic interest doubtless explain why the exchange is accorded so little significance by the English-speaking members of the Foucauldian cult.

2   Foucault's confession, in correspondence with Maher and Maher (1982: 759) that "The documentation which I have utilized for *L'Histoire de la folie* comes in large part from the library at Upsala [*sic*]" perhaps explains – though it scarcely excuses – the shortcomings of his scholarship and the weakness of the evidentiary basis on which he relies throughout the book.

3   Compare, too, Jean-Claude Guédon (1977: 273): "Moreover he generally uses a range of sources sufficiently wide to satisfy even the most demanding historian." (One might object that simply referring to a wide range of sources is not the same thing as using them in ways that would satisfy "the most demanding historian"; but in any event, the objection would be superfluous, for Guédon's claim is demonstrably false.)

4   Nicholls (1854) [Foucault cites the 1898 edition]; Nicholls (1856) [referred to in the text of Histoire de la folie, but omitted from the bibliography]. This tendency to rely on very selectively mined nineteenth-century sources of dubious provenance is a recurrent feature of Foucault's discussions. Indeed, Colin Gordon's defense of Foucault's scholarship refers on several occasions to his habit of plucking his "facts" from such sources, without displaying any sense of unease or concern about the implications of this practice for the reliability of the evidentiary foundation on which Foucault's flights of fancy purport to rest.

5   It is precisely the essentially tangential character of this passage which allowed for its entire and unnoticed excision from the abridged French edition and subsequent English translation. Note, too, that in Foucault's view, the differences are largely temporary and transitional. In less than a half dozen paragraphs, he

presents a brief discussion of Calvinist and Lutheran attitudes to poverty, and their impact in creating "une forme nouvelle de sensibilite a la misère" in northern Europe, then asserts that

> Par des chemins différents – et non sans de nombreuses difficultes – le catholicisme arrivera... à des resultats tout à fait analogues... Bientôt, le monde catholique va adopter un mode de perception de la misère qui s'etait developpé surtout dans le monde protestant.
>
> (Foucault 1972: 69, 70, 71)

6 "D'ailleurs, les nouveaux hôpitaux qui sont en train de s'ouvrir ne sont guère différents, dans leurs structure, de ceux qui les avaient précédés d'un siècle... pour être specialement destinés aux insensés, les hôpitaux nouveaux ne laissent guère plus de place a la médicine" (Foucault 1972: 406).

7 *Pace* Colin Gordon (1990b: 390–391), the difficulties here do not derive from the xenophobia of a bluff Anglo-Saxon historian, resistant to "foreign" ideology and unwilling grant "French facts" the same empirical weight as their English counterparts. It is not just that one can legitimately raise questions about the facticity of some of Foucault's facts (cf. Fairchilds 1976; Swain 1977; Gauchet and Swain 1980), and about the scholarly acceptability of what Jan Goldstein (1990: 334–336) suggests is "a deliberate rhetorical strategy on Foucault's part" of vacillation and ambiguity on the question of "whether [his book] is about France, or whether the France in its pages is supposed to represent the west." More importantly, I would argue that it is in good measure through this substitution of rhetorical gamesmanship for a serious comparative examination of the European encounter with madness that Foucault is able to circumvent the difficult but crucial task of providing a systematic examination of the relevance of the economic and the political realms to the understanding of the issues at hand.

8 "[D]epuis les grecs, [le médecine de l'esprit] n'était qu'un chapitre de la médecine, et nous avons vu Willis étudier les folies sous la rubrique des 'maladies de la tête'..." (Foucault 1965: 275, 1972: 527).

9 I have expanded on my discussion of this issue here (as compared with that offered in Scull 1990) in the first place because of the importance of spelling out the precise nature of Foucault's claims about the relationship between moral treatment and mental medicine; but also because Colin Gordon (1990b: 390–391) has objected that my earlier more truncated criticism had relied on selective quotation to prove its point (and had carelessly or stupidly failed to grasp that Foucault's analysis was actually identical to mine). In particular, he has claimed that in omitting the words "On croit" which immediately precede the phrase "Tuke et Pinel ont ouvert l'asile a la connaissance medicale" in *Histoire de la folie*, I have played fast and loose with Foucault's text for my own disreputable purposes. Not so. As the much more extended passages quoted here make clear (and the reader is also referred to the complete discussion in Foucault 1972: 523–527), Foucault is unquestionably one of those who "croit" that this is so. As for Gordon's claim that "Goldstein shows that Foucault's discussion of Tuke and Pinel, if read with a modicum of attentiveness, can be seen to expound the same view as Scull's on this matter" (Gordon 1990b: 390): I don't know whether to be flattered by the concession from a Foucauldian that I've at last got something right (albeit presumably by the neat trick of simultaneously misunderstanding and misappropriating the master); or bewildered by the creative (mis)reading of texts which allows him to make such a judgment. Goldstein, to my eyes, at least, claims nothing of the sort. She *does* suggest that Foucault was aware of Tuke's lay

status (though she concedes that he fails "to mention this seemingly important fact") (Goldstein 1990: 338); and I am sure she is correct on this point. (The lay origins of the English version of moral treatment are too blindingly obvious to be missed by anyone who reads the *Description of the Retreat* (Tuke 1813), as we know that Foucault did.) Her own creative account of what Foucault was up to (1990: 337–339) stresses his deliberate use of ambiguity as a tool "for breaking down conventional categories of analysis and thereby of defamiliarizing the past;" and, in a clever attempt to rescue a dubious line of argument, suggests that Foucault's strategy in emphasizing the way moral treatment transforms the asylum into "a medical space" depends upon a deliberate blurring of two distinct senses of medicine – medicine as the generic relief of suffering, and medicine as the application of physical remedies. Whether or not one chooses to accept her analysis (and one should recognize that its adoption would simultaneously require the dangerous concession that Foucault "revels" in ambiguity, but "never stops to analyse it or to provide us with a sober definition of terms that would clarify it" (Goldstein 1990: 338)), even Goldstein would concede the gulf between Foucault's project and my own attempt to provide a coherent and persuasive account of how professional control over madness was secured by physicians. Let me insist again: on the crucial issue of the *threat* moral treatment posed to the medical monopolization of the treatment of the mad, Foucault is utterly silent, and in my view, that silence cannot but be construed as a major misunderstanding of the significance of the events he purports to analyze.

10 See the more extended discussion in Scull (1989: 1–30).

11 An alternative text makes it abundantly clear that this is Foucault's central claim about madness in the pre-modern era. In 1962, a year after the publication of *Histoire de la folie*, Foucault's first book, *Maladie mentale et personalité* (1954) was reissued under the new title, *Maladie mentale et psychologie*. Its two new chapters on "Madness and Culture" contained Foucault's own précis of his argument, a text subsequently blessed by one of his epigones as "a stunning ten-page summary of [*Histoire de la folie*]" (Dreyfus 1987: xxvii). Having noted "the great prestige of madness" in the Renaissance, Foucault proceeds to stress that

> Generally speaking, madness was allowed free reign; it circulated throughout society, it formed part of the background and language of everyday life, it was for everyone an everyday experience that one sought not to exalt nor to control... Up to about 1650, Western culture was strangely hospitable to these forms of experience. About the middle of the seventeenth century a sudden change took place: the world of madness was to become the world of exclusion.... madness, which had for so long been present on the horizon, disappeared. It entered a phase of silence from which it was not to emerge for a long time; it was deprived of its language; and although one continued to speak of it, it became impossible for it to speak of itself.
>
> (Foucault 1987: 67–69)

12 "Il arrivait que certains insensés soient fouettes publiquement, et qu'au cours d'une sorte de jeu, ils soient ensuite poursuivies dans une course simulée et chassés de la ville à coups de verges" (Foucault 1965: 10, 1972: 21). So far as I can tell, this is the only reference Foucault makes to whipping, and the modifiers in the passage are not without interest: it *happens* that *certain* madmen... in the course of *a kind of game... a mock race*...find themselves subject to the whip; and the chasing out of town, so we are informed in the next sentence, is "un partage rituel," a *ritual* exile. There is material here for our semiotic friends to play with.

13 It is telling that even a participant in this debate who is relatively sympathetic to Gordon's position (LaCapra 1990: 32, 38) recognizes the weakness of his argument here. In response, Gordon (1990b: 388) has now been forced to concede that Foucault "elaborates his material with a certain degree of poetic license, at times blurring together the possible symbolic meanings of material practices and cultural motifs." But the same passage reveals a desperate attempt to rescue the reality of the ship of fools: I refer not just to the remarkable admission that Foucault may possibly have resorted to "slightly hyperbolic usage" (wishful thinking is more like it – as Midelfort (1990: 42) comments, "Foucault's few footnotes...do not substantiate a single ship of fools"); or even to the pathetic remark that "What Foucault is saying, by saying that there were actual ships of fools in the middle ages, is that some mad people travelled, for various reasons, in boats along European rivers in the course of the middle ages" (Gordon 1990b: 387); but also to the Alice-in-Wonderland attempts to reverse the plain meaning of Foucault's own text. Foucault (1965: 8, 1972: 19) writes: "Souvent, les villes d'Europe ont du voir aborder ces navires de fous" – "Often the cities of Europe must have seen these 'ships of fools' approaching their harbors." Gordon (1990b: 337–338) glosses: "This 'must' is probably one of the kind which actually...conveys a less than apodictic certainty." Where "must" is to be rendered "may just possibly have" one has indeed entered, in Gordon's (1990b: 393) own words, "a regime of commentary under which anything goes." Perhaps conscious of the frailty of this line of defense, Gordon (1990b: 388, 387) tries the alternative to downgrade the importance of the whole episode anyway: it lies, he suggests, "at the extreme initial margin of [Foucault's] theme and period" and the passages in question "cover six pages out of 600." But this won't do either, for the claimed marginality is a myth. Any unprejudiced reading of Foucault's text "must" (and I mean this in the ordinary, taken-for-granted, standard sense of the term) acknowledge the centrality of "the ship of fools,...given the metaphoric and argumentative role of Foucault's correlation of the Renaissance with embarkation in contrast to the linkage to the classical age with confinement and the house of confinement" (LaCapra 1990: 32).

14 For instance, following the appearance of inadequate English versions of Durkheim's *The Division of Labor in Society* and of his *Rules of Sociological Method* in 1933 and 1938 respectively, corrected versions did not appear in print until the 1980s (Durkheim 1982, 1984); and the haphazard appearance of translations of bits and pieces of Max Weber's *magnum opus*, *Wirtschaft und Gesellschaft* (poor as some of them were) meant that a translation of the whole was put off for something close to half a century (Weber 1968). Durkheim and Weber had the excuse of being dead, and hence of possessing no means of rectifying matters; but it was Foucault himself who licensed the production of an abbreviated version of his argument in *Histoire de la folie* for English-speaking audiences, and who made no move to alter this situation over the space of more than twenty years, long after his status as a cultural icon would have made the issue of the complete version a financially viable proposition.

15 Elswhere (Scull 1989: 15), I have pointed out that the reasons for the appearance of only an abridged text in English "remain obscure" and have suggested that "perhaps Foucault did not object too strenuously" to this state of affairs, since a truncated version of his argument, with its sometimes abrupt transitions, more readily accommodated itself to his later emphasis on historical discontinuities. I echoed here in tentative form a hypothesis first advanced by Erik Midelfort (1980). Colin Gordon (1990b: 386) attributes such suggestions to "moments of genuine intellectual disorientation" occurring in what he, with uncharacteristic

generosity, acknowledges to be "otherwise lucid minds." I do not want to make too much of this issue, since it is one on which I have always insisted that closure, or even a reasonable degree of certainty, is impossible. But I would point out that the idea that Foucault sought to influence the fate of his ideas through a strategic deployment and concealment of texts is more plausible than Gordon allows. One may instance several examples of him behaving in just this fashion: the suppression of the publication in French of his exchange with Lawrence Stone (see note 1 earlier); his repeated refusals to allow the republication of his first book, *Maladie mentale et psychologie*, in French, and his unsuccessful attempts to prevent the appearance of an English edition (Gordon 1990b: 386); his suppression of the original preface to *Histoire de la folie* in the second edition (Foucault 1972; see Sheridan 1980: 11, and Philo 2004: 36, 68, n. 147); and his written instruction that no posthumous manuscripts of his were to be published (Rabinow 1990: 56). Whatever one makes of these episodes, they certainly suggest that Foucault played a more active role in the management of his *oeuvre* and his image than Gordon is willing to acknowledge. Fortunately, the Foucault Archive has found a way around the master's injunction about the publication of posthumous manuscripts, and substantial portions of Foucault's unpublished work, including his lectures at the Collège de France, have begun to appear in print. One final point, correcting an earlier mis-statement of mine: in previous versions of this paper (Scull 1990, 1992), I had suggested that the Foucault Archive had adopted the notorious practices of the Freud Archive, screening who was to be allowed access, and censoring what was published. I was led to this conclusion by some comments in Rabinow (1990: 56), but I am delighted to have been proved wrong on this point and would like apologize for inadvertently making this claim in the first place.

16 One last comment: Gordon (1990b: 381–382, 393) repeatedly seeks to impugn the honesty and scholarly *bona fides* of Foucault's critics, frequently resorting to what I can only describe as smear tactics (while simultaneously protesting that he is not motivated by "the sad passions of the sectarian" and that he seeks to avoid "the stale and gloomy incriminatorial mode"). We critical voices, the unwashed and unconverted, are, it seems, poor "defensive" creatures, unwilling to face up to our own "insecurities" – feebly trying to practice "normal science . . . while teetering over an abyss." Called to account for our failings, we persist in egregious error "in ways which reveal an unusually drastic economizing of intellectual and scholarly means." Doubts are even expressed about whether (unspecified) particular individual participants in the debate have, "as a matter of fact, ever managed to find the necessary time to read [*Histoire de la folie*], let alone to reread it." And, in consequence, our judgments about the work in question are, it seems, "largely a matter of [in?]judicious guesswork." One cannot help at least feeling a twinge of admiration for the chutzpah all this represents. Astonishing and incredible as it may seem to Colin Gordon, however, one may be acquainted with the full panoply of Foucault's history of madness without being tempted to embrace his oracular utterances as revealed truth.

5 The mad-doctor and his craft

1 This essay, which originally appeared in the *Times Literary Supplement*, draws upon the text of the books I wrote with Jonathan Andrews (Andrews and Scull 2001, 2003), and though this particular synopsis is mine, it should properly be seen as the joint product of our labors.

6 Museums of madness revisited

1 A slightly revised version of the Presidential Address to the Society for the Social History of Medicine, All Souls College, Oxford University, June 1993.

2 Public visitation did not come to an abrupt end in 1770, but rather than Bethlem being open to all comers for a penny or tuppence a time, the hospital authorities now instituted a ticket system. Andrews suggests (1991: 93, 386) that "the graduate curtailment of visiting in the 1760s cannot simply be interpreted as a reaction to the mounting disenchantment of the educated public. It was partly an internal response to an escalation of the problems posed by visitors beyond the hospital's capacity to cope." Ironically, however, "the situation at the hospital appears to have markedly deteriorated [after] the exclusion of public visitors in 1770. Public access to Bethlem must have constituted both a diversion from, and a constraint upon the abuse of patients by staff, although carrying with it a whole host of other attendant ills."

3 In some distinguished company, I must confess to relying upon and helping to disseminate this myth in some of my earlier work, including the first edition of *Museums of Madness*.

4 On Bedlam patients as "curiosities," see *The Gentleman's Magazine*, May 18, 1748, p. 199. From Pepys to Boswell, seventeenth and eighteenth-century diarists recorded visits to Bethlem, often with family, friends from out of town and children in tow, in search of "extraordinarie" or "remarkable" spectacles.

5 As Jonathan Andrews reluctantly concedes, "The major enticement of Bedlamites was entertainment, pure and simple.... Visitors were essentially sightseers, for whom Bethlem was a "sight," and "a rare diversion"...a pleasure rather than a duty" (Andrews 1991: 38).

6 Other examples include Edward Long Fox's madhouse at Cleve, and later at Brislington House, near Bristol; Laverstock House near Salisbury, run by William Finch; Fishponds Asylum, founded in mid-century by the Baptist layman, George Mason (see Phillips 1973); and the Newington family's establishment at Ticehurst, Sussex (see MacKenzie 1987). For a description of another obscure provincial example, see Smith (1992).

7 As early as 1751, Henry Fielding (1751: 24) was complaining that "the introduction of trade...hath indeed given a new face to the whole nation, hath in great measure subverted the former state of affairs, and hath almost totally changed the manners, customs, and habits of the people, more especially of the lower sort."

8 As Keith Thomas (1983: 796) remarks, "Agriculture, after all, was the first sector of the British economy to become thoroughly capitalized and developed in a 'rational' manner. Magic was rejected by men who had faith in the potentiality of technical innovation but it must be remembered that in the sixteenth and seventeenth centuries much of this innovation was agricultural."

9 As Plumb notes (Brewer *et al.* 1982: 326),

> Tens of thousands of men and women, probably hundreds of thousands, were actively concerned in horticulture, eager for novelty and determined on improvement. The importance of this was the sense of modernity and novelty generated by this widespread activity, bent on changing nature. People no longer expected flowers, vegetables or trees to be static objects in the field of creation, but constantly changing, constantly improving, the change and the improvement due to the experimental activity of man.

10 Note the stress on esteem and disgrace, and the idea of putting them *into* children. Locke's educational doctrines acquired an ever greater popularity among the

upper and middle classes in the latter half of the eighteenth century. Plumb (1975: 70) draws attention to the fact that "by 1780 John Browne could make one the principal virtues of the expensive academy for gentlemen's sons that he proposed to set up a total absence of corporal punishment." (Interestingly enough, one of William Tuke's early philanthropic endeavors, prior to setting up the York Retreat, had been the establishment of Ackworth, a school for girls.) Seen in the context of these slightly earlier changes, Samuel Tuke's comment (Tuke 1813: 150) that "there is much analogy between the judicious treatment of children and that of insane persons" takes on a new significance. In practice, the analogy was to extend even further. When Locke's doctrines (and their intellectual descendants) were modified to accommodate the children of the poor, they spawned the rigidities of the monitorial system such as Andrew Bell's "steam engine of the moral world," and Joseph Lancaster's "new and mechanical system of education." When the techniques of the small, upper-middle class Retreat were adapted to the "requirements" of the mass of pauper lunatics, moral treatment, as we shall see, was simultaneously transformed into a set of management techniques for a custodial holding operation.

11 Andrews correctly emphasizes that one can find anticipations of this broader shift in sentiment even in the late seventeenth century (see, for example, Tryon 1689), and that "the percolation of the new philosophy" was spread out over several decades. Though still far from universal, even among the educated classes, such sentiments were becoming increasingly common and influential by the last third of the eighteenth century.

12 Female patients were particularly likely to be dealt with at home, while well-to-do lunatics of both sexes were funneled into a shadowy network of unlicensed and often illegal establishments specializing in single patients (see Hervey 1987, Vol. 1: 234–237, 242–262). Others were sent abroad, beyond the prying eyes of the Lunacy Commissioners, including, ironically enough, the son of the chairman of the commission, Lord Shaftesbury, packed off to confinement in private lodgings in Lausanne when his epilepsy rendered him mentally disturbed.

13 At Ticehurst, she was scarcely more manageable, being frequently "excited and restless...very talkative and annoying to those about her...throwing herself down when walking, endeavouring to meet men and looking at them in a wanton manner." After less than six months of this, and following complaints from her fellow patients, the Newingtons requested that her sister remove her to some alternative accommodation. Ticehurst Case Book 4, February 17, March 23, April 7, 25, June 6, 1857.

14 Ticehurst Asylum Case Book 5, July 2, 1858. Three days after Mrs F.'s admission, one of the attendants who had fetched her from her home in Blackheath still complained of sickness brought on by the experience of entering her room, "the atmosphere of it was so foul and the stench so great." The variety of eminent medical men dancing attendance on her sick bed had not done much for Mrs F.'s physical health. On admission, "her person was filthily dirty and her face and hands and other parts of her body were covered with boils. Her complexion was very yellow having just recovered from an attack of jaundice... vascular system weak, liver torpid, and its functions greatly deranged – bowels very obstinate, tongue white and much coated at the back, skin flabby and unhealthy."

15 As these facts suggest, and as the Newingtons' observations were subsequently to confirm, "Mrs. F. appears to have the power of inducing her husband to fall in with her wishes in everything." Ticehurst Asylum Case Book, August 28, 1858. Her certification as lunatic was signed by John Conolly, the doyen of English alienists.

16 On the role of violence to people or property, and threats or attempts at suicide in prompting certification as insane and admission into Ticehurst, cf. the discussion in MacKenzie 1992: 287–288.

17 In addition, a far higher fraction of the male patients were suffering from tertiary syphilis, which often produced dramatic psychiatric and neurological symptomatology, but also great and progressive physical debility, necessitating the sort of attentive and full-time nursing care which the elite private asylums were particularly well-placed to provide. Of 50 cases recorded in the Manor House Chiswick Male Case Book for 1884–1891, 11 were diagnosed as definite cases of General Paresis, and a further 6 possibly suffered from the same disorder. Even allowing for diagnostic imprecision prior to the introduction of the Wassermann test, these are striking figures. By contrast, GPI cases were extremely rare, verging on non-existent, among the female population. See Manor House Male Case Book, 1884–1891; and Female Case Book, 1884–1893, in manuscript at the Wellcome Institute for the History of Medicine, London.

18 Samuel Greg, a reformist mill-owner whose history is summarized by Charlotte MacKenzie, is a case in point. As she notes, he suffered a nervous breakdown in 1846, when the workforce at his mill in Cheshire opposed the introduction of new stretching machinery. Following this, he remained a total recluse for nine years, before essaying hydropathic treatment at Malvern and on the Continent. Failing to secure any relief, "he came at length to feel that he must sit down under his burden and live with it as best he could to the end" (MacKenzie 1985: 154, quoting Greg 1877). With considerable understatement, MacKenzie notes that "Such resignation could require tolerance and fortitude from family and friends."

19 Manor House Chiswick Male Case Book, 1884–1891, January 20, 1885. Walter M.S. to C. Molesworth Tuke, January 22, 1885. (His mother, Walter reported, "was horribly shocked when mention of certificates was made.") Almost two years later, on September 28, 1886, Albert S. was "Transferred to private care and discharged, relieved" (in fact, no better in any discernible respect). This may be an appropriate point to note that the term "relieved" covered a multitude of conditions. Any improvement in bodily health, in habits, or in mental state, however minor, was used to justify such a judgment, one all parties had an interest in reaching, since it provided reassurance to both physician and family that the expense of confinement had produced some tangible benefits, albeit not the hoped for cure. Consequently, only the most extraordinarily difficult and recalcitrant patients were discharged as "unimproved."

20 It would be self-serving to refer readers to my own work for the evidence that refutes such contentions. Instead, I suggest they consult the otherwise very different analyses of, for instance, Nancy Tomes (1984), David Rothman (1971), Ellen Dwyer (1987), Charlotte MacKenzie (1987, 1992), John Walton (1979, 1985) – even, dare I say it, Gerald Grob himself, whose two books dealing with nineteenth-century developments (Grob 1966, 1973a) admirably document the essential points, *malgré lui.*

21 Here, surely, is one source of historians' growing fascination with the rise of an extra-institutional psychiatry. See, for example, Showalter (1985); Stone (1985); Oppenheim (1991); Shorter (1992).

9 Psychiatry and social control in the nineteenth and twentieth centuries

1 In my view, this more positive view of the asylum in the last third of the nineteenth century and the first half of the twentieth century is largely mistaken.

The malign neglect that has masqueraded as "community care" in recent decades has encouraged a nostalgia for traditional mental hospitals that relies upon a rose-tinted and deeply distorted view of what they were like. Victorian bins and their twentieth-century counterparts were, for the most part, truly awful places that systematically dehumanized their patients and, very often, those who presided over them as well. The comparisons some well-informed observers made in the 1940s between American state hospitals and Nazi concentration camps were not necessarily hyperbole. See, for example, Maisel (1946); Orlans (1948); Wright (1947); Deutsch (1973). (Wright's volume, based on the experiences of conscientious objectors sent to work in mental hospitals to punish them for their pacifism deliberately omitted the most serious abuses these men had observed, lest they seemed too outlandish and cast doubt on the lesser parade of horrors they *did* include!) If the situation was not always and everywhere this bad, it was dreadful enough in all conscience. For a case study of how the profound power imbalances inherent in the relationship between certified lunatics and their captors could license literally deadly treatment, see Scull (2005).

2 For a sensitive exploration of this body of recent scholarship by a sympathetic participant, see Melling (1999).

3 I have drawn in this paragraph on a larger discussion of these issues in Scull (1999).

4 For an expanded version of this argument, see Scull (1989: ch. 1).

5 Perhaps the best discussion of the interaction of family and institution is Forsythe *et al.* (1996). See also Wright (1998); Walsh (1999); Michael (2003).

6 The best discussion and analysis of this novel arrangement and utilization of space in a systematic attempt to remoralize the dangerous and defective is to be found in Evans (1982). Foucault (1977), of course, develops much of his analysis of modern penalty and of the structures of social control with reference to the most famous architectural contrivance of this sort, Jeremy Bentham's Panopticon.

7 For a superb discussion of the multiple and overlapping interpretations of madness current in seventeenth-century England see MacDonald (1981).

8 In this case, there are quite literally two pictures of Pinel in action, painted some half century and more after the event they purport to record: "Pinel at the Bicêtre," painted by Charles Muller in 1849; and "Pinel Removes the Chains of the Insane Women at the Salpêtrière," painted in 1878 by Robert-Fleury. But the episode, as Dora Weiner (1984) and Jan Goldstein (1987) have documented at length, is wholly fictitious, the pictorial "records" completely spurious artifacts, and Pinel's presumed role as the author of moral treatment a major distortion of the historical record. As perhaps befits an Ur-myth, the claimed factual foundation dissolves under empirical scrutiny.

9 As George Orwell recognized, the ability to rewrite the past to provide an account supportive of the present powers that be is an extraordinarily useful ideological weapon. It thus comes as no surprise that psychiatrists have been unusually attentive to the need to police the writing of their own history: often writing it themselves; bestowing praise and whatever expert authority they can muster on writers who produce accounts they find congenial; and evincing violent hostility to historians whose work presents the history of psychiatry in a less than flattering light.

10 See the excellent discussion in Digby (1985: ch. 4); and the more general analysis in Scull (1979: chs 3–4).

11 On the roots and outcomes of such jurisdictional conflicts, and their sociological significance for the division of expert labor, see the superb discussion in Abbott (1988).

12 As Robert Nye (1984) has pointed out, alienists' views on the alarming spread of hereditary mental degeneracy resonated powerfully with the outlook of a French society increasingly both frightened and fascinated by visions of criminality, social pathology, and national decline. To the trained specialist, the existence of this underlying pathology was made manifest in a host of physical defects, often so subtle as to be overlooked by the unschooled – physical signs which were then seen, in circular fashion, as confirmation of the lunatic's degeneracy and as reaffirming medicine's jurisdictional claims.

13 For a detailed analysis and documentation of the shift of American psychiatric knowledge towards psychotherapy, cf. Abbott (1982: 324–330).

14 Gerald Grob (1983: 179–200, 234–322) has traced this abandonment of the chronic in considerable detail for the United States in the years leading up to the Second World War. Raw numbers tell the tale, for by 1956, only 17 percent of the members of the American Psychiatric Association were employed in state hospitals or Veterans Administration facilities (ibid.: 287).

15 Alienists had repeatedly expressed precisely these concerns throughout the nineteenth century, persistently tying their mandate to treat to a metaphysical embrace of the body, an incessantly reiterated insistence on the somatic basis of insanity, and an equally fierce rejection of psychological approaches to mental disorder. See Scull (1975); Clark (1981); Jacyna (1982); Dowbiggin (1985).

16 On the tactics employed by organized psychiatry as it sought "to retain a dominant position in the mental health professions," cf. Grob (1983: ch. 10).

17 The American Association of Psychiatric Social Workers even went so far as to treat supervision by psychiatrists as a central qualification for membership in the organization (Abbott 1988: 307). For discussions of psychiatric social work, see Lubove (1969) and Timms (1964). The demography of social work – its position as an almost exclusively female specialty – presented a further obstacle to any attempt to escape medical dominance. Cf. the discussion in Grob (1983: 249–257, *et passim*).

18 On the initial conflicts and tensions between psychology and psychiatry in the United States, cf. Grob (1983: 260–264).

19 For a sophisticated examination of perhaps the most prominent arena in which such jurisdictional issues are fought out, the seemingly irreconcilable debate over insanity and criminal responsibility, see Smith (1981).

10 Psychiatric therapeutics and the historian

1 Frederick Mott, who served as pathologist to London's mental hospitals, drew from repeated first-hand experience when he informed readers of his six volume *System of Syphilis* in 1910 that

> there is nothing more pitiable or degrading than the sight to a number of these wrecks of humanity sitting in a row, their heads on their breasts, grinding the teeth, saliva running out the angles of the mouth, oblivious to their surroundings, with expressionless faces and cold, livid, immobile hands.
>
> (quoted in Pennington 2003: 31)

2 A review of 35 studies in 1926 gave an average "complete" remission rate of 27.5 percent (Driver *et al.* 1926). Notwithstanding the substantial clinical consensus on the value of the malarial treatment, the intermittent and uncertain course of the underlying disease, the absence of any clear criteria of what constituted improvement, and the wholly uncontrolled character of the evaluations of

therapeutic outcomes make it very difficult at this remove to assess whether the therapy actually "worked." Contemporaries, however, were generally convinced of its efficacy, and, as we shall see, its existence dramatically altered the way doctors and patients afflicted with the disorder interacted with one another.

3 There were major ethical problems with this approach, not least the certainty, given the absence of a wholly reliable means of diagnosing general paresis, that misdiagnosed patients could be given syphilis as well as malaria. William Alanson White, the superintendent of St Elizabeth's Hospital in Washington, DC, was unusual in acknowledging the problem, and in refusing sometimes importunate requests from underlings who sought to embrace a clinical practice widely used elsewhere. See W. Watson Eldridge to W.A. White, June 21, 1930; White to Eldridge, June 24, 1930; Eldridge to White, June 27, 1930; White to Eldridge, June 28, 1930, William Alanson White Papers, Record Group 418, National Archives, Washington, DC. These letters are reproduced in Grob 1985: 124–125.

4 On July 7, 1941, for instance, White's successor as superintendent of St Elizabeth's Hospital, Winfred Overholser, noted that he had shipped quartan malarial blood, taken "from one of our paretics," in thermos flasks, and the same file records exchanges of malarial blood between state hospitals in Illinois, Tennessee, New Mexico, Pennsylvania, the Boston Psychopathic Hospital, Indiana, Maryland, and Connecticut, as well as Westbrook Sanatorium in Richmond, Virginia, and the mental hospital in Puerto Rico. Overholser to Ernesto Quintero, July 7, 1941; Seth Howes to W. Overholser, October 6, 1943, St Elizabeth's Hospital, Treatment Files, Entry 18, National Archives, Washington, DC (White's concerns about the ethical problems of injecting patients with paretic blood were evidently not shared by his successor).

5 Here, Cotton's key ally in the fight against focal sepsis, T.C. Graves, took the lead. See Graves 1919. One explanation offered at the time for the therapeutic effect of malarial therapy was that it somehow stimulated the immune system, a line of reasoning that may have commended fever therapy to Graves.

6 For the first report of the employment of such a device, see C.A. Neymann and S.L. Osborne, "Artificial Fever Produced by High-Frequency Currents, Preliminary Reports," *Illinois Medical Journal* 56, 1929: 199–203. Such devices were not without their hazards. The superintendent of the Arizona State Hospital complained to Winfred Overholser, superintendent of St Elizabeth's Hospital in Washington, DC, that at his establishment, "as sometimes happens, the first patient treated [in this fashion] died. Since that time the few graduate nurses we have have refused to operate the cabinet and I am in no position to force them to do so... [for the moment] we will be obliged to use malarial therapy." Seth Howes to Overholser, October 6, 1943, St Elizabeth's Hospital Treatment Files, Entry 18, National Archives, Washington, DC.

7 Pressman (1998: 15–16) in later chapters, for example, insists on "psychosurgery's actual contributions to the discipline's evolution. Controlled experiments, complete with "double-blind" protocols, matched samples, and sophisticated statistical analysis did not spontaneously arrive in psychiatry. Rather, psychiatry's scientific methodology itself slowly evolved. It was precisely through numerous lobotomy investigations and extensive conferences that psychiatrists learned important principles of experimental design, confronting problems that could not be foreseen but had to be experienced" (Pressman 1998: 366). This strikes me as a strained and unsatisfactory line of argument, since it rests upon a picture of psychiatry as a specialty so isolated from general medicine as to be unable to adopt improvements in research methodology that become the norm in medical

research more generally. Moreover, the research design even of the psychosurgical programs at major American universities remained so strikingly primitive as to render the "findings" produced quite useless as a guide to action and of dubious relevance to the methodological advance of psychiatric research. (See, for example, the so-called Columbia-Greystone study, reported in Mettler 1949.) And contrary to what Pressman here implies, the early studies of the efficacy of psychoactive drugs were generally uncontrolled or inadequately controlled, and seldom conducted under double blind conditions (an issue I discuss further later in this chapter). The importance of these methodologies for valid assessments of the therapeutic efficacy of the phenothiazines was a lesson slowly and painfully learned during the 1960s and 1970s. The experience with assessing lobotomies was thus of marginal relevance at best in arriving at suitable research designs for assessing new therapies.

8   To cite a handful of examples: the massive medical-commercial exploitation of new drugs and other treatments on the basis of flimsy scientific evidence is by no means confined to psychiatry, but the history of chlorpromazine would provide an ideal occasion for a case study of the phenomenon. Likewise, one of the most striking features of the history of chlorpromazine has been the way in which the so-called side-effects of these drugs (most notably irreversible extrapyramidal effects consequent upon organic impairment of patients' brains) were ignored by most professionals for well over a decade. See the discussion in Crane (1973a). I return to this issue below.

9   A simultaneous and more extensive review of 962 papers dealing with the use of chlorpromazine in psychiatric hospitals found that "only 10 papers mentioned controlled studies" (Bennett 1956: 19).

10   Twenty-one more papers were published on the subject between 1959 and 1966. See Crane (1968).

11   The very name "tardive dyskinesia" reflects the late onset of this particular disorder. Other disabling side-effects surface far more rapidly. A prospective study of the cumulative incidence of tardive dyskinesia in more than 850 patients with an average age of 29 (which is significant since the incidence of tardive dyskinesia increases markedly with age) revealed that it was 5 percent at one year, 10 percent at 2 years, 15 percent at 3 years, 19 percent at 4 years, 23 percent at 5 years, and 26 percent at 6 years – essentially a linear progression. See Kane *et al.* (1984); Kane (1986).

12

> Movements of the lips and tongue are grotesque, often socially objectionable, and thus are a source of profound embarrassment.... The neurological syndrome may cause a number of complications, such as hypertrophy of the tongue and ulcerations of the mouth. The speech may become incomprehensible. In extreme cases swallowing may become difficult.... Severe dystonia involving muscles controlling the balance of the body and of the head may be painful and thus greatly reduce the patient's activity.
>
> (Crane 1968: 41)

> The constant, and often grotesque, movements of the lips, cheeks, jaw, and tongue constitute a severe social handicap. The presence of these obvious and odd movements stigmatizes the patients. By causing embarrassment to family and friends and apprehension on the part of potential employers and coworkers, these movements can hinder the efforts being made to improve the ability of patients to function successfully within the community.
>
> (American Psychiatric Association 1992;
> see also Gardos and Cole 1976)

13 Crane 1973a: 124 – Remarkably, for instance, the NIMH Study Group which investigated phenothiazines was content with evidence drawn from a *six week* trial as "attesting to the safety of the active drugs" – though they were already commonly administered in "maintenance" doses for *years* at a time (cf. NIMH Study Group 1964). More than a decade and a half later, a blue ribbon task force set up by the American Psychiatric Association spoke of

> the frankly meager data base on which the long-term use of neuroleptic drugs has evolved... most of the outcome assessments made in the long-term evaluation of schizophrenic patients have been frankly crude, with an emphasis on the most easily measured changes, such as grossly psychotic behavior or the need for increased medication or hospital care. In fact, regarding the effects of all treatments of psychosis on finer levels of cognitive, psychological, and social function, little has been subjected to controlled scientific study.

They further warned that "In the rush to enjoy the benefits of the new technology, it is possible that some of its problems and limitations have been underemphasized" (American Psychiatric Association 1980: 114–115).

14 Healy records that "DSM-IV has over 350 [illness categories], where DSM-IIIR had only 292 and DSM-II had 180." More remarkably still, "Today's classification systems make it possible to have many different illnesses at the same time – something that happens nowhere else in medicine" (Healy 1997: 175).

11 "A Chance to Cut is a Chance to Cure": sexual surgery for psychosis in three nineteenth-century societies

1 The one obvious exception to this generalization is the treatment of cancer. Here, too, such standard treatments as chemotherapy, radiation, and surgery are viewed with great suspicion and fear by ordinary people. Significantly, as with mental illness, cancer is a disease whose etiology remains largely mysterious and whose treatment is both highly intrusive and of debatable efficacy.

2 For recent discussions of these developments, see Stephen Jacyna (1982) and Michael Clark (1982).

3 Compare Andrew Wynter (1875: 124–125): "There are epochs in all institutions at which a paralysis seems to seize upon those conducting them.... A miserable spirit of routine, without resources, spring, or energy, is sapping and destroying asylum life."

4 Most famously in the work of Hortatio Robinson Storer (1871).

5 We stress routine because even before either anesthesia or anti-sepsis were known, surgeons in desperation sometimes invaded the peritoneum (Ovariotomy, the surgical excision of the ovaries – with which we shall be extensively concerned below – was first successfully undertaken as early as 1809, by Ephraim McDowell (1771–1830), a backwoods surgeon from Kentucky, as he eventually reported in the [Philadelphia] Eclectic Repertory and Analytic Review 8 (1817: 242–244). And anesthesia alone, even in the absence of adequate understanding of (let alone means for combating) infection, sufficed to encourage the more aggressive surgeons to attack hitherto untreatable forms of pathology.

6 The extent of his "daring" if that is the appropriate word, is perhaps indicated by the fact that his fourth patient was his sister! She, at least, survived. According to the *British Medical Journal* (1866b: 231), he derived his operative technique from that used by veterinarians in the spaying of pigs.

7 The term masturbation never appears in Baker Brown's book; a tactic which he undoubtedly adopted from motives of professional prudence. As events were to demonstrate, it was a woefully inadequate defense.

8 See, for example: Burrows (1828); Esquirol (1838); Hare (1962); Comfort (1967).

9 Note too, that even the *British Medical Journal* (1866e: 439) otherwise one of Brown's sternest critics, conceded that his views about the dangers of masturbation were perfectly standard medical beliefs: "it has long been an established fact, that onanism practised to the extent supposed by Mr. Brown will occasion all the various disorders named by him."

10 For example, W. Tyler Smith (1848: 609) quoted in Showalter (1985: 65) suggested that the erotic and nervous systems of menopause be dealt with by "a course of injections of ice water into the rectum, introduction of ice into the vagina, and leeching of the labia and cervix." "The suddenness with which leeches applied to this part fill themselves," he writes admiringly, "considerably increases the good effect of their application, and for some hours after their removal there is an oozing of blood from the leech bites."

11 As one doctor scornfully remarked, "Fancy some innocent curate going about recommending his easy little operation for 'distressing cases of illness.'" For a further attack on Brown's self promotion, see *British Medical Journal* (1866f: 580).

12 At this time, it was illegal for a lunatic to be treated in any institution but a licensed asylum, so the involvement of the Lunacy Commissioners was a potentially ominous development for Brown, given his repeated boasts of having cured insanity through clitoridectomy. As we shall see, his efforts to wriggle out of this difficulty ultimately only compounded his problems with the profession at large.

13 For earlier examples of this accusation, see *British Medical Journal* (1866i: 729; 1867a: 42; 1867b: 61).

14 The entire correspondence on the matter was published in the *British Medical Journal* 1867c: 94.

15 Seymour Haden (*British Medical Journal* 1867g: 398) was even more pointed: either Brown had lied to the Lunacy Commissioners when he claimed never to have cured cases of insanity by clitoridectomy, or he had lied when he published his book claiming to have accomplished such cures. As for himself, he chose to accept the letter to the Commissioners, "and therefore I think we have convicted him of quackery, and that clitoridectomy is quackery."

16 Two of his defenders ruefully admitted as much as in the words of Dr Routh (*British Medical Journal* 1867g: 405), "I really do think, and am afraid, that Mr. Brown has damaged his cause by having spoken as he has done..." And Dr Savage (*British Medical Journal* 1867g: 404, 405) commented, "I am very sorry indeed that Mr. Brown undertook his own defense. I am sorry he ever uttered a word."

17 The entire proceedings were published in the *British Medical Journal* 1867g: 395–410.

18 As the *British Medical Journal* 1867g: 388 commented at the time of his expulsion from the Obstetrical Society, "So severe a punishment has not fallen upon any man holding a respectable position in our profession in the memory of any of us."

19 As Tait (1889a: 63) noted rather wistfully, Baker Brown's activities had "one disastrous result, the operation of clitoridectomy was absolutely discarded, and I have never heard a surgeon say he had performed it since 1867. Yet I am certain in many cases it would be useful."

20 The operation soon became known, eponymously, as Battey's operation.

21 In the words of William Goodell, Professor of Clinical Gynecology at the University of Pennsylvania,

> By the aid of Listerism, abdominal surgery has reached such a pass that many formidable operations involving the hitherto sacred peritoneal cavity are daily undertaken, with a success and a degree of safety as much assured as in surface surgery.... Hence, it is that oophorectomy, or the extirpation of the ovaries – not for any intrinsic disease, but merely to bring on the climacteric – has been placed on a firm basis.
>
> (1881a: 638)

George Engelmann (1882: 2) Professor of Obstetrics at the Missouri Medical College, went further, drawing attention to the remarkable contrast between the reception accorded Baker Brown's "harmless" operation for "unsexing women" and the free acceptance of "the bolder, more dangerous, and far more important operation recently given to the world by Robert Battey."

22 Looking back on this period, Thomas Kelly (1909 quoted in Longo 1979: 278) recalled that "one might see in almost any hospital numbers of normal organs sacrificed...so rabid were gynecologists to do surgery that there was nearly a wholesale wiping out of gynecological therapeutics."

23 On another occasion, (Goodell 1881b: 295) he went even further: "I am not sure but that, in this progressive age, it may not in future be deemed political economy to stamp out insanity by removing the ovaries of insane women."

24 For a series of skeptical comments on the value of ovariotomy as a treatment for female insanity, see the responses of Pennsylvania asylum superintendents surveyed by Wharton Sinkler (1891: 184–185).

25 On psychiatrists' "intellectual aloofness...[tendency] to regard themselves as men apart...[and isolation] from the newer trends in medicine" during the 1870s and 1880s, see Barbara Sicherman (1967) and Ruth Caplan (1969, especially 154–168, 212–223).

26 Perhaps the key document of this "new realism" was Pliny Earle's *The Curability of Insanity: A Series of Studies* (1887), which claimed to demolish the factual foundation of the earlier cult of curability and, not-so-incidentally, to rescue his fellow alienists from the charge that they were vastly less competent and successful than their predecessors. Representative of the new therapeutic nihilism is John Chapin's (1877: 7) comment to the Conference of Charities: "The majority of the insane are not likely to, and, as a matter of fact, do not recover."

27 One should also point out that state lunatic asylums, unlike other arenas of medical practice, were subject to a whole range of professional and extra-professional controls over their activities, making them in some respects an unpropitious site in which to introduce controversial new therapies.

28 Not that this situation precluded extravagant claims that "Few facts in medicine are so well established as, that scores of women are being rescued from insanity and some of the protean forms of hysteria, by the gynecologist..." (Stone 1890: 307), coupled with complaints that many more women now languishing in asylums could be cured if only psychiatric obstructionism ceased (Kitto 1891: 517).

29 When James Russell, Superintendent at the Asylum for the Insane, Hamilton, Ontario, Canada (1898: 587), sent a mail questionnaire to "one hundred and twenty of the principal alienists in America," almost all the state hospital superintendents reported that few or none of their patients had been operated upon prior to admission to the asylum. By contrast, among the few private institutions he surveyed were the Mount Hope Retreat in Maryland, and the Butler Hospital

for the Insane in Rhode Island. At the former, the superintendent noted that "The majority of the females who come to us here have been treated or operated upon without avail;" while at the Butler Hospital, "Our patients, all coming from the higher rank of society, have passed through the hands of the gynecologist, neurologist, and every other ologist before we see them." Clearly, this reflected desperate attempts by upper-class patients and their families to avoid the social defacement associated with institutionalization in an asylum.

30 Physicians' characteristic responses included a mixture of threats, intimidation, and punishments barely disguised as "therapy." See Showalter (1985, esp. ch. 5) and Clark (1981).

31 "It cannot be denied that the temptation to use the knife in these cases is very strong, and even though the gynecological surgeon may have doubts of the appropriateness of the treatment, he is urged by the despondent and desperate friends of the patient, who received little hope either from previous neurological treatment or the prognosis given by well-informed physicians." Morantz and Zschoche (1980: 568–588) have provided additional evidence that gynecological surgeons "were often pressured by female patients." Marie Zakrzewska, for example, wrote to Elizabeth Blackwell in 1891 of the numerous women who came to the New England Hospital, begging for such operations "on the slightest cause."

32 In the hierarchical world of British medicine, such ex-cathedra condemnation seems swiftly to have had a chilling effect. Lawson Tait (1886: 853), perhaps the leading provincial British gynecologist and on other occasions bitterly critical of Wells, acknowledged that he was "really much disposed to agree" that the operation was inadmissible in cases of insanity. And just over a decade later, Dr Yellowlees (quoted in Russell 1898: 589), superintendent of the Glasgow Royal Asylum, commented sharply that "the reckless way in which the ovaries are removed on your side of the Atlantic [is] quite wrong."

33 There were as it happens, very occasional reports in the literature of castration being used a remedy for the mental problems of the male. See, for example, J.H. Marshall, 1865: 363–364. (The patient in this instance was a 36-year-old chronic masturbator who, following operative interference, was reported as becoming "quiet, kind, and docile.") And some gynecologists were *theoretically* in favor of dispensing their surgical assistance to male and female alike. David Gilliam (1896: 319–321) for instance, confessed

> I believe in the castration of epileptics and the insane. I believe in it on broad humanitarian grounds. Insanity is hereditary. Epilepsy is hereditary. They constitute the greatest curse to humanity. An insane father or an insane mother will bring more misery into the world than any other father or mother.
>
> (1896: 319–321)

Still, he was not prepared actually to operate on such a grand scale. And in practice, women alone were in receipt of his attention, something he rationalized to himself by noting that "Women are by nature more nearly neutral than men, and the deprivation of sexual glands is less felt by them..."

34 Those denouncing this "most flagrant and pernicious form...of...mutilation" included Archibald Church (1861–1952), Professor of Neurology at the Chicago Polyclinic and Professor of Mental Diseases and Jurisprudence at the Chicago Medical College (after whom the medical library at Northwestern University Medical School is now named); Robert Thaxter Edes (1838–1923), Jackson Professor of Clinical Medicine at Harvard, President (in 1883) of the American

Neurological Association, and one of the seven founders of Association of American Physicians; and Allan McLane Hamilton and Wharton Sinkler, who were among the most prominent neurologists in New York and Philadelphia respectively. Leading gynecologists were not as uniformly aroused by the excesses of their colleagues who provided surgical treatment for mental disorder, but in general, the most eminent were also the most highly critical. Their ranks included William Goodell, one of the founders of the American Gynecological Society and Professor of Gynecology at the University of Pennsylvania (and someone who had originally supported the operation); Howard A. Kelly (1858–1943), Professor of Gynecology at Johns Hopkins, President of the AGS (in 1912), and the leading American gynecologist of his generation; Ely Van de Warker (1841–1910), President of the AGS (in 1901); Alexander Skene (1838–1900), Professor of Gynecology at the New York Post-Graduate Medical School, and President of the AGS (in 1887) and of the New York Obstetrical Society, and William Playfair (1836–1903) and Robert Barnes (1817–1907), of London, both past Presidents of the (English) Obstetrical Society.

35 See also Hamilton (1893: 183):

> I undertake to say that if these patients had been subjected to the same care, solicitude, attention, change, and watchfulness, without operation, as they received under it, there might have been secured as much improvement as followed this heroic treatment.

36 McMurty (1897: 212–213): "I venture to say that if we were to take forty healthy women as they walked along the street, and if it were admissible to open their abdomens, lesions... would be found which had never produced symptoms of serious importance."

37 "We [gynecologists] know nothing of physiology.... It is due to this want of knowledge that, surgically speaking, we have been led into many errors. It was this ignorance that caused the false position of Battey and the evil influence of Tait" (Van de Warker 1906: 366).

38 See B. Sherwood-Dunn (1897) and the ensuing discussion, especially the comments of Matthew D. Mann and Albert Goldspohn. The side effects reported included a number of cases where it was alleged that the operation had produced insanity. See Ill 1888: 1–5; Manton 1889: 262–265; Thomas 1889: 396–399.

39 As Magali Larson (1977) has argued on a more general level, this "conquest of public confidence" was perhaps the central ideological task facing nineteenth-century professionals.

40 Howard A. Kelly (1896: 251) quoting "a distinguished physician, the leading practitioner in one of our large cities, and a man of national reputation." Compare also William Goodell (quoted in Mitchinson):

> The majority of physicians and all laymen look upon women deprived on their ovaries as unsexed. Just as castration in the male, so castration in the female is deemed a sexual mutilation to which common consent attaches a stigma. No woman would marry a eunuch, and few men would wed a woman deprived of her ovaries.
>
> (1984: 141–142)

41 Arnold Praeger was a Los Angeles physician; other defenders of normal ovariotomy included Joseph Meyer, a practitioner in Honey Grove, Texas; and David Todd Gilliam of Columbus, Ohio. Perhaps the best-known figure advocate of this form of sexual surgery was W.P. Manton of Detroit, though even he could not pretend

to move in the elevated circles occupied by his opponents; and besides, his advocacy of ovariotomy was characteristically the most cautious and circumspect of those arguing in favor of operative treatment.

42 This "reform" movement is discussed in John A. Pitts (1978) and in Ruth B. Caplan (1969: 170–183).

43 Morton was the chairman of the State Committee on Lunacy, Surgeon to the Pennsylvania Hospital, and a leading member of the Philadelphia medical elite. John B. Chapin, President of the alienists' professional association, superintendent of the (private) Pennsylvania Hospital for the Insane, and probably the prime mover in the whole enterprise, thanked the Board for putting a stop to

> a scandalous proceeding.... To erect a hospital, or propose one, where women were to be castrated in companies of fifties, with the hope of a cure of insanity, would be generally regarded, in the present state of meager knowledge upon the subject, as revolting.
>
> (quoted in Anonymous 1893: 136)

Chapin was the protégé of Thomas Story Kirkbride, one of the founders of the Association of Medical Superintendents of American Hospitals for the Insane, and had absorbed the latter's highly conservative outlook. See Nancy Tomes (1984). There is some discussion of the Norristown episode in Constance McGovern (1981).

44 One unsurprising result of this eclecticism was frequent teasing by his associates, "asking what his 'latest specialty' was" Robinson (1952: 18).

45 Bucke's activities have recently received considerable attention from two Canadian historians of medicine, Wendy Mitchinson and Samuel Shortt. We are grateful to Professor Shortt for sharing his as yet unpublished findings with us. For fuller published discussion of Bucke's work, see Mitchinson 1980, 1981, 1982.

46 For his acknowledgment of Rohé's influence, see A.T. Hobbs 1898: 513. Like Rohé and the staff at the Norristown State Hospital Hobbs and Bucke claimed to operate only to relieve physical disability and disease, and both the forms of disease and the types of operations undertaken were extended to encompass much more than ovarian disorders and oophorectomy. Hobbs' first five cases, for instance, included "an ovarian tumor, a subinvoluted uterus, a perineum torn to the sphincter, a retroverted enlarged uterus, and a cervix hypertrophied and lacerated" (Hobbs 1898: 514).

47 In a subsequent report, Bucke (1900: 99) indicated that he and Hobbs had found evidence of diseases of the reproductive organs in 219 of the 256 women they had examined.

48 Retrospective study of the records of the London Asylum indicates that the skepticism was well merited. In 1913, the case records were reviewed by an assistant physician at the asylum. Dr John H. Stead (1913: 132, 135). His conclusion was that the results following surgery were as bad or worse than those consequent on doing nothing, and that such temporary improvement as was reported at the time derived, not from operative interference, but from the additional "careful, sympathetic and considerate attention...these patients received." Wendy Mitchinson's (1982: 476) review of the case records uncovered marked discrepancies between these and Bucke's published claims to a combined cure and improvement rate of 60–70 percent. And Samuel Shortt's more systematic statistical review of the same evidence demonstrates that the outcome for those operated upon was actually significantly *worse* than for a group of matched controls drawn from the asylum population (personal communication).

49 One of Bucke's few supporters, the Vancouver physician Ernest Hall, did continue to agitate on behalf of sexual surgery for several more years. See, for example, Hall 1903: 301–312, 1906: 597–604, 1908: 147–151. But he never had any chance of success. Henceforth, the only advocates and practitioners of sexual surgery as a remedy for mental disorders were to be found among such fringe elements as the followers of E.H. Pratt who apparently viewed "orificial surgery" as an almost universal panacea for all the ills to which [female] flesh was heir. Pratt himself, for example, advocated female circumcision as a remedy for "the dangers of infantile convulsions, of hip-joint disease, of kidney disease, of paralysis, of eczema universalis, of stammering, of dyspepsia, of pulmonary tuberculosis, of constipation, of locomotor ataxia, of rheumatism, of idiocy and insanity, and of lust and all its consequences."

50 We suggest that the mere advance of knowledge, important as it undoubtedly was, did not necessarily entail the abandonment of surgical intervention. Under other circumstances, and absent the effects of the larger social and professional forces we have analyzed here, the incorporation of knowledge of the endocrine system might equally well have provided (as had the doctrines of reflex physiology a generation earlier) a new and yet more sophisticated rationale for operative interference. That this is not just an idle sociological speculation is intimated by the attempt by Bucke and Hobbs of the London Asylum to make just such a rhetorical move. Defending his actions before his skeptical, even hostile fellow alienists in 1898, Bucke (1898: 87) argued that his institution's activities were justified by the most esoteric advances of the new scientific medicine. In particular, "it seems to me that the recent physiological theory of so-called internal secretions will furnish the clue we want." Evidently, gynecological troubles were productive of mental disorders at least in part through their impact on the fluids that served as chemical regulators of the body. For example, the body might cease to secrete "testicular juice" or might secrete an altered, pathological fluid which would then serve as "a toxic agent of unknown but probably great virulence."

12 Focal sepsis and psychosis: the career of Thomas Chivers Graves (1883–1964)

1 The younger Graves was virtually disowned by his father when he had the presumption to marry an Irish Catholic nurse during the Second World War. How these prejudices may subsequently have affected T.C. Graves' actions as head of mental hospitals which contained large numbers of Irish Catholics we simply do not know.

2 Though Graves at this time had no interest in a psychiatric career, the scholarship he now depended upon had been endowed, coincidentally, by the eminent nineteenth-century alienist, Sir John Charles Bucknill (founding editor of the *Journal of Mental Science* and, in the 1880s, one of the four co-editors of *Brain*). Himself a graduate of University College, Bucknill had left one-third of his residuary estate in trust to its President and Council in his will in 1897, to establish "a Medical Scholarship . . . to be awarded at least once in three years as the President and Council may from time to time decide."

3 Indeed, the Committee's proposed remedies for the problems it had uncovered were extraordinarily threadbare. Appeals to the superintendents to modify the restrictive regulations which made the lives of their junior officers so unattractive and, most particularly, to permit their subordinates to marry, met with resistance and ridicule as one superintendent commented, "Marriage meant to a medical

officer, a diminution of his value to the service for a time; in some it amounted to an observable post-nuptial inertia or dementia, a condition whose course was about twelve months. £700 a year would have a tendency, he feared, to make this condition chronic" (Anonymous 1914: 689). As for the committee's other major proposal, the establishment on the German model of university-affiliated clinics for outpatient treatment and research on mental disorder, there was widespread and well-warranted skepticism about whether the necessary funds would be forthcoming from either local or central coffers.

4 Not that a few psychiatrists didn't make the attempt. See, for example, Sir Robert Armstrong Jones' attempt to blame the outbreak on "tainted heredity" (Jones 1917a: 1–3) – a stance which was unlikely to sit well with either the politicians or the public, and which opened him up to the devastating riposte that he was committing "a slur upon the noblest of our race" (Smith and Pear 1917: 65).

5 I am very grateful to Dr Ogden for sharing this most helpful survey with me, and I have drawn upon his lecture at a number of points in this essay. Through his kindness, I was also able to inspect the operating theatre and other facilities at Rubery Hill in June 1987, as well as to talk with a number of former members of staff who had worked under T.C. Graves.

6 The appointment of an outsider to such a post must obviously have come as a bitter blow to aspiring assistant physicians. Three such doctors had once ruefully compared their situation with that of "dutiful relatives, most patiently await[ing] the falling in of their estate." They felt that the contrast of "the fat salaries of the Superintendents with the lean ones of the assistants" had perhaps been bearable "when the Assistant Medical Officers were few and superintendencies ripened in four or five years, but [their elders' counsel to be patient] loses all its sweet reasonableness when we have to wait ten, twelve, or more years for the golden fruit, and even run the risk [they prophetically added] of its being plucked by some outsider from over the wall just as we thought it about to drop" (Dodds *et al.* 1890).

7 His obituarists discreetly termed him "stimulating, but at times overwhelming" (Anonymous 1964a: 1711). His daughter-in-law (V. Graves 1986) more bluntly informed me that he was "a bit of a bully," and Dr D.W. Millard (personal communication), who became consultant psychiatrist at Rubery a few years after Graves' retirement found that "T.C. seemed to have been capable of inducing real terror among the staff" – a reaction Millard attributes to the "fact that he was an absolute tyrant."

8 Billings was dean of the Rush Medical School in Chicago, and past president of both the American Medical Association and the American Association of Physicians. This book was his Lane Lectures, delivered at Stanford Medical School in 1915. See also Billings 1914; Barker 1920. Leading American physicians who embraced focal infection included Edward Rosenow and Charles Mayo of Minnesota, and William Thayer and Llewellys Barker at Johns Hopkins. British adherents included Sir William Wilcox, Sir Arbuthnot Lane, William Hunter, and Chalmers Watson.

9 For some chronic diseases whose etiology remained poorly understood, focal sepsis continued to be suspected as the culprit even into the 1950s.

10 These views were reiterated at greater length in later papers, where he was to make a particular point of its role in the genesis of "dementia praecox, manic depressive insanity, paranoid conditions, psychoneurosis, and toxic insanities" (Hunter 1927, 1929).

11 In his Morison Lectures two years later, Bruce was still more emphatic, and had widened the potential source of trouble: "There are … many links in the chain of

evidence wanting, but such evidence as is already in my possession is sufficient to warrant the general conclusion being drawn that the disease known as mania is due to bacterial toxaemia, which is in many ways comparable to the bacterial toxaemia of rheumatism."

12 Later in his paper, Cotton (1923: 458–459) contrasted the recovery rate at Trenton between 1908 and 1918 (38 percent), with the rate between 1918 and 1922, which corresponded to the implementation of a radical program of eliminating sepsis (87 percent, or "a total of 1,412 successfully treated cases").

13 Elsewhere, he had claimed that "Modern biological research tends to show that the inheritance of mental disorders ... is next to impossible" (Cotton 1922: 158).

14 For his contributions, see Pickworth (1935, 1952) I am grateful to Dr John Pickworth for information on his father's work at Rubery Hill.

15 The study had been undertaken over an 18-month period by one of Meyer's assistants, Phyllis Greenacre. Her work had meticulously documented the spurious character of Cotton's claims, demonstrating, for example, that the death rate from his abdominal surgery approached 43 percent, and that the more extensive the treatment a patient received for focal sepsis, the lower his or her chance of recovery. For details of this episode, and Meyer's unsavory role in covering up a major medical scandal, see Scull (2005).

16 This is still the routine procedure when treating difficult sinus infections.

17 Dr Millard (personal communication, see Note 21) confirms that stories of Graves extracting teeth sans anaesthetic were still circulating in hospital mythology in the 1950s, and suggests, not implausibly, that sporadic instances of recovery following this procedure may have followed upon cases of toxic confusion being mistaken for psychosis – raising "the possibility of occasional misdiagnosis ... conferring enough spurious credibility to help [sustain belief in the focal infection hypothesis]."

18 Hunter's work was hailed in the *Times* (July 21, 1927) as the "work of a new Lister." It approvingly quoted his dictum that "All the public authorities responsible for the mental hospitals should issue an order that every mental hospital under their charge should ... be forthwith supplied with every arrangement for surgical work" while warning its readers of the dangers of sepsis, whose "foci were small, hidden, chronic, and generally caused no local effect drawing attention to themselves."

19 The *Daily Telegraph*'s report of the occasion (July 21, 1927) indicates that these encomiums were greeted with "loud cheers." Further symbolizing the endorsement of focal sepsis theory by the Establishment, during the meeting Moynihan and Hunter were recognized for their contributions to its triumph by the award of honorary Doctorates of Law from Edinburgh University.

20 *Daily Telegraph*, July 21, 1927. The following day, the *Telegraph* left no doubt where its sympathies lay in the debate. In an editorial on "Mind and Body," it hailed "a new and hopeful vista in the prevention, amelioration, and cure of mental disorders." "It is not," the leader pointed out, "the layman who will find any difficulty in accepting as reasonable the conclusions presented by Dr. William Hunter.... The effect of septic poison coming from diseased teeth or from pockets of infection at their roots is by this time thoroughly well known. All sorts of bodily ailments are now attributed to this cause, and there is no reason why the brain should not suffer from the same cause, however the poison may be conveyed thither."

21 In fact, Cotton continued to employ abdominal surgery on an extensive scale right up to his death in 1933. See Cotton (1930, 1933).

22 Their article contains detailed blueprints for psychiatrists wishing to construct their own colonic machines. This less drastic alternative to colectomies was

perhaps motivated by concern at the mortality associated with Cotton's more drastic abdominal interventions. Graves subsequently visited Cotton at Trenton to examine his procedures at first hand, and in 1929, he visited Norway, where Gjessing had become one of Cotton's most devoted disciples.

23 General paralytics were subjected to the same series of treatments, "with the addition of a course of tryparsamide, frequent lumbar punctures, malaria, if they are considered well enough, or an extended course of colsul if not."

24 For example, in his official address to his professional colleagues, Daniel Rambaut, President of the RMPA from 1934–1935 and Superintendent of St Andrew's Hospital, Northampton, was critical of some of Graves' claims, but nonetheless conceded that the somatic treatments he had introduced had "seen a complete change introduced into the spirit of the mental hospital." He "look[ed] upon it as our duty to make every attempt to improve the physical health of our patients, in the hope that by doing so we may remove some obstacle to mental recovery." And he insisted that "Even if one agrees with Dr. D.K. Henderson that several forms of physical treatment derive their benefit from faith and suggestion, they are worth pursuing empirically" (Rambaut 1934: 638).

25 The Superintendent at Powick, H.F. Fenton, was, in the words of Frederick Graves, "a mouse of a man" completely intimidated by T.C. Graves, who "kept him up to the mark" (F. Graves 1986). Fenton used the profits from patients boarded at Powick by other local authorities to underwrite the construction of a treatment center modeled on Rubery and Hollymoor. Cf. Ogden (1983: 5); and Fenton (1938).

26 The successive editions of D.K. Henderson's and R.D. Gillespie's *Textbook of Psychiatry* routinely surveyed these criticisms. See, for example, 1st edn, 1927, pp. 50–53; 5th edn, 1940, pp. 60–63; 6th edn, 1944, 61–65; 7th edn, 1950, pp. 66–71.

27 The relative popularity of these new therapies is readily seen from the rapid rise in the space devoted to them in the *Journal of Mental Science* during these years. Where before, focal sepsis had been the source of a whole series of somatic treatments, now it had many rivals, at the same time as faith was waning in many quarters about its scientific merits.

28 Symptomatic of his growing isolation was his loss of control over one of the hospitals that formerly formed part of his empire. The appointment of J.J. Reilly as superintendent at the Winson Green Mental Hospital in 1939 was rapidly followed by the abandonment of the routine investigation and treatment of focal sepsis, and their replacement by ECT and occupational therapy, to both of which Graves was fiercely opposed. Cf. Ogden (1983: 6).

29 For a similar verdict on this address, see A.H. Ogden (1983: 5–6).

30 These included Bedford Russell of St Bartholomew's Hospital in London, Patrick Watson Williams of Bristol, James Hogg and Samuel Birdsall of London, and R.S. Strang (Visiting ENT Surgeon to the Birmingham Mental Hospitals), together with F.A. Pickworth, the pathologist on Graves' staff.

31 The production and use of crude penicillin filtrates was quite widely attempted in these years. For an overview, see Wainwright (1987), which, however, contains no mention of Graves' experiments.

32 There is one very odd exception to this generalization, which Dr D.W. Millard has kindly drawn to my attention: from the late 1920s onwards, as we have seen, D.K. Henderson had been one of the most vocal and persistent critics of the focal infection doctrine, and he had made a point of roundly dismissing Graves' and Cotton's claims in successive editions of his textbook. In the eighth edition of

1956, however, a far more favorable assessment is offered (Henderson and Batchelor 1956: 66), for the first and last time. The authors point out that "belief in the aetiological importance of focal infection has become greatly modified" but continue in a very different vein: "That, however, does not mean that we can afford to neglect its possible significance . . . we should never neglect in every case of nervous and mental illness to carry out physical examinations with the same meticulous care and standard as if the patient were in a general hospital. Failure to do so may lead to disaster both in relation to diagnosis and treatment. We are, therefore, indebted to Cotton in the U.S.A. and to Ford Robertson and Graves in this country who did so much to promote the view that the toxaemic aetiology of nervous disorder was of paramount importance."

Quite what explains this extraordinary *volte-face* is unclear. Perhaps the passage was written by Henderson's new co-author, Ivor Batchelor, and simply escaped his attention. The respectful tone remains, however, an isolated example of the doctrine being treated seriously at this late date, an ironic exception that proves the rule. Indeed, as Dr Millard notes (personal communication), this passage "was probably the final salute in the serious [psychiatric] literature to T.C."

Bibliography

Abbott, Andrew (1982), "The Emergence of American Psychiatry," unpublished doctoral dissertation, University of Chicago.

Abbott, Andrew (1988), *The System of Professions*. Chicago, IL: University of Chicago Press.

Alexander, Franz D. and Selesnick, Sheldon T. (1966), *The History of Psychiatry: An Evaluation of Psychiatric Thought and Practice from Pre-Historic Times to the Present*. New York: Harper and Row.

Alexander, Mark D. (1976), "The Administration of Madness and Attitudes Towards the Insane in Nineteenth-Century Paris," unpublished PhD dissertation, Johns Hopkins University.

Allderidge, Patricia (1985), "Bedlam: Fact or Fantasy?" in Bynum, W.F., Porter, R., and Shepherd, M. (eds), *The Anatomy of Madness*, Volume 2, London: Tavistock: 17–33.

American Psychiatric Association (1980), *Tardive Dyskinesia: Report of the American Psychiatric Association Task Force on Late Neurological Effects of Antipsychotic Drugs*. Washington, DC: American Psychiatric Association.

American Psychiatric Association (1992), *Tardive Dyskinesia: A Task Force Report of the American Psychiatric Association*. Washington, DC: American Psychiatric Association.

Andrews, Jonathan (1991), "Bethlem Revisited: A History of Bethlem Hospital c. 1634–1770," unpublished PhD dissertation, London University.

Andrews, J. and Scull, A. (2001), *Undertaker of the Mind: John Monro and Mad-Doctoring in Eighteenth Century England*. Berkeley, CA: University of California Press.

Andrews, J. and Scull, A. (2003), *Customers and Patrons of the Mad Trade: The Management of Lunacy in Eighteenth Century London* Berkeley, CA: University of California Press.

Andrews, J., Briggs, A., Porter, R., Tucker, P., and Waddington, K. (1997), *The History of Bethlem*. London: Routledge.

Anonymous (1794), *Some Particulars of the Royal Indisposition of 1788 to 1789*. London: Printed for the editor by R. Taylor.

Anonymous (1836–1837), "Review of *What Asylums Were, Are, and Ought to Be*," *Phrenological Journal*, 10: 53.

Anonymous (1836–1837), Miscellaneous Notices – Dundee and Montrose Lunatic Asylums, *Phrenological Journal*, 10: 156.

Anonymous (1857), Lunatic Asylums, *Quarterly Review*, 101: 353–393.

Anonymous (1881–1882), The American System of Public Provision for The Insane and Despotism in Lunatic Asylums," *American Journal of Insanity*, 38: 113–139.

Anonymous (1893), "Editorial: Removal of the Ovaries as a Therapeutic Measure in Public Institutions for the Insane," *Journal of the American Medical Association*, 20: 135–137.

Anonymous (1913), "Interim Report," *Journal of Mental Science*, 59: 688–706.

Anonymous (1914), "Report of the Committee re Status of British Psychiatry and of Medical Officers," *Journal of Mental Science*, 60: 667–694.

Anonymous (1922), "Discussion – Functional Psychosis," *American Journal of Psychiatry*, 79: 195–210.

Anonymous (1923), "Discussion," *Journal of Mental Science*, 69: 553–558.

Anonymous (1927), "Discussion: Chronic Sepsis as a Cause of Mental Disorder," *British Medical Journal*, ii, November 5: 817.

Anonymous (1931), "Aural Sepsis in Relation to Mental Disorder," *Journal of Mental Science*, 77: 193–195.

Anonymons (1933), "Meetings of the Society," *Journal of Mental Science*, 79: 222.

Anonymous (1941), "Symposium on Ear, Nose and Throat Disease in Mental Disorder," *Journal of Mental Science*, 87: 477–528.

Anonymous (1949), "Lobotomy Disappointment," *Newsweek*, December 12: 51.

Anonymous (1964a), "Obituary Notice: T.C. Graves," *British Medical Journal*, i: 1711.

Anonymous (1964b), "Obituary: T.C. Graves,"*The Lancet*, i: 1400.

Armstrong, David (1980), "Madness and Coping," *Sociology of Health and Illness*, 2: 293–316.

Aviram, U. and Cohen, J.B. (1976), "Policy Decisions and The Reduction of Mental Hospitalization of The Aged," *Mental Health and Society*, 3: 315–325.

Aviram, U., Syme, S.L., and Cohen, J.B. (1976), "The Effects of Policies and Programs on The Reduction of Mental Hospitalization," *Social Science and Medicine*, 10: 571–577.

Baiter, M.B. and Levine, J. (1969), "The Nature and Extent of Psychotropic Drug Usage in The United States," *Psychopharmacological Bulletin*, 5: 3–13.

Bakewell, Thomas (1805), *The Domestic Guide in Cases of Insanity*, Stafford, for the author.

Barker, Llewellys, F. (1920), "Oral Sepsis and Internal Medicine," *Journal of Dental Research*, 2: 43–58.

Bartlett, Peter (1999), *The Poor Law of Lunacy*. London: Cassells.

Bartlett, Peter and Wright, David (eds) (1999), *Outside The Walls of The Asylum: The History of Care in the Community 1750–2000*. London: Athlone Press.

Barton, Russell (1965), *Institutional Neurosis*, 2nd edition. Bristol: Wright.

Battey, Robert (1872), "Normal ovariotomy: Case," *Atlanta Medical and Surgical Journal*, 10: 321–339.

Battey, Robert (1873), "Normal ovariotomy," *Atlanta Medical and Surgical Journal*, 11: 1–22.

Battey, Robert (1886), "Antisepsis in Ovariotomy and Battey's Operation," 197–240.

Battie, William (1758), *A Treatise on Madness*. London: Whiston and White.

Beard, George M. (1881), *A Practical Treatise on Nervous Exhaustion (Neurasthenia), Its Symptoms, Nature, Sequences, Treatment*. New York: Treat.

Belknap, Ivan (1956), *Human Problems of The State Mental Hospital*. New York: McGraw-Hill.

Bennett, I.F. (1956), *Chemotherapy in Psychiatric Hospitals: A Critical Review of The Literature and Research Trends*. Washington, DC: Veterans' Administration.

Berger, Bennett (1981), *The Survival of a Counter-Culture*. Berkeley, CA: University of California Press.

Berrios, G. and Freeman, H. (eds) (1991), *150 Years of British Psychiatry 1841–1991*. London: Gaskell.

Berrios, G. and Porter, R. (1995), *A History of Clinical Psychiatry: The Origin and History of Psychiatric Disorders*. London: Athlone.

Billings, Frank (1914) "Focal Infection: Its Broader Application in The Etiology of General Disease," *Journal of the American Medical Association*, 63: 899–903.

Billings, Frank (1916), *Focal Infection*. New York: Appleton.

Blackmore, (Sir)Richard (1724), *A Treatise of The Spleen or Vapours*. London: Pemberton.

Blandford, J. Fielding (1871), *Insanity and Its Treatment: Lecture on The Treatment, Medical and Legal, of Insane Patients*. Philadelphia, PA: Henry C. Lea.

Bloch, A.J. (1894), "Sexual Perversion in The Female," *New Orleans Medical and Surgical Journal*, 22: 1–7.

Blustein, Bonnie Ellen (1979), "New York Neurologists and the Specialization of American Medicine," *Bulletin of the History of Medicine*, 53: 170–183.

Blustein, Bonnie Ellen (1981), " 'A Hollow Square of Psychological Science': American Neurologists and Psychiatrists in Conflict," in Scull, Andrew (ed.), *Madhouses, Mad-doctors, and Madmen: The Social History of Psychiatry in The Victorian Era*. Philadelphia, PA: University of Pennsylvania Press/London: Athlone: 241–270.

Blustein, Bonnie Ellen (1991), *Preserve Your Love for Science: Life of William A. Hammond, American Neurologist*. Cambridge: Cambridge University Press.

Bockoven, J. Sanbourne (1963), *Moral Treatment in American Psychiatry*. New York: Springer.

Borrell, Morriley (1976), "Brown-Sequard's Organotherapy and, Its Appearance in America at The End of The Nineteenth Century," *Bulletin of the History of Medicine*, 50: 309–320.

Borus, J.F. (1981), "Deinstitutionalization of The Chronically Mentally Ill," *New England Journal of Medicine*, 305: 339–342.

Braslow, Joel (1996a), "In the Name of Therapeutics: The Practice of Sterilization in a California State Hospital," *Journal of the History of Medicine and the Allied Sciences*, 51: 29–51.

Braslow, Joel (1996b), "The Influence of a Biological Therapy on Doctors' Narratives and Interrogations: The Case of General Paralysis of the Insane and Malaria Fever Therapy, 1910–1950," *Bulletin of the History of Medicine*, 70: 577–608.

Braslow, Joel (1997), *Mental Ills and Bodily Cures: Psychiatric Treatment in the First Half of the Twentieth Century*. Berkeley, CA: University of California Press.

Breggin, Peter (1991), *Toxic Psychiatry*. New York: St Martin's Press.

Brewer, John, McKendrick, Neil, and Plumb J.H. (1982), *The Birth of a Consumer Society: The Commercialization of Eighteenth Century England*. Bloomington, IN: Indiana University Press.

British Medical Journal (1866a), "The Week," January 20: 77–78.

British Medical Journal (1866b), "Local Anaesthesia," March 3: 231.

British Medical Journal (1866c), "Reviews and Notes: On The Curability of Certain Forms of Insanity, Epilepsy, Catalepsy, and Hysteria, in Females," April 28: 433–440.

British Medical Journal (1866d), "Medical News: Spiritual Advice," April 28: 456.

British Medical Journal (1866e), "Medical News: Mr. Baker Brown's Operation," April 28: 478.

British Medical Journal (1866f), "A Proposed Testimonial," June 2: 579–581.

British Medical Journal (1866g), "Clitoridectomy," December 15: 664–665.

British Medical Journal (1866h), "A Hint to The Lunacy Commissioners," December 22: 702.

British Medical Journal (1866i), "Letter From Robert Greenhalgh," December 29: 729–730.

British Medical Journal (1867a), "Letter From Robert Greenhalgh," January 12: 41–42.

British Medical Journal (1867b), "The Obstetrical Society," January 19: 61.

British Medical Journal (1867c), "Correspondence: The Lunacy Commissioners and The Surgical Home for Women," January 26: 94.

British Medical Journal (1867d), "Surgery for Lunatics," February 2: 119.

British Medical Journal (1867e), "Surgery for Lunatics," February 9: 144.

British Medical Journal (1867f), "Correspondence: Clitoridectomy," February 9: 154.

British Medical Journal (1867g), "The Debate at The Obstetrical Society," April 6: 387–388.

Brooks, C.M. (1962), *Humors, Hormones and Neurosecretions*. New York: State University of New York Press.

Brown, Isaac Baker (1866), *On The Curability of Certain Forms of Insanity, Epilepsy, Catalepsy, and Hysteria in Females*. London: Harwicke.

Brown, Theodore M. (1987), "Alan Gregg and The Rockefeller Foundation's Support of Franz Alexander's Psychosomatic Research," *Bulletin of The History of Medicine*, 61: 155–182.

Browne, Thomas (1730), *The Third Volume of the Works of Mr. Thomas Browne: Being Amusements Serious and Comical, Calculated fort The Meridian of London*, 7th edition. London: Edward Midwinter.

Browne, William Alexander Francis (1837), *What Asylums Were, Are, And Ought to Be*. Edinburgh: Black.

Bruce, Lewis (1906), *Studies in Clinical Psychiatry*. London: Macmillan.

Bryant, J.H., Moss, B.M., and Hine, F.R. (1956), "Drug Therapy – A Survey of The Literature," *Research Report # 3*, Baton Rouge, LA: Department of Institutions.

Bucke, R.M. (1898), "Surgery Among The Insane in Canada" (The Presidential Address to the Association), in *Proceedings of the American Medico-Psychological Association*, 5: 71–88.

Bucke, R.M. (1900), "Two Hundred Operative Cases – Insane Women," in *Proceedings of the American Medico-Psychological Association*, 7: 99–105.

Bucknill, John Charles (1860), "President's Address," *Journal of Mental Science*, 7: 1–23.

Bucknill, John Charles (1880), *The Care of The Insane and Their Legal Control*. London: Macmillan.

Bucknill, John Charles and Tuke, Daniel Hack (1858), *A Manual of Psychological Medicine*. London: Churchill.

Bucks County Asylum, *Annual Reports 1854–1890*.

Bucks County Asylum, *Superintendent's Diary* 2 volumes, 1853–1856 and 1856–1879, in manuscript, St John's Hospital, Stone, Bucks.

Burdett, H.C. (1891), *Hospitals and Asylums of The World*, Volumes 2. London: Churchill: 263–264.

Burgh, James (1775), *Political Disquisitions*, Volume 3. London: Dilly.

Burlingame, Charles to Adolf Meyer, 1938, Meyer Archive, Chesney Medical Archives, Johns Hopkins University, 1/557/2.

Burrows, George Man (1828), *Commentaries on The Causes, Forms, Symptoms and Treatment, Moral and Medical, of Insanity*. London: Underwood.

Burt, Cyril (1977) (original edition 1935), *The Subnormal Mind*, 3rd reprint edition. Oxford: Oxford University Press.

Bynum, W.F. (1974) "Rationales for Therapy in British Psychiatry, 1780–1835," *Medical History* 18: 317–334.

Bynum, W.F. (1981), "Rationales for Therapy in British Psychiatry, 1770–1835," in Scull, Andrew (ed.), *Madhouses, Mad-Doctors, and Madmen: The Social History of Psychiatry in the Victorian Era*. London/Philadelphia, PA: Athlone/University of Pennsylvania Press: 35–57.

Bynum, William F., Porter, Roy, and Shepherd, Michael (1985), "Introduction," to *The Anatomy of Madness*, Volume 1. London: Tavistock.

Bynum, W.F., Porter, R. and Shepherd, M. (1985), *The Anatomy of Madness*, Volumes 1 and 2. London: Tavistock.

Bynum, W.F., Porter, R., and Shepherd, M. (1988), *The Anatomy of Madness*, Volume 3. London: Routledge.

Byrd, Max (1974), *Visits to Bedlam*. Columbia, CA: University of South Carolina Press.

Callender, H. (1883–1884), "Presidential Address: History and Work of The Association of Medical Superintendents of American Institutions," *American Journal of Insanity*, 40: 1–32.

Caplan, Eric (1998), *Mind Games: American Culture and The Birth of Psychotherapy*. Berkeley, CA: University of California Press.

Caplan, Ruth (1969), *Psychiatry and The Community in The Nineteenth Century*. New York: Basic Books.

Carkesse, James (1679), *Lucida Intervalla: Containing Divers Miscellaneous Poems*. Berkeley, CA: University of California Press, 1979 (first edition, London, 1679).

Carstens, J. Henry (1897), "Commentary on Conservation of The Ovary by B. Sherwood-Dunn," *Transactions of The American Association of Obstetrics and Gynecology*, 10: 207–234.

Castel, Robert (1976), *L'Ordre psychiatrique. L'Age d'or d'alienisme*. Paris: Minuit.

Castel, Robert (1988), *The Regulation of Madness: Origins of Incarceration in France*. Berkeley, CA: University of California Press.

Castel, Françoise, Castel, Robert, and Lovell, Anne (1979), *La société psychiatrique avancée*. Paris: Editions Grasset, translated as *The Psychiatric Society*. New York: Columbia University Press, 1982.

Chapin, John (1877), "Address," in *Proceedings of The Conference of Charities*, 4: 7.

Chapin, John (1883–1884), "Public Complaints Against Asylums for The Insane, and The Commitment of The Insane," *American Journal of Insanity*, 40: 33–49.

Chapin, John (1893), Quoted in "Editorial: Removal of The Ovaries as a Therapeutic Measure in Public Institutions for The Insane," *Journal of the American Medical Association*, 20: 136.

Charcot, J.-M. (1971), *L'Hystérie* (E. Trillat ed.). Toulouse: Edouard Privat.

Chu, Franklin and Trotter, Sharland (1974), *The Madness Establishment*. New York: Grossman.

Church, Archibald (1893), "Removal of Ovaries and Tubes in The Insane and Neurotic," *American Journal of Obstetrics and Diseases of Women and Children*, 28: 491–498.

Clark, Daniel (1899), "Reflexes in Psychiatry," *Canadian Journal of Medicine and Surgery*, 5: 86–93.

Clarke, L.D. (1957), "Evaluation of Therapeutic Effects of Drugs in Psychiatric Patients," *Diseases of the Nervous System*, 17: 282–286.

Clark, Michael (1981), "The Rejection of Psychological Approaches to Mental Disorder in Late Nineteenth Century British psychiatry," in Scull, Andrew (ed.), *Madhouses, Mad-doctors, and Madmen: The Social History of Psychiatry in The Victorian Era*. Philadelphia, PA: University of Pennsylvania Press/London: The Athlone Press: 271–312.

Clark, Michael (1982), " 'The Data of Alienism': Evolutionary Neurology, Physiological Psychology, and The Reconstruction of British Psychiatric Theory, c. 1850–c.1900," unpublished DPhil. dissertation, Oxford University.

Cochrane, David (1988), " 'Humane, Economical, and Medically Wise': The LCC as Administrators of Victorian Lunacy Policy," in Bynum, W.F., Porter, R., and Shepherd, M. (eds), *The Anatomy of Madness*, Volume 3. London: Routledge: 247–272.

Cohen, Stanley (1985), *Visions of Social Control*. Cambridge: Polity.

Cohen, Stanley and Scull, Andrew (eds) (1983), *Social Control and the State: Historical and Comparative Essays*. Oxford: Martin Robertson.

Cokenower, James W. (1904), "A Plea for Conservative Operations on The Ovaries," *Transactions of The Section on Obstetrics and Diseases of Women of The American Medical Association*, 1: 293–300.

Comfort, Alex (1967), *The Anxiety Makers*. Bristol: Thomas Nelson & Son.

Commissioners in Lunacy (1876), *30th Annual Report*. London: HMSO.

Conolly, John (1849), *On The Construction and Government of Lunatic Asylums*. London: Churchill.

Conrad, Peter and Schneider, Joseph (1980), *Deviance and Medicalization: From Badness to Sickness*. St Louis: Mosby.

Cotton, Henry A. (1922), "The Etiology and Treatment of The So-Called Functional Psychoses," *American Journal of Psychiatry*, 79: 152–210.

Cotton, Henry A. (1923), "The Relationship of Chronic Sepsis to The So-Called Functional Mental Disorders," *Journal of Mental Science*, 69: 434–465.

Cotton, Henry A. (1927), "European Rambles of a Psychiatrist," unpublished typescript, Trenton State Hospital Archives, Trenton, NJ.

Cotton, Henry A. (1930), "Gastro-intestinal Stasis in The Psychoses," in *Proceedings of the Fifth International Congress of Physiotherapy*, Liege, Belgium.

Cotton, Henry A. to Adolf Meyer, April 29, May 8, 1933, Meyer Archive, Johns Hopkins University.

Coulter, Jeff (1973), *Approaches to Insanity*. Oxford: Martin Robertson.

Cowper, William (1816), *Memoir of the Early Life of William Cowper, Esq. Written by Himself*. London: Edwards.

Cox, Joseph Mason (1813), *Practical Observations on Insanity*, 3rd edition. London: Baldwin and Underwood.

Crammer, John L. (1990), *Asylum History: Buckinghamshire County Pauper Lunatic Asylum – St. John's*. London: Gaskell.

Crammer, John L. (1994), "English Asylums and English Doctors: Where Scull is Wrong," *History of Psychiatry* 5: 103–115.

Crane, George (1968), "Tardive Dyskinesia in Patients Treated With Major Neuroleptics: a Review of The Literature," *American Journal of Psychiatry*, 124, Supplement: 40–48.

Crane, George (1973a), "Clinical Psychopharmacology in Its Twentieth Year," *Science* 181, July 13: 124–128.

Crane, George (1973b), "Persistent Dyskinesia," *British Journal of Psychiatry*, 122: 399–400.

Creer, C. and Wing, J.K. (1974), *Schizophrenia at Home*. London: Institute of Psychiatry.

Crichton Royal Asylum (1857), *17th Annual Report*. Dumfries: At the Asylum.

Cruden, Alexander (1739), *The London Citizen Exceedingly Injured, Or, A British Inquisition Displayed*. London: Cooper and Dodd.

Cruden, Alexander (1754), *The Adventures of Alexander the Corrector, With an Account of The Chelsea Academies, Or The Private Places of Such As Are Supposed to Be Deprived of The Exercise of Their Reason*. London: for the author.

Cullerre, A. (1888), *Les frontières de la folie*. Paris: Baillère.

Culpin, Millais (1931), *Recent Advances in the Study of the Psychoneuroses*. London: Churchill.

Curran, J.P. (1973), "Tardive Dyskinesia: Side Effect or Not?" *American Journal of Psychiatry*, 130: 406–410.

Dain, Norman (1981), *Clifford W. Beers: Advocate for The Insane*. Pittsburgh, PA: University of Pittsburgh Press.

Dana, Charles L. (1913). "The Future of Neurology," *Journal of Nervous and Mental Diseases*, 40: 755.

Davis, J.M. (1965), "Efficacy of Tranquillizing and Anti-Depressant Drugs," *Archives of General Psychiatry*, 13: 552–572.

Defoe, Daniel (1728), *Augusta Triumphans*. London: Roberts.

Department of Health and Social Security (1971), *Better Services for The Mentally Handicapped*, Cmnd 4683. London: HMSO.

Deutsch, Albert (1973), *The Shame of The States*. Reprint edition (1948), New York: Arno.

Devine, Henry (1924), "Presidential Address on Psychiatry and Medicine," *British Medical Journal*, ii, December 6: 1033–1035.

Digby, Anne (1985), *Madness, Morality, and Medicine: A Study of The York Retreat, 1796–1914*. Cambridge: Cambridge University Press.

Dobb, Maurice (1963), *Studies in The Development of Capitalism*. New York: International Publishers.

Dodds, Dr, Strahan, Dr, and Greenlees, Dr (1890), "Assistant Medical Officers in Asylums: Their Status in The Specialty," *Journal of Mental Science*, 36: 43–50.

Doerner, Klaus (1969), Bürger und Irre. Munich: Europaische Verlagsanstalt.

Doerner, Klaus (1981), *Madmen and the Bourgeoisie*. Oxford: Blackwell.

Donzelot, Jacques (1977), *La Police des familles*. Paris: Editions de Minuit.

Dowbiggin, Ian (1985) "French Psychiatry, Hereditarianism and Professional Legitimacy 1840–1900," in Spitzer, Steven and Scull, Andrew (eds), *Research in Law, Deviance and Social Control* Volume 7, Greenwich, CT: JA1 Press: 135–165.

Dowbiggin, I. (1986), "The Professional, Sociopolitical, and Cultural Dimensions of Psychiatric Theory in France, 1840–1890," unpublished PhD dissertation. Rochester University.

Dowbiggin, Ian (1991), *Inheriting Madness: Professionalization and Psychiatric Knowledge in Nineteenth Century France*. Berkeley, CA: University of California Press.

Dowbiggin, I. (1997), "Review of Andrew Scull, *The Most Solitary of Afflictions: Madness and Society in Britain, 1700–1900*," *Victorian Studies*, 40: 360–362.

Dreyfus, H. (1987), "Foreword to The California Edition" of Michel Foucault, *Mental Illness and Psychology Berkeley* Berkeley, CA: University of California Press: vii–xliii.

Driver, J.R., Gammel, J.A., and Karnosh, L.J. (1926), "Malarial Treatment of Central Nervous System Syphilis," *Journal of the American Medical Association*, 87: 1821–1827.

Durkheim, E. (1982), *The Rules of Sociological Method*. New York: Free Press.

Durkheim, E. (1984), *The Division of Labor in Society*. New York: Free Press.

Dwyer, Ellen (1987), *Homes for the Mad: Life Inside Two Nineteenth Century Asylums*. New Brunswick, NJ: Rutgers University Press.

Earle, Pliny (1887), *The Curability of Insanity: A Series of Studies*. Philadelphia, PA: Lippincott.

Eaton, Dorman B. (1881), "Despotism in Lunatic Asylums," *North American Review*, 132: 263–275.

Edes, Robert T. (1896), "Points in The Diagnosis and Treatment of Some Obscure Common Neuroses," *Journal of the American Medical Association*, 27: 1077–1082.

Edes, Robert T. (1898), "The relations of pelvic and nervous diseases," *Journal of the American Medical Association*, 31: 1133–1136.

Englemann, George (1882), "Clitoridectomy," *The American Practitioner*, 25: 1–12.

Esquirol, J.E.D. (1838), *Des Maladies Mentales*. Paris: Baillière.

Evans, Robin (1974), "'A Rational Plan for Softening the Mind': Prison Design, 1750–1842," unpublished PhD dissertation, Essex University.

Evans, Robin (1982), *The Fabrication of Virtue: English Prison Architecture 1750–1842*. Cambridge: Cambridge University Press.

Fairchilds, C.C. (1976), *Poverty and Charity in Aix-en-Provence 1640–1789*. Baltimore, MD: Johns Hopkins University Press.

Falconer, William (1788), *A Dissertation on The Influence of The Passions upon Disorders of The Body*. London: Dill.

Fenton, H.F. (1938), "Enhancement of Physical and Mental Capacity Following Treatment of Chronic Infective Disease," *Journal of Mental Science*, 84: 544–551.

Fielding, Henry (1751), *An Enquiry into The Causes of The Late Increase of Robbers*. London: Millar.

Fine, Bob (1977), "Objectification and The Bourgeois Contradictions of Consciousness," *Economy and Society*, 6: 408–435.

Finnane, Mark (1981), *Insanity and The Insane in Post-Famine Ireland*. London: Croom Helm.

Forster, Nathaniel (1767), *An Enquiry into The Causes of The Present High Price of Provisions*. London: Fletcher.

Forsythe, Bill, Melling, Joseph, and Adair, Richard (1996), "The New Poor Law and The County Pauper Lunatic Asylum – The Devon Experience, 1834–84," *Social History of Medicine*, 9: 335–356.

Foucault, Michel (1954), *Maladie Mentale et personalité*. Paris: Presses universitaires de France.

Foucault, Michel (1961), *Folie et déraison: L'histoire de la folie à l'âge classique*. Paris: Plon.

Foucault, M. (1965), *Madness and Civilization: A History of Insanity in the Age of Reason*. New York: Vintage.

Foucault, M. (1972), *Histoire de la folie*. Paris: Gallimard.

Foucault, Michel (1977), *Discipline and Punish: The Birth of The Prison*. London: Allen Lane/New York: Pantheon.

Foucault, M. (1987), *Mental Illness and Psychology*. Berkeley, CA: University of California Press.

Fox, B. (1961), "The Investigation of The Effects of Psychiatric Treatment," *Journal of Mental Science*, 107: 493–502.

Fox, Richard (1976), "Beyond 'Social Control': Institutions and Disorder in Bourgeois Society," *History of Education Quarterly*, 16: 203–207.

Foyster, Elizabeth (1999), "Wrongful Confinement in Eighteenth Century England: A Question of Gender?," unpublished paper delivered to the Conference on Social and Medical Representations of the Links Between Insanity and Sexuality, University of Wales, Bangor.

Freeman, Hugh (1993), "The Constraints of History," *Nature*, 364: 200–201.

Freidson, Eliot (1970), *The Profession of Medicine: A Study in the Sociology of Applied Knowledge*. New York: Dodd, Mead.

Gairdner, W.T. (1982), "Presidential Address," *Journal of Mental Science*, 28: 321–332.

Gardos, G. and Cole, J.O. (1976), "Maintenance Antipsychotic Therapy: Is The Cure Worse Than The Disease?," *American Journal of Psychiatry*, 133: 32–36.

Garland, David (1985), *Punishment and Welfare: A History of Penal Strategies*. Aldershot: Gower.

Garland, David (2001), *The Culture of Control: Crime and Social Order in Contemporary Society*. Chicago, IL: University of Chicago Press.

Gauchet, M. and G. Swain (1980), *La Pratique de l'esprit humain. L'Institution asilaitre et la revolution democratique*. Paris: Gallimard.

Gay, Peter (1969), *The Enlightenment: An Interpretation*, Volume 2, *The Science of Freedom*. New York: Knopf.

Gijswijt-Hofstra, Marijke and Porter, Roy (1998), *Cultures of Psychiatry and Mental Health Care in Postwar Britain and The Netherlands*. Amsterdam: Rodopi.

Gilman, Sander, King, Helen, Porter, Roy, Rousseau, George, and Showalter, Elaine (1993), *Hysteria Beyond Freud*. Berkeley, CA: University of California Press.

Gilliam, David Tod (1896), "Oophorectomy for The Insanity and Epilepsy of The Female," *Transactions of the American Association of Obstetrics and Gynecology*, 9: 315–321.

Gittleman, R.K., Klein. D.F., and Pollack, M. (1964), "Effects of Psychotropic Drugs on Long-Term Adjustment: A Review," *Psychopharmacology*, 5: 317–338.

Glick, B. and Margolis, R. (1962), "A Study of The Influence of Experimental Design on Clinical Outcome in Drug Research," *American Journal of Psychiatry*, 118: 1087–1096.

Goffman, Erving (1961), *Asylums: Essays on The Social Situation of Mental Patients and Other Inmates*. New York: Doubleday.

Goffman, Erving (1969), "The Insanity of Place," *Psychiatry*, 32: 357–387.

Goffman, Erving (1971), "The Insanity of Place," Appendix to *Relations in Public: Microstudies of the Public Order*. New York: Basic Books: 335–390.

Goldhamer, Herbert and Marshall, Andrew (1953), *Psychosis and Civilization: Two Studies in The Frequency of Mental Disease*. Glencoe, IL: Free Press.

Goldstein, J. (1987), *Console and Classify: The French Psychiatric Profession in The Nineteenth Century*. Cambridge: Cambridge University Press.

Goldstein, J. (1990), " 'The Lively Sensibility of The Frenchman': Some Reflections on the Place of France in Foucault's *Histoire de la folie*," *History of the Human Sciences*, 3: 333–341.

Goodall, E. (1932), "The Existence of Certain States, at Present Classified under 'Schizophrenia' by Psychiatrists, May Be Infection," *Journal of Mental Science*, 78: 746–750.

Goodell, William (1881a), "Clinical Notes on The Extirpation of The Ovaries for Insanity," *Transactions of the Medical Society of the State of Pennsylvania*, 13: 638–643.

Goodell, William (1881b), *Discussion of International Medical Congress*, Seventh Session. London: J.W. Kolckmann.

Goodell, William (1890), *Lessons in Gynecology*, Philadelphia, PA: F.A. Davis.

Gordon, C. (1990a), "*Histoire de la folie*: An Unknown Book by Michel Foucault," *History of the Human Sciences*, 3: 3–26.

Gordon, C. (1990b), "History, Madness, and Other Errors," *History of the Human Sciences*, 3: 381–396.

Grad de Alcaron, Jacqueline and Sainsbury, Peter (1963), "Mental Illness and The Family," *The Lancet*, i: 544–547.

Graves, Frederick (1986), Interview With The Author, July 31, 1986.

Graves, Thomas Chivers (1919), "A Short Note on The Use of Calcium in Excited States," *Journal of Mental Science*, 65: 109.

Graves, T.C. (1922), "Colloidal Calcium in Malnutrition, Chronic Sepsis, and Emotional Disturbance," *The Lancet*, ii: 957.

Graves, T.C. (1923), "The Relation of Chronic Sepsis to So-Called Functional Mental Disorder," *Journal of Mental Science*, 69: 465–471.

Graves, T.C. (1929), "The Relation of Unresolved Infective Processes Following Acute Infective Diseases to The Causation of Mental Disorder," *Journal of Mental Science*, 75: 31–44.

Graves, T.C. (1931), "Observations on Some of The Disturbances Referable to The Principal Sensory Fields in Oso-Naso-Pharyngeal Sepsis with Mental Disorder," *Journal of Mental Science*, 77: 67–83.

Graves, T.C. (1932a), "Non-Specific Therapy in Mental Disorder," *The Lancet*, ii: 57–60, 115–121.

Graves, T.C. (1932b), "Sinusitis and Mental Disorder: Clinical Manifestations," *Journal of Mental Science*, 78: 459–464.

Graves, T.C. (1938), "Head Injuries and Mental Disorder," *Journal of Mental Science*, 84: 552–562.

Graves, T.C. (1940), "The Common Cause in the Functional Insanities," *British Medical Journal*, i, April 13: 608–611.

Graves, T.C. (1941a), "Head Injuries: Their Psychiatric Sequelae," *Journal of Mental Science*, 87: 552–562.

Graves, T.C. (1941b), "Contribution to The Discussion of Major Palmer's Paper by The President, T.C. Graves, M.D.," *Journal of Mental Science*, 81, Supplement: 10–14.

Graves, T.C. (1946), "Penicillin in The Psychoses," *The Medical Press and Circular*, March 13: 172–178.

Graves, T.C. and Turner, D.E. (1930), "A Method of Continuous Colon Irrigation," *Journal of Mental Science*, 76: 306–317.

Graves, Valerie (1986), Interview With The Author, July 28, 1986.

Greene, Richard (1889) "The Care and Cure of The Insane," *The Universal Review*, July: 493–508.

Greg, Samuel (1877), *A Layman's Legacy*. London: Macmillan.

Gregg, Alan (unpublished) Manuscript Diaries. Rockfeller Foundation Archives, Tarrytown, New York.

Griffiths, Sir Roy (1988), *Community Care: Agenda for Action: A Report to the Secretary of State*. London: HMSO.

Grob, Gerald (1966), *The State and the Mentally Ill: A History of Worcester State Mental Hospital*. Chapel Hill, NC: University of North Carolina Press.

Grob, Gerald (1973a), *Mental Institutions in America: Social Policy to 1875*. New York: Free Press.

Grob, Gerald N. (1973b), "Welfare and Poverty in American History," *Reviews in American History*, 1: 43–52.

Grob, Gerald (1977), "Rediscovering Asylums: The Unhistorical History of The Mental Hospital," *Hastings Center Report* 7, 4: 33–41.

Grob, Gerald (1978), "Public Policymaking and Social Policy," unpublished paper delivered at the Conference on the History of Public Policy, Cambridge, MA, November 3–4.

Grob, Gerald (1983), *Mental Illness and American Society, 1875–1940*. Princeton, NJ: Princeton University Press.

Grob, Gerald N. (1985), *The Inner World of American Psychiatry: Selected Correspondence*. New Brunswick, NJ: Rutgers University Press.

Grob, Gerald (1990), "Marxian Analysis and Mental Illness," *History of Psychiatry*, 1: 33–41.

Grob, Gerald (1991), *From Asylum to Community: Mental Health Policy in Modern America*. Princeton, NJ: Princeton University Press.

Gronfein, William (1984), "From Madhouse to Main Street: The Changing Place of Mental Illness in Post World War II America," unpublished PhD dissertation, State University of New York at Stony Brook.

Gronfein, William (1985a), "Psychotropic Drugs and The Origins of Deinstitutionalization," *Social Problems*, 32: 437–453.

Gronfein, William (1985b), "Incentives and Intentions in Mental Health Policy: A Comparison of The Medicaid and Community Mental Health Programs," *Journal of Health and Social Behavior*, 26: 192–206.

Gruenberg, E. and J. Archer (1979), "Abandonment of Responsibility for The Seriously Mentally Ill," *Milbank Memorial Fund Quarterly*, 57: 485–506.

Guédon, J.-C. (1977), "Michel Foucault: The Knowledge of Power and The Power of Knowledge," *Bulletin of the History of Medicine*, 51: 245–277.

Gwillim, C.M. (1962), "A Meeting of The Royal Medical and Chirurgical Society in The Session 1862," in *Proceedings of the Royal Society of Medicine*, 55: 87–91.

Hacking, I. (1986), "The Archeology of Foucault," in D.C. Hoy (ed.), *Foucault: A Critical Reader*. Oxford: Blackwell.

Hale, Nathan G. Jr (1971), *Freud and the Americans*. New York: Oxford University Press.

Hall, Ernest (1903), "Experiences of The Treatment of Pelvic Diseases in The Female Insane," *The Canadian Lancet*, 37: 301–312.

Hall, Ernest (1906). "Additional Experience in The Treatment of Pelvic Disease Associated with Psychosis," *The Canadian Lancet*, 39: 597–604.

Hall, Ernest (1908), "Gynecological Treatment in The Insane," The Canadian Practitioner, 33: 147–151.

Hall, Marshall (1837), *Memoirs on the Nervous System*. London: Sherwood, Gilbert, and Piper.

Hamilton, Allan McLane (1893), "The Abuse of Oophorectomy in Diseases of The Nervous System," *New York Medical Journal*, 57: 180–183.

Hammond, William A. (1879), "The Non-Asylum Treatment of The Insane," *Transactions of the Medical Society of New York*, 280–297.

Hare, E.H. (1962), "Masturbatory Insanity: The History of an Idea," *Journal of Mental Science*, 108: 1–25.

Haughton, R.E. (1896), "Hysterectomy, its Legitimacy, When and How," *Journal of the American Medical Association*, 26: 254–257.

Hawkes, J.M. (1871), *On the General Management of Public Lunatic Asylums in England and Wales*. London: Churchill.

Haywood, Eliza (1726), *The Distress'd Orphan, or Love in a Madhouse*, 2nd edition. London: Roberts.

Healy, David (1990), "The Psychopharmacological Era: Notes Toward a History," *Psychopharmacology*, 4: 152–167.

Healy, David (1997), *The Anti Depressant Era*. Cambridge, MA: Harvard University Press.

Henderson, D. and Gillespie, R.D. (1927), *Textbook of Psychiatry*. London: Oxford University Press.

Henderson, D.K. and Batchelor, I. (1956), *Textbook of Psychiatry*. Oxford: Oxford University Press.

Hervey, Nicholas (1986), "Advocacy or Folly? The Alleged Lunatics' Friend Society," *Medical History*, 30: 254–275.

Hervey, Nicholas (1987), "The Lunacy Commission, 1845–60," unpublished PhD dissertation, 2 volumes, Bristol University.

Hinshelwood, R.D. (1991), "Psychodynamic Psychiatry Before World War I," in G.E. Berrios, G.E. and Freeman, H. (eds), *150 Years of British Psychiatry*. London: Gaskell, 197–205.

Hobbs, A.T. (1898), "Some Present Methods of Treatment," *The Canadian Practitioner*, 23: 513–525.

Hobbs, A.T. (1899), "Surgical Gynecology Among The Insane: Right or Wrong?" *The Canadian Practitioner*, 24: 379–384.

Hoffman, Jay (1949) "Clinical Observations Concerning Schizophrenic Patients Treated With Prefrontal Leucotomy," *New England Journal of Medicine*, 241: 233–236.

Horn, Margo (1989), *Before It's Too Late: The Child Guidance Movement in the United States*. Philadelphia, PA: Temple University Press.

House of Commons (1763), *A Report from The Committee Appointed to Enquire into The State of The Private Madhouses in This Kingdom*. London: Whiston.

House of Commons (1877), *Select Committee on the Operations of the Lunacy Law*.

Howard, John (1778), *The State of the Prisons*. Warrington: Egres.

Howell, Joel (1995), *Technology in the Hospital: The Transformation of Patient Care in The Early Twentieth Century*. Baltimore, MD: Johns Hopkins University Press.

Hughes, A.F.W. (1977), "A History of Endocrinology," *Journal of the History of Medicine and Allied Sciences*, 32: 292–313.

Hunter, William (1900), "Oral Sepsis as a Cause of Disease," *British Medical Journal*, ii: 215–216.

Hunter, William (1927), "Chronic Sepsis as a Cause of Mental Disorder," *Journal of Mental Science*, 73: 549–563.

Hunter, William (1929), "The Relation of Focal Infection to Mental Diseases," *Journal of Mental Science*, 75: 464–466.

Hunter, Michael and Schaffer, Simon (eds) (1989), *Robert Hooke: New Studies Woodbridge*, Suffolk: Boydell Press.

Hunter, Richard and Macalpine, Ida (1963), *Three Hundred Years of Psychiatry*. Oxford: Oxford University Press.

Hunter, Richard and Macalpine, Ida (eds) (1964a), *Description of the Retreat* facsimile edition with a new introduction. London: Dawsons.

Hunter, Richard and Macalpine, Ida (eds) (1964b), *Inquiry Concerning The Indications of Insanity* by John Conolly, facsimile edition with a new introduction. London: Dawsons.

Hurd, Henry M. (1916), *The Institutional Care of The Insane in The United States and Canada*, Volume 1, Baltimore, MD: Johns Hopkins University Press.

Ignatieff, Michael (1976), "Prison and Factory Discipline, 1770–1800: The Origins of an Idea," unpublished paper presented at the Annual Meeting of the American Historical Association.

Ignatieff, Michael (1978), *A Just Measure of Pain: The Penitentiary in the Industrial Revolution in England*. New York: Pantheon.

Ignatieff, Michael (1983), "State Civil Society and Total Institutions: A Critique of Recent Social Histories of Punishment," in Cohen, Stanley and Scull, Andrew (eds), *Social Control and the State: Historical and Comparative Essays*. Oxford: Martin Robertson: 75–105.

Ill, Edward J. (1888), "Acute Psychoses Following Gynecological Operations," *The Pittsburgh Medical Review*, 2: 1–5.

Illinois Department of Public Welfare (1927–1929), *Annual Reports*, 11, 12.

Ingleby, David (1973), "The Psychology of Child Psychology," *The Human Context*, 5: 557–568.

Ingleby, David (1982), "The Social Construction of Mental Illness," in Treacher, A. and Wright, P. (eds), *The Problem of Medical Knowledge: Towards a Social Constructivist View*. Edinburgh: Edinburgh University Press, 123–143.

Ingleby, David (1983), "Mental Health and the Social Order," in Cohen, Stanley and Scull, Andrew (eds), *Social Control and the State: Historical and Comparative Essays*. Oxford: Martin Robertson: 141–188.

Ingleby, David (1985), "Professionals as Socializers: The 'Psy Complex,'" *Research in Law, Deviance, and Social Control*, 7: 79–109.

Jackson, Mark (2000), *The Borderland of Imbecility: Medicine, Society, and The Fabrication of The Feeble Mind in Late Victorian and Edwardian England*. Manchester: Manchester University Press.

Jacyna, Stephen (1982), "Somatic Theories of Mind and The Interests of Medicine in Britain, 1850–1879," *Medical History*, 26: 233–258.

Joint Commission on Mental Illness and Health (1961), *Action for Mental Health: The Final Report of the Joint Commission on Mental Illness and Health*. New York: Basic Books.

Jones, Kathleen W. (1988), "As The Twig Is Bent: American Psychiatry and The Troublesome Child 1890–1940," unpublished PhD dissertation, Rutgers University.

Jones, Kathleen (1994), *Asylums and After*. London: Athlone.

Jones, Sir Robert Armsrong (1917a), "Correspondence," *Nature*, 100, September 6: 1–3.

Jones, R.A. (1917b), "Shell Shock," *Nature*, 100, September 6, 7: 1–3.

Journal of the American Medical Association (1893), "Editorial: Removal of the Ovaries as a Therapeutic Measure in Public Institutions for the Insane," 20: 135–137.

Jowett, R.E. (1936), "Sinus Sepsis and Mental Disorder," *Journal of Mental Science*, 82: 28–37.

Kane, J., Woerner, M., and Weinhold, (1984), "Incidence of Tardive Dyskinesia: Five Year Data from a Prospective Study," *Psychopharmacology Bulletin*, 20: 387–389.

Kane, J., Woerner M., and Borenstein, M. (1986), "Integrating Incidence and Prevalence of Tardive Dyskinesia," *Psychopharmacology Bulletin*, 2: 254–258.

Kaplan, Harold and Saddock, Benjamin (eds) (1995), *Comprehensive Textbook of Psychiatry*, 6th edition. Baltimore, MD: Williams and Wilkins.

Keay, Julia (2004), *Alexander the Corrector: The Tormented Genius Who Unwrote the Bible*. New York: Harper-Collins.

Kelly, Howard A. (1893), "The Ethical Side of the Operation of Oophorectomy," *American Journal of Obstetrics*, 27: 206–208.

Kelly, Howard A. (1896), "Conservatism in Ovariotomy," *Journal of the American Medical Association*, 6: 249–257.

Kelly, Howard A. (1908), *Medical Gynecology*, New York: Appleton.

Kelly, Thomas, J. (1909), "How far is The So-Called Conservative Pelvic Surgery Conservative?" *American Journal of Obstetrics and Diseases of Women and Children*, 60: 94–100, *Journal of the American Medical Association*, 16: 516–517.

Kirk, S. and Thierren M. (1975), "Community Mental Health Myths and The Fate of Formerly Hospitalized Patients," *Psychiatry*, 38: 209–217.

Kitto, Robert A. (1891), "Ovariotomy as a Prophylaxis and Cure for Insanity," *Journal of the American Medical Association*, 16: 516–517.

Kittrie, Nicholas (1972), *The Right to be Different: Deviance and Enforced Therapy*, Baltimore, MD: Johns Hopkins University Press.

LaCapra, D. (1990), "Foucault, History, and Madness," *History of the Human Sciences*, 3: 31–38.

Laffey, Paul (2002), "Two Registers of Madness in Enlightenment Britain: Part I," *History of Psychiatry*, 3: 419–431.

Laffey, Paul (2003), "Two Registers of Madness in Enlightenment Britain: Part II," *History of Psychiatry*, 14: 63–81.

Laing, R.D. (1969), *Self and Others*. New York: Pantheon.

Laing, R.D. and Esterson, A. (1965), *Sanity, Madness, and the Family*. New York: Basic Books.

Lalor, Joseph (1860), "Observations on The Size and Construction of Lunatic Asylums," *Journal of Mental Science*, 7: 104–111.

Lancet (1873a), "Mr. Isaac Baker Brown," January 25: 151–152.

Lancet (1873b), "Obituary: Isaac Baker Brown, F.R.C.S.," February 8: 222–223.

Langsley, Donald G. (1980), "The Community Mental Health Center: Does It Treat Patients?" *Hospital and Community Psychiatry*, 31: 815–819.

Larson, Magali (1977), *The Rise of Professionalism: A Sociological Analysis*. Berkeley, CA: University of California Press.

Lasch, Christopher (1977), *Haven in a Heartless World: The Family Beseiged*. New York: Basic Books.

Laycock, Thomas (1840), *A Treatise on The Nervous Diseases of Women*. London: Longman, Orme, Brown, Green, and Longmans.

Laycock, Thomas (1876), "Reflex, Automatic, and Unconscious Cerebration: A History and Criticism," *Journal of Mental Science*, 21, 1876: 477–498 and 22, 1876: 1–17.

Leary, D. (1976), "Michel Foucault: an Historian of the *Sciences Humaines*," *Journal of the History of Behavioral Sciences*, 12: 286–293.

Lerman, Paul (1982), *Deinstitutionalization and the Welfare State*, New Brunswick, NJ: Rutgers University Press.

Leveton, A.F. (1958), "The Evaluation and Testing of Psychopharmaceutical Drugs," *American Journal of Psychiatry*, 115: 232–238.

Levillain, Fernard (1891), *La neurasthénie*. Paris: Maloine.

Lewis, Aubrey (1959), "The Impact of Psychotropic Drugs on The Structure, Function, and Future of The Psychiatric Services," in Bradley, P.B., Deniker, P. and Radouco-Thomas, C. (eds), *Neuropsychopharmacology*, 1: 207–212.

Locke, John (1968), *Educational Writings*. Cambridge: Cambridge University Press.

Lomax, Montague (1922), *The Experiences of an Asylum Doctor*. London: George Allen and Unwin.

Longo. Lawrence D. (1979), "The rise and Fall of Battey's Operation: a Fashion in Surgery," *Bulletin of the History of Medicine*, 53: 244–267.

Lowe, Louisa (1883), *The Bastilles of England, or The Lunacy Laws at Work*. London: Crookende.

Lubove, Roy (1969), *The Professional Altruist*. New York: Atheneum.

Lunbeck, Elizabeth (1994), *The Psychiatric Persuasion: Knowledge, Gender, and Power in Modern America*. Princeton, NJ: Princeton University Press.

Macalpine, Ida and Hunter, Richard (1969), *George III and the Mad Business*. London: Allen Lane.

MacBride, David (1772), *A Methodical Introduction to The Theory and Practice of Physick*. London: Strahan.

MacDonald, Michael (1981), *Mystical Bedlam: Madness, Anxiety, and Healing in Seventeenth Century England*. Cambridge: Cambridge University Press.

McDowell, Ephraim (1817), "Three Cases of Extirpation of Diseased Ovaries," *Eclectic Repertory and Analytic Review*, 8: 242–244.

McGovern, Constance (1981), "Doctors or Ladies? Women Physicians in Psychiatric Institutions. 1872–1900," *Bulletin of the History of Medicine*, 55: 88–107.

McKendrick, Neil (1961), "Josiah Wedgwood and Factory Discipline," *Historical Journal*, 4: 30–55.

MacKenzie, Charlotte (1985), "Social Factors in the Admission, Discharge, and Continuing Stay of Patients at Ticehurst Asylum, 1845–1917," in Bynum, W.F., Porter, R., and Shepherd, M. (eds), *The Anatomy of Madness* Volume 2. London: Tavistock: 147–174.

MacKenzie, Charlotte (1987), "A Family Asylum: A History of the Private Asylum at Ticehurst in Sussex, 1792–1917," unpublished PhD thesis, University of London.

MacKenzie, Charlotte (1992), *Psychiatry for The Rich: A History of Ticehurst Private Asylum*. London: Routledge.

MacKenzie, Henry (1771), *The Man of Feeling*. London: Cadell.

Maclean, D. (1894), "Sexual Mutilation," *California Medical Journal*, 15: 382–384.

McMurtry, Lewis (1897), "Commentary on 'Conservation of The Ovary' by B. Sherwood-Dunn," *Transactions of the American Association of Obstetrics and Gynecology*, 10: 212–213.

Maher, W.B. and Maher B. (1982), "The Ship of Fools: *Stultifera Navis* or *Ignis Fatuus?*," *American Psychologist*, 37: 756–761.

Maisel, Albert Q. (1946), "Bedlam 1946," *Life* 20, May 6: 102–118.

Manor House Chiswick, *Male Case Book*, 1884–1891, in manuscript at the Wellcome Institute for the History of Medicine, London.

Manor House Chiswick, *Female Case Book*, 1884–1893, in manuscript at the Wellcome Institute for the History of Medicine, London.

Manton, W.P. (1889), "A Contribution to The History of Ovariotomy on The Insane," *Transactions of the American Association of Obstetricians and Gynecologists*, 2: 262–265.

Manton, W.P. (1900), "Discussion of R. M. Bucke, Two Hundred Operative Cases-Insane Women," in *Proceedings of the American Medico-Psychological Association*, 7: 99–105.

Marcy, Henry O. (1887), "Recent Advances in Abdominal Surgery," *The Medical Register*, i: 6–10.

Marks, Harry (1997), *The Progress of Experiment: Science and Therapeutic Reform in the United States, 1900–1990*. Cambridge: Cambridge University Press.

Marshall, J. H. (1865), "Insanity Cured by Castration," *Medical and Surgical Reporter* (Philadelphia), 13: 363–364.

Massachusetts State Board of Charities (1867), *4th Annual Report*.

Maudsley, Henry (1867), *The Physiology and Pathology of Mind*. London: Macmillan.

Maudsley, Henry (1870), *Body and Mind*. London: Macmillan.

Maudsley, Henry (1871), *The Physiology and Pathology of the Mind*. New York: Appleton.

Maudsley, Henry (1879), *The Pathology of Mind*. London: Macmillan.

Maudsley, Henry (1895), *The Pathology of Mind*. London: Macmillan.

Mayer-Gross, W., Slater, E., and Roth, M. (1960), *Clinical Psychiatry*. London: Cassell.

Mead, Richard (1751), *Medical Precepts and Cautions*. London: Brindley.

Meigs, Charles (1847), A Lecture on Some of The Distinctive Characteristics of The Female." Delivered before the class of the Jefferson Medical College. January 5, 1847, Philadelphia/London: Macmillan.

Melling, Joseph and Forsythe, Bill (eds), (1999), *Insanity, Institutions, and Society: A Social History of Madness in Comparative Perspective*. London: Routledge.

Mercier, Charles (1914), *A Textbook of Insanity*, 2nd edition. London: Allen and Unwin.

Merquior, J. G. (1985), *Foucault*. London: Fontana.

Merskey, Harold (1994), "Somatic Treatments, Ignorance, and the Historiography of Psychiatry," *History of Psychiatry*, 5: 387–391.

Metcalf, Urban (1818), *The Interior of Bethlem Hospital*. London: for the author.

Mettler, F.A. (ed.) (1949), *Selective Partial Ablation of The Frontal Cortex: A Correlative Study of Its Effects on Human Psychotic Subjects*. New York: Hoeber.

Meyer, Joseph (1894), "A case of Insanity, Caused by Diseased Ovaries, Cured by Their Removal: a Phenomenal Triumph for Operative Treatment," *Transactions of the American Association of Obstetricians and Gynecologists*, 7: 503–504.

Micale, Mark and Lerner, Paul (2001), *Traumatic Pasts: History, Psychiatry, and Trauma in The Modern Age, 1870–1930*. Cambridge: Cambridge University Press.

Micale, Mark and Porter, Roy (eds) (1993), *Discovering The History of Psychiatry*. Oxford: Oxford University Press.

Michael, Pamela (2003), *Care and Treatment of The Mentally Ill in North Wales 1800–2000*. Cardiff: University of Wales Press.

Midelfort, H.C.E. (1980), "Madness and civilization in early modern Europe," in Malament, B.C. (ed.), *After The Reformation: Essays in Honor of J.H. Hexter*. Philadelphia, PA: University of Pennsylvania Press: 247–265.

Midelfort, Erik (1990), "Comment on Colin Gordon," *History of the Human Sciences*, 3: 41–45.

Miller, Peter (1980), "The Territory of The Psychiatrist," *Ideology and Consciousness*, 7: 63–106.

Mitchell, Silas Weir (1894), *Address Before The American Medico-Psychological Association*. Philadelphia, PA: for the author.

Mitchell, J.J. and Smith, G.M. (1930), *History of the Great War Medical Services*, Volume 2. London: HMSO.

Mitchell, S. Weir (1894), "An Address Before The American Medico-Psychological Association," *Journal of Nervous and Mental Disease*, 21: 411–437.

Mitchinson, Wendy (1980), "Gynecological Operations on The Insane," *Archivaria*, 10: 125–144.

Mitchinson, Wendy (1981), "R, M. Bucke: a Victorian Asylum Superintendent," *Ontario History*, 73: 239–254.

Mitchinson, Wendy (1982), "Gynecological Operations on Insane Women: London, Ontario, 1895–1901," *Journal of Social History*, 15: 467–484.

Mitchinson, Wendy (1984), "A Medical Debate in Nineteenth Century English Canada: Ovariotomies," *Histoire Sociale/Social History*, 17: 125–144.

Mollica, Richard (1983), "From Asylum to Community: The Threatened Disintegration of Public Psychiatry," *New England Journal of Medicine*, 308: 267–273.

Monro, John (1758), *Remarks on Dr. Battie's Treatise on Madness*. London: Clarke.

Morantz, Regina and Sue Zschoche (1980), "Professionalism, Feminism, and Gender Roles: A Comparative Study of Nineteenth Century Medical Therapeutics," *Journal of American History*, 67: 568–588.

Morel, B.A. (1857), *Traité des dégénérescences physiques, intellectuelles, et morales de l'espèce humaine*. Paris, Masson.

Morel, B.A. (1869), *Annales médico-psychologiques*, 2: 282–283.

Morgan David (1975), "Explaining Mental Illness," *European Journal of Sociology*, 16: 262–280.

Morton, Thomas (1893), "Removal of the Ovaries as a Cure for Insanity," *American Journal of Insanity*, 49: 397–401.

Moynihan, Sir Berkeley (1927), "Relation of Aberrant Mental States to Organic Disease," *British Medical Journal*, ii, November 5: 815–817.

Müller, Johannes (1839–1842), *Elements of Physiology*, 2 volumes. London: Taylor and Walton.

Muraskin, William (1976), "The Social Control Theory in American History, A Critique," *Journal of Social History*, 9: 559–565.

Newington, Herbert Hayes (1989), "Presidential Address," *Journal of Mental Science*, 35: 293–315.

N.I.M.H. Study Group (1964), "Phenothiazine Treatment in Acute Schizophrenia – Effectiveness," *Archives of General Psychiatry*, 10: 246–261.

Nicholls, G. (1854), *A History of The English Poor Law in Connection with The Legislation and Other Circumstances Affecting The Condition of The People*, 2 volumes. London: Murray.

Nicholls, G. (1856), *A History of the Irish Poor Law*. London: Murray.

Nye, Robert A. (1984), *Crime, Madness and Politics in Modern France: The Medical Concept of National Decline*. Princeton, PA: Princeton University Press.

Ogden, A.H. (1983), "T.T. Graves and Focal Sepsis Theory," unpublished paper delivered at the Regional Meeting of the Midlands Division of the Royal College of Psychiatrists.

Oppenheim, Janet (1991), *"Shattered Nerves": Doctors, Patients, and Depression in Victorian England*. New York: Oxford University Press.

Orlans, Harold (1948), "An American Death Camp," *Politics*, 5: 162–168.

Packard, Elizabeth (1873), *Modern Persecution, or Insane Asylums Unveiled*, 2 volumes, Hartford, CT: Case, Lockwood, and Brainard.

Paget, Sir George (1866), *The Harveian Oration*. Cambridge: Deighton and Bell.

Pargeter, William (1792), *Observations on Maniacal Disorders*. Reading: for the author.

Parry-Jones, William Ll. (1972), *The Trade in Lunacy: A Study of Private Madhouses in England in The Eighteenth and Nineteenth Centuries*. London: Routledge.

Parry-Jones, William Ll. (1981), "The Model of the Geel Lunatic Colony and its Influence on The Nineteenth Century Asylum System in Great Britain," in Scull, Andrew (ed.), *Madhouses, Mad-Doctors, and Madmen: The Social History of Insanity in the Victorian Era*. Philadelphia, PA: University of Pennsylvania Press/London: Athlone: 201–217.

Peaslee, E.R. (1872), *Ovarian Tumors: Their Pathology, Diagnosis, and Treatment, Especially by Ovariotomy*. New York: Appleton.

Pennington, Hugh (2003), "Can You Close Your Eyes Without Falling Over?" *London Review of Books*, September 11: 31.

Perceval, John Thomas (1839, 1840), *A Narrative of the Treatment Received by a Gentleman, During a State of Mental Derangement*, 2 volumes. London: Effingham Wilson.

Pernick, Martin (1985) *A Calculus of Suffering: Pain, Professionalism, and Anesthesia in Nineteenth Century America*. New York: Columbia University Press.

Peters, M. (1971), "Extended review of Michel Foucault, *Madness and Civilization*, and of Jean Piaget, *Structuralism*," *Sociological Review*, 19: 634–638.

Peterson, M. Jeanne (1978), *The Medical Profession in Mid-Victorian London*. Berkeley, CA: University of California Press.

Phillips, H. Temple (1973), "The History of the Old Private Lunatic Asylum at Fishponds Bristol, 1740–1859," unpublished MSc thesis, Bristol University.

Philo, Chris (2004), *A Geographical History of Institutional Provision for the Insane from Medieval Times to the Present in England and Wales: The Space Reserved for Insanity*. Lampeter, Wales: Edwin Mellen.

Pickworth, F.A. (1935), *Chronic Nasal Sinusitis & Its Relation to Mental Disorder*. London: Lewis.

Pickworth, F.A. (1952), *A New Outlook on Mental Disease*. Bristol: Wright.

Pinel, Philippe (1806), *A Treatise on Insanity* (translated by D.D. Davis). Sheffield: Cadell and Davies.

Pinel, P. (1962), *A Treatise on Insanity*, trans. D.D. Davis, 1806; facsimile edition, New York: Haffner.

Pines, Malcolm (1991), "The Development of The Psychodynamic Movement," in Berrios, G. and Freeman, H. (eds), *150 Years of British Psychiatry*. London: Gaskell: 206–231.

Pitts, John (1978), "The Association of Medical Superintendents of American Institutions for The Insane, 1844–1892," unpublished PhD dissertation, University of Pennsylvania.

Plumb, J.H. (1975), "The New World of Children in Eighteenth Century England," *Past and Present*, 67: 64–95.

Pollard, S. (1965), *The Making of Modern Management*. Harmonsworth, Middlesex: Penguin.

Porter, Roy (1977), *The Making of Geology: Earth Science in Britain, 1660–1815*. Cambridge: Cambridge University Press.

Porter, Roy (1981–1982), "Was There a Moral Therapy in The Eighteenth Century?" *Lychnos*: 12–26.

Porter, Roy (1982), *English Society in The Eighteenth Century*. London: Allen Lane.

Porter, Roy (1983), "The Rage of Party: A Glorious Revolution in English Psychiatry?" *Medical History*, 27: 35–50.

Porter, Roy (1987a), *Mind Forg's Manacles: A History of Madness in England from The Restoration to the Regency*. London: Athlone.

Porter, Roy (1987b), *A Social History of Madness: Stories of The Insane*. London: Weidenfeld and Nicolson.

Porter, Roy (1988a), *Edward Gibbon: Making History*. London: Weidenfeld and Nicolson.

Porter, Roy (ed.) (1988b), Thomas Trotter, *An Essay, Medical, Philosophical, and Chemical on Drunkenness and its Effects on the Human Body*. London: Routledge.

Porter, Roy (ed.) (1988c), John Haslam, *Illustrations of Madness*. Routledge: London.

Porter, Roy (1990), *Health for Sale: Quakery in England, 1660–1850*. Manchester: Manchester University Press.

Porter, Roy (ed.) (1991), George Cheyne, *The English Malady*. London: Routledge.

Porter, Roy (1994), *London: A Social History*. London: Hamish Hamilton.

Porter, Roy (1997), *The Greatest Benefit to Mankind: A Medical History of Humanity from Antiquity to the Present*. London: Fontana.

Porter, Roy (2000), *Enlightenment Britain and The Creation of The Modern World*. London: Allen Lane.

Porter, Roy (2001), "Review of *Undertaker of The Mind*," *Social History of Medicine*, 14: 348–349.

Porter, Roy (2002), *Madness: A Brief History*. Oxford: Oxford University Press.

Porter, Roy and Hall, Lesley (1995), *The Facts of Life: The Creation of Sexual Knowledge in Britain, 1650–1950*. New Haven, CT: Yale University Press.

Porter, Roy and Porter, Dorothy (1988), *In Sickness and in Health: The English Experience, 1650–1850*. London: Fourth Estate.

Porter, Roy and Porter, Dorothy (1989), *Patient's Progress: Doctors and Doctoring in Eighteenth Century England*. Oxford: Polity.

Porter, Roy and Wright, David (eds) (2003), *The Confinement of The Insane: International Perspectives*. Cambridge; Cambridge University Press.

Potts, W.A. (1935), "The Diagnosis and Treatment of Some Physical Factors in Nervous Breakdown and Incipient Mental Disorder," *Journal of Mental Science*, 81: 260–264.

Powell, Enoch (1961), "Speech to The National Association for Mental Health," *Report of the Annual Conference*. London: Mind.

Praeger, E. Arnold (1895), "Is So-Called Conservatism in Gynecology Conducive of the Best Results to the Patient?" *Transactions of the American Association of Obstetrics and Gynecology*, 2: 320–329.

Pratt, E.H. (1898), "Circumcision of Girls," *Journal of Oroficial Surgery*, 6: 385–392.

Pressman, Jack (1986), "Uncertain Promise: Psychosurgery and The Development of Scientific Psychiatry in America, 1935 to 1955," unpublished PhD dissertation, University of Pennsylvania.

Pressman, Jack (1998), *Last Resort: Psychosurgery and The Limits of Medicine*. Cambridge: Cambridge University Press.

Putnam, James Jackson (1908), "Discussion of Edward Wyllys Taylor, 'The Attitude of The Medical Profession Toward The Psychotherapeutic Movement,'" *Journal of Nervous and Mental Diseases*, 35: 405–420.

Quen, Jacques (1974), "David Rothman's *Discovery of the Asylum*," *Journal of Psychiatry and the Law*, 2: 105–120.

Rabinow, P. (1990), "Truth and society," *History of the Human Sciences*, 3: 55–56.

Ray, Gordon (ed.) (1945), *The Letters and Private Papers of William Makepeace Thackeray*. London: Oxford University Press.

Ray, Laurence (1981), "Models of Madness in Victorian Asylum Practice," *European Journal of Sociology*, 22: 229–264.

[Rayner Report] (1981), *Government Statistical Services*. Cmnd 8236 London: H.M.S.O.

Reade, Charles (1864), *Hard Cash: A Matter of Fact Romance*. London: Ward Locke.

Rees, T.P. (1957), "Some Observations on the Psychiatric Patient, The Mental Hospital, and the Community," in Greenblatt, M., Levinson, D.J., and Williams, R.H. (eds), *The Patient and The Mental Hospital*. Glencoe, IL: Free Press.

Richardson, Samuel (1754), *The History of Six Charles Grandison*. London: for the author.

Rieder, R.O. (1974), "Hospitals, Patients, and Politics," *Schizophrenia Bulletin*, 11: 9–15.

Robinson, Harry M. (1952), "A Short History of Dermatology as it Progressed in Baltimore," *Bulletin of the University of Maryland School of Medicine*, 9–23.

Rohé, George H. (1892), "The Relation of Pelvic Disease to Insanity," *American Journal of Insanity*, 49: 327.

Rohé, George H. (1893), "Further Observations on The Relation of Pelvic Disease and Psychical Disturbances in Women," *Transactions of the American Association of Obstetricians and Gynecologists*, 6: 249–264.

Rosanoff, Aaron J. (1917), "Psychiatric Problems at Large," in *Proceedings of the American Medico-Psychological Association*, 24: 257–261.

Rose, Nikolas (1985), *The Psychological Complex: Psychology, Politics, and Society in England 1869–1939*. London: Routledge and Kegan Paul.

Rose, Nikolas (1986), "Psychiatry: The Discipline of Mental Health," in Miller, P. and Rose, N. (eds), *The Power of Psychiatry*. Oxford: Polity Press: ADD.

Rose, Stephen (1979), "Deciphering Deinstitutionalization: Complexities in Policy and Program Analysis," *Milbank Memorial Fund Quarterly*, 57: 429–460.

Rosenberg, Charles (1962), "The Place of George M. Beard in Nineteenth Century Psychiatry," *Bulletin of the History of Medicine*, 36: 245–259.

Rosenberg, Charles (1975), "The Crisis of Psychiatric Legitimacy," in Kreigman, George (ed.), *American Psychiatry: Past, Present, and Future*. Charlottesville: University of Virginia Press: 135–148.

Rosenberg, Charles (1979) "The Therapeutic Revolution: Medicine, Meaning, and Social Change in Nineteenth Century America," in Morris J. Vogel and Charles Rosenberg (eds), *The Therapeutic Revolution: Essays in the Social History of American Medicine*. Philadelphia, PA: University of Pennsylvania Press: 3–25.

Ross, James (1897), "Commentary on 'Conservation of the Ovary' by B. Sherwood-Dunn," *Transactions of the American Association of Obstetrics and Gynecology*, 10: 229–230.

Roth, Sir Martin (1973), "Psychiatry and its Critics," *British Journal of Psychiatry*, 122: 374–402.

Rothman, David J. (1971), *The Discovery of the Asylum*. Boston, MA: Little, Brown.

Rothman, David J. (1976), "Review of *Mental Institutions in America*," *Journal of Interdisciplinary History*, 7: 534–536.

Rothman, David J. (1980), *Conscience and Convenience: The Asylum and Its Alternatives in Progressive America*. Boston, MA: Little, Brown.

Rothman, David J. and Sheila M. Rothman (1984), *The Willowbrook Wars*. New York: Harper and Row.

Rumbaut, Daniel (1934), "Some Recent Forms of Mental Treatment," *Journal of Mental Science*, 80: 630–638.

Russell, James (1898), "The After-Effects of Surgical Procedures on The Generative Organs of Females for The Relief of Insanity," *The Canadian Practitioner*, 23: 577–589.

Sainz, A.N., Bigelow, N., and Barwise, C. (1957), "On a Methodology for The Clinical Evaluation of 'Psychopraxic Drugs'," *Psychiatric Quarterly*, 31: 10–16.

Salmon, Thomas W. (1917), "Some New Fields in Neurology and Psychiatry," *Journal of Nervous and Mental Diseases*, 46: 90–99.

Salmon, Thomas W. (1920), "Some New Problems for Psychiatric Research in Delinquency," *Mental Hygiene*, 4: 29–42.

Salmon, Thomas W. (1924), "Presidential Address," *American Journal of Psychiatry*, 81: 1–11.

Scheff, Thomas (1966), *Being Mentally Ill*. Chicago: Aldine.

Scott, Francis (1879), "English County Asylums," *Fortnightly Review*, 26: 114–143.

Scull, Andrew (1975), "From Madness to Mental Illness: Medical Men as Moral Entrepreneurs," *European Journal of Sociology*, 16: 219–261.

Scull, Andrew (1976), "The Decarceration of the Mentally Ill: A Critical View," *Politics and Society*, 6: 173–211.

Scull, Andrew (1977), *Decarceration: Community Treatment and The Deviant*. Englewood Cliffs, NJ: Prentice-Hall.

Scull, Andrew (1979), *Museums of Madness: The Social Organization of Insanity in Nineteenth Century England*. London: Allen Lane/Penguin Books.

Scull, Andrew (1981a), "The Discovery of The Asylum Revisited: Lunacy Reform in The New American Republic," in Scull, Andrew (ed.), *Madhouses, Mad-Doctors, and Madmen: The Social History of Psychiatry in The Victorian Era*. Philadelphia, PA: University of Pennsylvania Press/London: The Athlone Press: 144–165.

Scull, Andrew (1981b), *Madhouses, Mad-Doctors, and Madmen: The Social History of Psychiatry in The Victorian Era*. Philadelphia, PA: University of Pennsylvania Press/London: The Athlone Press.

Scull, Andrew (1981c), "A New Trade In Lunacy: The Recommodification of The Mental Patient," *American Behavioral Scientist*, 24: 741–754.

Scull, Andrew (1984a), "A Brilliant Career? John Conolly and Victorian Psychiatry." *Victorian Studies*, 27: 203–235.

Scull, Andrew (1984b), *Decarceration: Community Treatment and the Deviant: A Radical View*, 2nd edition. Oxford: Polity Press/New Brunswick, NJ: Rutgers University Press.

Scull, Andrew (1987), "Desperate Remedies: A Gothic Tale of Madness and Modern Medicine," *Psychological Medicine*, 17: 561–577.

Scull, A. (1988), "Keepers," *London Review of Books*, September 29: 21–23.

Scull, Andrew (1989), *Social Order/Mental Disorder: Anglo-American Psychiatry in Historical Perspective*. Berkeley, CA: University of California Press.

Scull, A. (1990), "Michel Foucault's History of Madness," *History of the Human Sciences*, 3: 57–67.

Scull, Andrew (1991), *The Asylum as Utopia: W.A.F. Browne and The Mid-Nineteenth Century Consolidation of Psychiatry*. London: Routledge.

Scull, Andrew (1992), "A Failure to Communicate?' On The Reception of Foucault's *Histoire de la folie* by Anglo-American Historians," in Arthur Still and Irving Velody (eds), *Rewriting the History of Madness*. London: Routledge: 150–163.

Scull, Andrew (1993), *The Most Solitary of Afflictions: Madness and Society in Britain, 1700–1900*. New Haven, CT and London: Yale University Press.

Scull, Andrew (1994), "Somantic Treatments and the Historiography of Psychiatry," *History of Psychiatry*, 5: 1–12.

Scull, Andrew (1999), "Rethinking The History of Asylumdom," in Melling, Joseph, Forsythe, Bill, and Adair, Richard (eds), *Insanity, Institutions, and Society: New Approaches to The Social History of Insanity*, London: Routledge: 294–314.

Scull, Andrew (2005), *Madhouse: A Tragic Tale of Megalomania and Modern Medicine*. London and New Haven, CT: Yale University Press.

Scull, Andrew, MacKenzie, Charlotte, and Hervey, Nicholas (1996), *Masters of Bedlam: The Transformation of the Mad-Doctoring Trade*. Princeton, NJ: Princeton University Press.

Sedgwick, Peter (1982), *Psychopolitics*. London: Pluto Press.

Segal, S. and Aviram, U. (1978), *The Mentally Ill in Community Based Sheltered Care*. New York: Wiley.

Shapin, Steven (1989), "Who was Robert Hooke?" in Hunter, M. and Schaffer, S. (eds), *Robert Hooke: New Studies*. Woodbridge, Suffolk: Boydell Press: 253–285.

Shera, Geoffrey (1930), "A Special Method of Investigating the Streptococcal and Acidophilus Intestinal Flora: With Results in Fifty Three Mental Patients," *Journal of Mental Science*, 76: 56–65.

Sheridan, Alan (1980), *Michel Foucault: The Will to Truth*. London: Tavistock.

Sherwood-Dunn, B. (1897), "Conservation of The Ovary," *Transactions of the American Association of Obstetrics and Gynecology*, 10: 195–234.

Shorter, Edward (1975), *The Making of The Modern Family*. New York: Basic Books.

Shorter, Edward (1982), *A History of Women's Bodies*. New York: Basic Books.

Shorter, Edward (1992), *From Paralysis to Fatigue: A History of Psychosomatic Illnesses in the Modern Era*. New York: Free Press.

Shorter, Edward (1994), *From The Mind into The Body: The Cultural Origins of Psychosomatic Symptoms*. New York: Free Press.

Shorter, Edward (1996), "C.B. Farrar: A Life," in Shorter, Edward (ed.), *TPH: History and Memories of The Toronto Psychiatric Hospital, 1925–1966*. Toronto: Wall and Emerson: 59–96.

Shorter, Edward (1997), *A History of Psychiatry: From the Era of The Asylum to The Age of Prozac*. New York: Free Press, Chichester: John Wiley and Sons.

Shorter, Edward and Tilly, Charles (1974), *Strikes in France, 1830–1968*. London: Cambridge University Press.

Showalter, Elaine (1985), *The Female Malady: Madness and English Culture, 1830–1980*. New York: Pantheon, 1985.

Sicherman, Barbara (1967), "The Quest for Mental Health in America, 1880–1917," unpublished PhD dissertation, Columbia University.

Sicherman, Barbara (1977), "The Uses of a Diagnosis: Doctors, Patients, and Neurasthenia," *Journal of the History of Medicine and Allied Sciences*, 32: 33–54.

Sinkler, Wharton (1891), "The Remote Results of Removal of The Tubes and Ovaries," *University Medical Magazine*, 4: 173–186.

Skene, Alexander (1895), *Medical Gynecology*. New York: Appleton and Co.

Skey, F.C. (1867), *Hysteria*, 2nd edition, London: Longmans.

Smith, Charlotte (1798), *The Young Philosopher*. London: Cadell and Davies.

Smith, Leonard D. (1992), "Eighteenth Century Madhouse Practice: The Prouds of Bilston," *History of Psychiatry*, 3: 45–52.

Smith, Roger (1981), *Trial by Medicine: Insanity and Responsibility in Victorian Trials*. Edinburgh: Edinburgh University Press.

Smith, Tyler W. (1848), "The Climacteric Disease in Women," *London Journal of Medicine*, 1: 609.

Smith, C.J. and Hanham, R.Q. (1981), "Deinstitutionalization of The Mentally Ill: A Time Path Analysis of The American States," *Social Science and Medicine*, 15D: 361–378.

Smith, G.E. and Pear, T.H. (1917), "Shell Shock," *Nature*, 100, September 27: 65.

Smith-Rosenberg, Carroll (1972), "The Hysterical Woman: Sex Roles and Role Conflict in 19th Century America," *Social Research*, 39: 652–678.

Smith-Rosenberg, Carroll and Rosenberg, Charles (1973), "The Female Animal: Medical and Biological Views of Woman and her Role in Nineteenth Century America," *Journal of American History*, 60: 332–356.

Smollett, Tobias (1762), *The Adventures of Sir Lancelot Greaves*. London: Coote.

Southard, Elmer E. (1916), "The Psychopathic Hospital's Function of Early Intensive Service for Persons Not Legally Insane," in *Proceedings of the National Conference of Social Work*, 43: 277.

Spitzer, Steven and Andrew Scull (eds) (1985), *Research in Law, Deviance and Social Control*, Volume 7. Greenwich, CT: JAI Press.

Spitzka, Edward C. (1878), "Reform in the Scientific Study of Psychiatry," *Journal of Nervous and Mental Disease*, 5: 201–229.

Stafford, Richard (1692), *Because to Many People, I have Seemed to Falsify My Word and Promise, Which I made Upon My Being Discharged Out of Bethlehem Hospital*. London: for the author.

Stanton, Alfred H. and Schwartz, Morris S. (1954), *The Mental Hospital: A Study of Institutional Participation in Mental Illness and Treatment*. New York: Basic Books.

Stead, John H. (1913), "End Results of Surgical Operations Upon Two Hundred and Fifty One Insane Women," *Bulletin of the Ontario Hospitals for the Insane*, 6: 129–136.

Stevenson, Christine (1996), "Robert Hooke's Bethlem," *Journal of the Society of Architectural Historians*, 55: 254–275.

Stevenson, Christine (1997), "The Architecture of Bethlem at Moorfields," in Andrews, Jonathan, Briggs, Asa, Porter, Roy, Tucker, Penny, and Keir Waddington, *The History of Bethlem*. London: Routledge: 230–259.

Stevenson, Christine (2000), *Medicine and Magnificence: British Hospital and Asylum Architecture, 1660–1815*. London and New Haven, CT: Yale University Press.

Stevenson, George S. and Smith, Geddes (1934), *Child Guidance Clinics: A Quarter Century of Development*. New York: Commonwealth Fund.

Stone, I.S. (1890), "Psychical Results of Gynecological Operations," *Journal of the American Medical Association*, 15: 305–307.

Stone, Lawrence (1987), *The Past and Present Revisited*. London: Routledge & Kegan Paul.

Stone, Martin (1985a), "Shellshock and the Psychiatrists," in Bynum, W.F., Porter, R., and M. Shepherd, M. (eds), *The Anatomy of Madness*, Volume 2. London: Tavistock: 242–271.

Stone, Martin (1985b), "The Military and Industrial Roots of Clinical Psychology in Britain, 1900–1945," unpublished PhD dissertation, London School of Economics and Political Science.

Storer, Horatio Robinson (1871), *The Causation, Course, and Treatment of Reflex Insanity in Women*. Reprint edition: New York: Arno, 1972.

Strahan, S.A.K. (1890), "The Propagation of Insanity and Other Neuroses," *Journal of Mental Science*, 36: 325–338.

Sturdy, Harriet and Parry-Jones, William (1999), "Boarding-out insane patients: the significance of the Scottish System 1857–1913," in Bartlett, Peter and Wright, David (eds), *Outside the Walls of the Asylum*, London: Athlone: 86–114.

Suzuki, Akihito (1991), "Lunacy in Seventeenth and Eighteenth Century England: Analysis of Quarter Sessions Records, Part I," *History of Psychiatry*, 2: 437–456.

Suzuki, Akihito (1992a), "Mind and its Disease in Enlightenment Medicine," unpublished PhD thesis, University of London.

Suzuki, Akihito (1992b), "Lunacy in Seventeenth and Eighteenth Century England: Analysis of Quarter Sessions Records, Part II," *History of Psychiatry*, 3: 29–44.

Suzuki, Akihito (1998), "The Household and Care of Lunatics in Eighteenth Century London," in Horden, P. and Smith, R. (eds), *The Locus of Care: Families, Communities, Institutions, and the Provision of Welfare Since Antiquity*. London: Routledge: 153–175.

Suzuki, Akihito (2006), *Domestic Psychiatry: The Doctor, The Patient, and the Family in England, 1820–1860*. Berkeley, CA: University of California Press.

Swain, G. (1977), *La sujet de la folie: naissance de la psychiatrie*. Toulouse: Privat.

Swazey, Judith (1974), *Chlorpromazine in Psychiatry: A Study of Therapeutic Innovation*. Cambridge, MA: MIT Press.

Sykes, Kathleen A. (1933), "The Routine Investigation and Treatment of Cases Admitted to Rubery Hill Hospital," *Journal of Mental Science*, 79: 223–224.

Szasz, Thomas (1961), *The Myth of Mental Illness*. New York: Dell.

Szasz, Thomas (1970), *The Manufacture of Madness*. New York: Dell.

Tait, Lawson (1886), "On The General Principles Involved in The Operation of Removal of The Uterine Appendages," *British Medical Journal*, November 6: 852–853.

Tait, Lawson (1889a), *Diseases of Women and Abdominal Surgery*. Philadelphia, PA: Lea Brothers and Co. Thomas, T. Gaillard.

Tait, Lawson (1889b), "Acute Mania and Melancholia as sequelae of Gynecological Operations," *Medical News*, April 13: 396–399.

Tenon, J. (n.d.), "Journal d'observations sur les principaux hôpitaux et prisons d'Angleterre," *Papiers sur les hôpitaux* III, folios 11–16 (*c.* 1790).

Tepper, S.J. and Haas, J.F. (1979) "Prevalence of Tardive Dyskinesia," *Journal of Clinical Psychiatry*, 40: 508–516.

Thomas, Keith (1983), *Religion and The Decline of Magic*. London: Allen Lane.

Thomas, T. Galliard (1889), "Acute Manai and Melancholia as a Sequelac of Gynaecological Operation," *Medical News*, April 13: 396–399.

Thompson, David G. (1890) "Letter to The Editor," *Journal of Mental Science* 36, ADD.

Ticehurst Asylum (n.d.), *Patient Case Books*, in manuscript, Contemporary Medical Archives, Wellcome Institute for the History of Medicine, London.

Timms, N. (1964), *Psychiatric Social Work in Great Britain 1939–1962*. London: Routledge.

Tomes, Nancy (1984), *A Generous Confidence: Thomas Story Kirkbride and The Art of Asylum Keeping, 1840–1833*. Cambridge: Cambridge University Press.

Tomes, Nancy (1988), "The Anglo-American Asylum in Historical Perspective," in Giggs, J. and Smith, C. (eds), *Location and Stigma*. London: Unwin Hyman.

Tryon, Thomas (1689), *A Treatise of Dreams and Visions, to Which Is Added, a Discourse of The Causes, Nature, and Cure of Phrensie, Madness, or Distraction*. London: Sowle.

Tuke, Daniel Hack (1878), *Insanity in Ancient and Modern Life, With Chapters on Its Prevention*. London: Macmillan.

Tuke, Daniel Hack (1882), *Chapters in The History of The Insane in The British Isles*. London: Kegan Paul and Trench.

Tuke, Samuel (1813), *Description of the Retreat*. York: Alexander.

Turek, I.S. (1975), "Drug-Induced Dyskinesia: Reality or Myth?" *Diseases of the Nervous System*, 36: 397–399.

Turner, Trevor (1988), "Henry Maudsley, Psychiatrist, Philosopher, and Entrepreneur," in Bynum, W.F., Porter, R., and Shepherd, M. (eds), *The Anatomy of Madness*, Volume 3. London: Routledge: 151–189.

Upson, Henry (1907), "Nervous Disorders Due to The Teeth: A Preliminary Report," *Cleveland Medical Journal*, 6: 458–459.

Upson, Henry (1909), "Dementia Praecox Caused by Dental Impaction," *Monthly Cyclopedia and Medical Bulletin*, 648–651.

Upson, Henry (1910), "Serious Mental Disturbances Caused by Painless Dental Lesions," *American Quarterly of Roentgenology*, 11: 223–243.

US Department of Commerce, Bureau of the Census (1971), *Pharmaceutical Preparations*, 1969, Washington, DC: Government Printing Office.

Valenstein, Elliot (1986), *Great and Desperate Cures: The Rise and Decline of Psychosurgery and Other Radical Treatments for Mental Illness*. New York: Basic Books.

Van de Warker, E. (1906), "The Fetish of the Ovary," *American Journal of Obstetrics*, 54: 366–373.

Von Meduna, Ladislas (1938), "General Discussion of Cardiazol Therapy," *American Journal of Psychiatry*, 94 (Supplement): 50.

Wagner von Jauregg, Julius (1946), "The History of The Malaria Treatment of General Paralysis," *American Journal of Psychiatry*, 102: 577–582.

Wainwright, Milton (1987), "The History of the Therapeutic Use of Crude Penicillin," *Medical History*, 31: 41–50.

Walsh, Oonagh (1999), "'The Designs of Providence': Race, Religion and Irish Insanity," in Melling, J. and Forsythe, B. (eds), *Insanity, Institutions, and Society, 1800–1914*. London: Routledge: 223–242.

Walton, John (1979), "Lunacy in The Industrial Revolution: A Study of Asylum Admissions in Lancashire, 1848–50," *Journal of Social History*, 13: 13–18.

Walton, John (1985), "Casting Out and Bringing Back in Victorian England: Pauper Lunatics, 1840–70," in Bynum, W.F., Porter, R. and Shepherd, M. (eds), *The Anatomy of Madness*, Volume 2. London: Tavistock: 132–146.

Ward, Mary Jane (1946), *The Snake Pit*. New York: Random House.

Ward, Ned (1709), *The London Spy*. 4th edition, reprinted edition, East Lansing, MI: Colleagues Press, 1993.

Warner, John Harley (1980), "The Edinburgh Bloodletting Controversy," *Medical History*, 24: 241–258.

Warner, John Harley (1986), *The Therapeutic Perspective: Medical Practice, Knowledge, and Identity in America, 1820–1885*. Cambridge, MA: Harvard University Press.

Watson, Chalmers (1923), "The Role of Auto-Intoxication or Auto-Infection in Mental Disorders," *Journal of Mental Science*, 69: 52–77.

Weber, Max (1968), *Economy and Society*. Totowa, NJ: Bedminster Press.

Weiner, D. (1984), "The Origins of Psychiatry: Pinel or The Zeitgeist," in Baur, O. and Glandien, O. (eds), *Zussammenhang: Festschrift für Marielene Putscher*, Volume 2. Köln: Wienand: 611–631.

Weiner, D. (1999), *Comprendre et soigner: Philippe Pinel (1746–1826): La medicine de l'esprit*. Paris: Fayard.

Wells, Sir Thomas Spencer (1886), "Castration in Nervous and Mental Diseases," *American Journal of the Medical Sciences*, 91–92: 455–471.

West, Charles (1866), "Clitoridectomy," *British Medical Journal*, November 24: 585.

West Riding Lunatic Asylum (1873), *Annual Report*. Wakefield.

White, William Alanson (1936) to Smith Ely Jelliffe, 7 August, Jelliffe Papers, Library of Congress, Washington, DC.

Willis, Thomas (1684), *The Practice of Physick*. London: Dring, Harper, and Leigh.

Windle, Charles and Scully, D. (1976), "Community Mental Health Centers and the Decreasing Use of State Mental Hospitals," *Community Mental Health Journal*, 12: 239–243.

Wing, J.K. (1962), "Institutionalism in mental hospitals," *British Journal of Social and Clinical Psychiatry*, 1: 38.

Wing, J.K. and Brown, G.W. (1970), *Institutionalism and Schizophrenia*. Cambridge: Cambridge University Press.

Winkworth, Susanna (1883), *Letters and Memorials of Catherine Winkworth*. Clifton, for the author.

Winslow, Lionel Forbes (1910), *Recollections of Forty Years*. London: Ouseley.

Woerner, M., Kane, J.M. and Lieberman, J. (1991), "The Prevalence of Tardive Dyskinesia," *Journal of Clinical Psychopharmacology*, 11: 34–42.

Wollstonecraft, Mary (1788), *Mary, A Fiction*. London: Joseph.

Wright, David (1998), "Family Strategies and The Institutional Commitment of Idiots in Victorian England," *Journal of Family History*, 23: 189–208.

Wright, David (1999), "The Discharge of Pauper Lunatics from County Asylums in Mid-Victorian England: The Case of Buckinghamshire, 1853–1872," in Melling, J. and Forsythe, B. (eds), *Insanity, Institutions and Society, 1800–1914*. London: Routledge: 93–112.

Wright, Frank L. (1947), *Out of Sight, Out of Mind*. Philadelphia, PA: National Mental Health Foundation.

Wynter, Andrew (1875), *The Borderlands of Insanity*. London: Hardwicke.

Wynter, Andrew (1877), *The Borderlands of Insanity*, 2nd edition. London: Renshaw.

Yellowlees, David (1890), "Presidential Address [to the Medico-Psychological Association]," *Journal of Mental Science*, 36: 473–489.

Zilboorg, Gregory (1941), *A History of Medical Psychology*. New York: Norton.

Zola, Irving K. (1972), "Medicine as an Institution of Social Control," *The Sociological Review*, 20: 487–504.

Index